T0324798

Cardio-oncology Related to Heart Failure

Guest Editors

DANIEL J. LENIHAN, MD
DOUGLAS B. SAWYER, MD, PhD

HEART FAILURE CLINICS

www.heartfailure.theclinics.com

Consulting Editors
RAGAVENDRA R. BALIGA, MD, MBA
JAMES B. YOUNG, MD

Founding Editor
JAGAT NARULA, MD, PhD

July 2011 • Volume 7 • Number 3

SAUNDERS an imprint of ELSEVIER, Inc.

W.B. SAUNDERS COMPANY
A Division of Elsevier Inc.

1600 John F. Kennedy Boulevard • Suite 1800 • Philadelphia, Pennsylvania 19103-2899

http://www.theclinics.com

HEART FAILURE CLINICS Volume 7, Number 3
July 2011 ISSN 1551-7136, ISBN-13: 978-1-4557-1101-7

Editor: Barbara Cohen-Kligerman
Developmental Editor: Donald Mumford

Heart Failure Clinics (ISSN 1551-7136) is published quarterly by Elsevier Inc., 360 Park Avenue South, New York, NY 10010-1710. Months of publication are January, April, July, and October. Business and editorial offices: 1600 John F. Kennedy Boulevard, Suite 1800, Philadelphia, PA 19103-2899. Periodicals postage paid at New York, NY, and additional mailing offices. Subscription prices are USD 207.00 per year for US individuals, USD 326.00 per year for US institutions, USD 70.00 per year for US students and residents, USD 248.00 per year for Canadian individuals, USD 374.00 per year for Canadian institutions, USD 264.00 per year for international individuals, USD 374.00 per year for international institutions, and USD 89.00 per year for Canadian and foreign students/residents. To receive student and resident rate, orders must be accompanied by name of affiliated institution, date of term, and the *signature* of program/residency coordinator on institution letterhead. Orders will be billed at individual rate until proof of status is received. Foreign air speed delivery is included in all *Clinics* subscription prices. All prices are subject to change without notice. **POSTMASTER:** Send address changes to *Heart Failure Clinics*, Elsevier Health Sciences Division, Subscription Customer Service, 3251 Riverport Lane, Maryland Heights, MO 63043. **Customer Service: 1-800-654-2452 (US and Canada). From outside of the US and Canada, call 314-447-8871. Fax: 314-447-8029. For print support, e-mail: JournalsCustomerService-usa@elsevier.com. For online support, e-mail: JournalsOnlineSupport-usa@elsevier.com.**

Reprints. For copies of 100 or more of articles in this publication, please contact the Commercial Reprints Department, Elsevier Inc., 360 Park Avenue South, New York, NY 10010-1710. Tel.: 212-633-3812; Fax: 212-462-1935; E-mail: reprints@elsevier.com.

Heart Failure Clinics is covered in *MEDLINE/PubMed (Index Medicus).*

Printed in the United States of America.

Cover artwork courtesy of Umberto M. Jezek.

Contributors

CONSULTING EDITORS

RAGAVENDRA R. BALIGA, MD, MBA
Vice-Chair, Division of Cardiovascular
Medicine; Professor of Internal Medicine, The
Ohio State University Medical Center,
Columbus, Ohio

JAMES B. YOUNG, MD
Professor of Medicine and Executive Dean,
Cleveland Clinic Lerner College of Medicine;
George and Linda Kaufman Chair, Chairman,
Endocrinology and Metabolism Institute,
Cleveland Clinic, Cleveland, Ohio

GUEST EDITORS

DANIEL J. LENIHAN, MD
Director, Clinical Research Program,
Vanderbilt Heart and Vascular Institute,
Nashville, Tennessee

DOUGLAS B. SAWYER, MD, PhD
Chief, Division of Cardiovascular Medicine;
Physician-in-Chief, Vanderbilt Heart and
Vascular Institute, Vanderbilt University
Medical Center, Nashville, Tennessee

AUTHORS

ROBERT S. BENJAMIN, MD
Chairman, Departments of Cardiology and
Sarcoma Medical Oncology, The University
of Texas MD Anderson Cancer Center,
Houston, Texas

JOHN L. BERK, MD
Associate Professor and Clinical Director,
Amyloidosis Treatment and Research
Program and Section of Pulmonary Medicine,
Department of Medicine, Boston University
School of Medicine and Boston Medical
Center, Boston, Massachusetts

JOSEPH R. CARVER, MD
Clinical Professor of Medicine, Division
of Cardiovascular Medicine; Chief of Staff,
Abramson Cancer Center, University
of Pennsylvania School of Medicine,
Philadelphia, Pennsylvania

ALICE CHEN, MD, FACP
Senior Investigator, Investigational Drug
Branch, Cancer Therapy Evaluation Program,
Division of Cancer Treatment and Diagnosis,
National Cancer Institute, Rockville, Maryland

CAROL L. CHEN, MD
Assistant Clinical Member, Director of Cardiac
Intermediate Care Unit, Cardiology Division,
Memorial Sloan-Kettering Cancer Center,
New York, New York

KELLI S. DEMPSEY, MSN, APRN-BC, AOCNP
Oncology Nurse Practitioner, American Cancer
Care, Evansville, Indiana

MICHAEL S. EWER, MD, JD
Professor of Medicine, Departments
of Cardiology and Sarcoma Medical Oncology,
The University of Texas MD Anderson Cancer
Center, Houston, Texas

MICHAEL B. FOWLER, MB, FRCP
Professor of Medicine, Division of
Cardiovascular Medicine, Stanford University
Medical Center, Stanford, California

AKM HOSSAIN, MD, MPH
Assistant Professor of Medicine, Departments
of Medicine, Hematology and Oncology, Ellis
Fischel Cancer Center, University of Missouri,
Columbia, Missouri

PERCY IVY, MD
Associate Chief, Investigational Drug Branch,
Cancer Therapy Evaluation Program, Division
of Cancer Treatment and Diagnosis, National
Cancer Institute, Rockville, Maryland

JONATHAN KALTMAN, MD
Medical Officer, Division of Cardiovascular
Sciences, National Heart, Lung, and Blood
Institute, Bethesda, Maryland

AARIF Y. KHAKOO, MD, MBA
Associate Professor, Department of
Cardiology, University of Texas MD Anderson
Cancer Center, Houston, Texas

BONNIE KY, MD, MSCE
Assistant Professor of Medicine, Division
of Cardiovascular Medicine; Assistant
Professor of Epidemiology, Department of
Biostatistics and Epidemiology; Senior
Scholar, Center for Clinical Epidemiology and
Biostatistics; Member, Abramson Cancer
Center, University of Pennsylvania School
of Medicine, Philadelphia, Pennsylvania

DANIEL J. LENIHAN, MD
Director, Clinical Research Program,
Vanderbilt Heart and Vascular Institute,
Nashville, Tennessee

ALLEN J. NAFTILAN, MD, PhD
Associate Professor of Medicine, Hematology
Division, Department of Medicine, Vanderbilt
Heart and Vascular Institute, Vanderbilt
University, Nashville, Tennessee

JUAN CARLOS PLANA, MD
Staff, Section of Imaging, Department of
Cardiovascular Medicine, The Cleveland Clinic
Foundation, Cleveland, Ohio

CHARLES PORTER, MD, FACC, FACP
Associate Professor of Medicine - Cardiology,
University of Kansas Medical Center
in Kansas City, Kansas City, Missouri

CAROL S. PORTLOCK, MD
Department of Medicine, Memorial
Sloan-Kettering Cancer Center,
New York, New York

MEREDITH L. REES, BA
PhD Graduate Student, Department
of Cardiology, University of Texas MD
Anderson Cancer Center, Houston, Texas

SCOT C. REMICK, MD, FACP
Director and Professor of Medicine, Laurence
and Jean DeLynn Chair of Oncology,
Department of Medicine, West Virginia
University School of Medicine, Mary Babb
Randolph Cancer Center, Morgantown,
West Virginia

MARC A. ROZNER, MD, PhD
Professor of Anesthesiology and Perioperative
Medicine, Professor of Cardiology, The
University of Texas MD Anderson Cancer
Center, Houston, Texas

SUNIL K. SAHAI, MD
Associate Professor of Medicine,
Department of General Internal Medicine;
Medical Director, Internal Medicine
Perioperative Assessment Center,
The University of Texas MD Anderson
Cancer Center, Houston, Texas

FLORA SAM, MD
Associate Professor, Amyloidosis Treatment
and Research Program and Division
of Cardiology, Whitaker Cardiovascular
Institute, Department of Medicine, Boston
University School of Medicine and Boston
Medical Center, Boston, Massachusetts

VAISHALI SANCHORAWALA, MD
Professor and Director, Stem Cell Transplant
Program, Amyloidosis Treatment and
Research Program and Section of
Hematology-Oncology, Department
of Medicine, Boston University School
of Medicine and Boston Medical Center,
Boston, Massachusetts

HELOISA SAWAYA, MD, PhD
Research Fellow, Division of Cardiology, Cardiac Ultrasound Laboratory, Massachusetts General Hospital, Harvard Medical School, Boston, Massachusetts

MARIELLE SCHERRER-CROSBIE, MD, PhD
Associate Professor of Medicine, Division of Cardiology, Cardiac Ultrasound Laboratory, Massachusetts General Hospital, Harvard Medical School, Boston, Massachusetts

FRIEDRICH G. SCHUENING, MD
Professor of Medicine, Hematology Division, Department of Medicine, Vanderbilt Heart and Vascular Institute, Vanderbilt University, Nashville, Tennessee

DAVID C. SELDIN, MD, PhD
Professor, Program Director, and Section Chief, Amyloidosis Treatment and Research Program and Section of Hematology-Oncology, Department of Medicine, Boston University School of Medicine and Boston Medical Center, Boston, Massachusetts

DAVID SLOSKY, MD
Assistant Professor of Medicine, Vanderbilt Heart and Vascular Institute, Vanderbilt University, Nashville, Tennessee

RICHARD STEINGART, MD, FACC
Professor of Medicine and Chief, Cardiology Division, Memorial Sloan-Kettering Cancer Center, New York, New York

WENDY TADDEI-PETERS, PhD
Clinical Trial Specialist, Office of the Director, Division of Cardiovascular Sciences, National Heart, Lung, and Blood Institute, Bethesda, Maryland

MELINDA L. TELLI, MD
Assistant Professor of Medicine, Division of Medical Oncology, Stanford University Medical Center, Stanford, California

DANIEL D. VON HOFF, MD
Senior Investigator and Head of Translational Research, Translational Drug Development Division, Translational Genomics Research Institute (TGen); Head, Pancreatic Cancer Research Program in Phoenix; Chief Scientific Officer, US Oncology and the Scottsdale Clinical Research Institute, Phoenix, Arizona

RONALD M. WITTELES, MD, FACC
Assistant Professor of Medicine, Division of Cardiovascular Medicine, Stanford University Medical Center, Stanford, California

JOACHIM YAHALOM, MD
Attending and Member, Department of Radiation Oncology, Memorial Sloan-Kettering Cancer Center; Professor of Radiation Oncology, Weill Medical College of Cornell University, New York, New York

ALI ZALPOUR, PharmD, BCPS
Clinical Pharmacist, Department of General Internal Medicine, The University of Texas MD Anderson Cancer Center, Houston, Texas

Contents

Targeted antiangiogenic cancer therapies have revolutionized the treatment of highly vascularized cancers such as metastatic renal cell carcinoma and gastrointestinal stromal tumors. Such agents act by inhibiting the actions of proangiogenic growth factors and their receptor tyrosine kinases, which are known to be overexpressed in cancer. However, these factors also play an important role in normal cardiovascular physiology. This article summarizes the incidences of cardiovascular toxicities (namely hypertension and heart failure) associated with the most commonly used antiangiogenic therapies, and then presents data from preclinical and clinical studies to provide some insight into the underlying molecular mechanisms.

Chemotherapy-induced cardiotoxicity has become a significant public health issue. Left ventricular ejection fraction is routinely used to monitor cardiotoxicity but fails to detect subtle alterations in cardiac function. Improvements in the measurement of left ventricular ejection fraction, physical or pharmacologic stressors, and novel cardiac functional indices may be useful in the detection of cardiotoxicity. The improvements in the detection and therapy of cancer have led to the emergence of chemotherapy-induced cardiotoxicity. New echocardiographic techniques may be useful in the detection of patients undergoing chemotherapy treatments who could benefit from alternative cancer treatments, therefore decreasing the incidence of cardiotoxicity.

Treatment of cancer patients with anthracycline chemotherapy has resulted in significant improvements in the overall survival of this population. These regimens, however, are associated with important cardiotoxic side effects. As the incidence and prevalence of cancer rises, there is a need to decrease the cardiotoxic risks associated with chemotherapy. Biomarkers targeting early identification of patients at risk for anthracycline-induced cardiotoxicity and effective cardioprotective therapeutics can fulfill this need and are a priority in the field of cardio-oncology. This review highlights the current evidence regarding the use of biomarkers in anthracycline-treated patients and presents the available literature on prophylactic cardioprotective strategies.

Cardiotoxicity remains the limiting factor for many forms of cancer therapy and is the focus of growing research and clinical emphasis. This article outlines the current clinical evidence for left ventricular dysfunction and heart failure for the two most important classes of cardiotoxic chemotherapeutic agents, examines the potential pitfalls that have led to underestimated rates of left ventricular dysfunction from these agents, and reviews strategies for screening for and providing prophylaxis against chemotherapy-associated left ventricular dysfunction.

Hematopoietic stem cells (HSCs) are the most well-characterized and studied stem cells. They have been used to treat various benign and malignant hematologic disorders. Most stem cell transplant recipients survive more than 5 years without any evidence of their original clinical disease. Early animal trials have demonstrated the ability to improve cardiac function by transfer of HSCs into the myocardium, and early human studies have demonstrated the feasibility and safety of this approach. Trials in patients after myocardial infarction and with chronic heart failure have seen limited and mixed success, probably because of the various cell types and methods used.

The care of patients with cancer who have cardiac disease is dispersed both sequentially and concurrently across multiple providers, and an important goal of education is communication among the providers regarding change of therapy, toxicity of therapy, and symptom assessments. Changes must be made to improve the delivery of cardiac care in patients with cancer and cancer survivors. Therefore, the authors propose a multilevel approach that includes short, targeted curriculum for housestaff training programs in internal medicine, family medicine, pediatrics, cardiology and oncology; increasing presence at national meetings of internists, oncologists and cardiologists; and an Internet-based repository of core information.

Anthracyclines remain important agents in the treatment of solid and hematological malignancy. Early experience with these drugs reported cardiac failure as an adverse event. Later, clinical recognition of cell injury at the time of administration was appreciated. This article explores the evolution of our understanding about anthracycline-associated cardiotoxicity, including the various strategies for the pretreatment assessment of patients for whom anthracyclines are contemplated, the frustrations associated with the lack of specific tests that could identify patients at risk of developing problems with their next 1 or 2 cycles, the concept of balancing oncologic benefit with cardiac risk in the treatment of cancer patients, and the newer strategies for reducing the potentially devastating complications of the treatment of malignant disease with anthracyclines.

The Importance of Clinical Grading of Heart Failure and Other Cardiac Toxicities During Chemotherapy: Updating the Common Terminology Criteria for Clinical Trial Reporting

373

Akm Hossain, Alice Chen, Percy Ivy, Daniel J. Lenihan, Jonathan Kaltman, Wendy Taddei-Peters, and Scot C. Remick

Although the use of chemotherapy and targeted therapy has improved the clinical benefit, progression-free survival, and overall survival of various cancers in recent years, old and new toxicities have limited their use. To balance the risk with the benefit of treatment, Common Toxicity Criteria and now Common Terminology Criteria for Adverse Events (CTCAE) have been used by the oncology community for more than 20 years to assess toxicity from cancer treatment. This article details the description and grading of cardiac toxicities reported in association with cancer treatment and the use of CTCAE to assess them.

Amyloidotic Cardiomyopathy: Multidisciplinary Approach to Diagnosis and Treatment

385

David C. Seldin, John L. Berk, Flora Sam, and Vaishali Sanchorawala

Amyloidotic cardiomyopathy (ACMP) occurs in the setting of rare genetic diseases, blood dyscrasias, chronic infection and inflammation, and advanced age. Cardiologists are on the front lines of diagnosis of ACMP when evaluating patients with unexplained dyspnea, congestive heart failure, or arrhythmias. Noninvasive detection of diastolic cardiac dysfunction and unexplained left ventricular hypertrophy should be followed by biopsy to demonstrate the presence of amyloid deposits and appropriate genetic, biochemical, and immunologic testing to accurately define the type of amyloid. Growing numbers of treatment options exist for these diseases, and timely diagnosis and institution of therapy is essential for preservation of cardiac function.

Interventional Strategies to Manage Heart Failure in Patients with Cancer

395

Charles Porter and David Slosky

The unique clinical circumstances that are typically encountered by cardiology providers when caring for patients undergoing treatment for cancer require an in-depth understanding of the recommended treatments for the diagnosis and management of heart failure and ischemic heart disease. It is also recognized that there is not a broadly described clinical research basis from which to provide guidance when specific clinical decision making is required. Thus, it is imperative that cardiology and oncology closely collaborate when difficult patient decisions arise. Engaging each discipline together with active patient involvement in clinical care will undoubtedly provide optimal care for our patients.

Special Articles

Long-Term Cardiac and Pulmonary Complications of Cancer Therapy

403

Joachim Yahalom and Carol S. Portlock

Cardiac complications resulting from chemotherapy and radiation pose a significant risk for morbidity and mortality to the cancer survivor. Cardiac side effects may progress over time and are a concern for patients treated during childhood. Long-term pulmonary complications are relatively infrequent, and acute respiratory effects of drugs (mostly bleomycin) or radiation normally resolve early after therapy. Although most cardiovascular risk statistics and clinical experience are derived from patients treated before 1985, the modern radiation approach that limits the exposure of the heart and reduces the total dose seems to attenuate the previously observed cardiovascular risk. Potential preventive measures for high-risk patients are of increasing interest but remain experimental.

This review focuses on the unique perioperative concerns of patients with cancer undergoing surgery. Importantly, not all surgical procedures are intended as cures: some patients who have cancer also undergo surgery for noncancer issues. Also, many of these patients have undergone prior chemotherapy and/or radiation therapy that can introduce perioperative concerns. These previous treatments, unique to patients with cancer, can adversely affect their cardiovascular, pulmonary, gastrointestinal, renal, and endocrine systems. This article also summarizes many important effects of a wide variety of chemotherapy agents in use today.

Chemotherapy-induced cardiotoxicity (CIC) is a major complication found with some life-saving medications used to treat breast and other cancers. Cardiotoxicity may present immediately during treatment or years later. These patients need education, screening, preventive measures, prompt interventions, and proper follow-up. This article focuses on CIC in patients who have breast cancer, but the process of evaluation and treatment design applies to all types of cancer and organ toxicities. Comprehensive pretreatment history, examination, and testing are needed for proper diagnosis and staging. CIC and other toxicities need to be considered in drug selection, treatment sequencing, testing, and appropriate follow-up.

Heart Failure Clinics

VISIT THE CLINICS ONLINE!

Access your subscription at:
www.theclinics.com

Editorial

Early Detection and Monitoring of Vulnerable Myocardium in Patients Receiving Chemotherapy: Is It Time to Change Tracks?

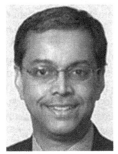 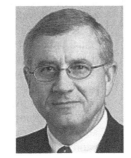

Ragavendra R. Baliga, MD, MBA   James B. Young, MD
Consulting Editors

Even if you're on the right track, you'll get run over if you just sit there.

—*Will Rogers*[1]

The development of novel chemotherapeutic agents[2–4] in the past 2 decades has substantially improved survival for patients with cancer. For example, 5-year relative survival rates for leukemia and non-Hodgkin lymphoma increased from 42% in 1977 to 58% in 2004, and for breast cancer the rates have risen from 75% in 1977 to 89% in 2004.[5] However, several of these agents have significant cardiotoxicity (**Table 1**).[6] Additionally, if radiation therapy is also employed, with the heart in the target zone, additive toxicity can be noted. The long-term survival of cardiomyopathy in patients receiving aggressive cancer therapies depends on many things, including underlying cardiac condition[7] (**Fig. 1**) and type of chemotherapeutic agent employed.[8] Cardiomyopathy caused by anthracyclines has been reported to be permanent. However, recent data suggest that early initiation of cardioprotective therapy may actually salvage at-risk myocardium,[9] whereas cardiomyopathy caused by trastuzumab has been reported to be reversible, although this conclusion has recently been disputed.[10] Early detection of mild asymptomatic left ventricular (LV) dysfunction is important because it is associated with a 5-fold increased risk of subsequent heart failure.[11] Reducing morbidity and mortality caused by LV dysfunction, therefore, requires early detection of patients whose myocardium is vulnerable to chemotherapy. It includes frequent monitoring of cardiovascular function (**Table 2**); prompt discontinuation of the offending chemotherapeutic regimen; and rapid initiation of therapy, including angiotensin-converting enzyme inhibitors (and perhaps angiotensin receptor antagonists),[12] beta-blockers[13] (**Fig. 2**), and aldosterone receptor antagonists.[14,15] The current monitoring regimens for LV ventricular systolic function require serial estimation of LV ejection fraction (LVEF), either by radionuclide scintigraphy, echocardiography, or cardiac magnetic resonance imaging (CMR).[16] The quantitation of LVEF may vary by interpreter or by institution, when based on the commonly used visual estimation technique in echocardiography,[17] and can also vary as a function of the imaging modality (ie, echocardiography vs radionuclide ventriculography). The suitability of a given technique is largely determined by the local availability and expertise.

Radionuclide techniques to measure LVEF include planar multiple-gated radionuclide angiography (MUGA) and quantitative gated blood-pool

Heart Failure Clin 7 (2011) xiii–xix
doi:10.1016/j.hfc.2011.05.001
1551-7136/11/$ – see front matter © 2011 Published by Elsevier Inc.

heartfailure.theclinics.com

Table 1
Partial list of cardiovascular adverse effects of chemotherapeutic agents

Therapeutic Agent	Cardiac Effect
Anthracycline, trastuzumab, alemtuzumab, cyclophosphamide, cisplatin, mitomycin	Heart Failure
Interleukin-2, cisplatin, capecitabine, vinca alkaloids, bevacizumab, 5-fluorouracil	Cardiac ischemia
Cyclophosphamide, busulfan	Myocarditis
Bevacizumab, cisplatin, interferon-alpha	Systemic Hypertension
Interleukin-2, interferon-alpha, paclitaxel, etoposide, alemtuzumab, cetuximab, rituximab	Hypotension
Paclitaxel	Bradyarrhythmia
Paclitaxel, bevacizumab	Thromboembolism

electrocardiography-based triggering, which often occurs in patients with cardiac failure. GBPS is not as accurate as MUGA for LVEF measurement because it requires detection of myocardial contours rather than quantification of the cardiac blood pool, and, thus, is limited by potential spillover effects from the myocardium in the LV cavity, resulting in the underestimation of either cardiac volumes. Radionuclide techniques are also limited by the need for ionizing radiation,[18] particularly in pediatric patients. One recent study reported that multiple radionuclide imaging tests were associated with a cumulative estimated effective dose of more than 100 mSv in more than 30% of patients.[18] Although the effects of cumulative doses of radiation are unclear, it can be argued that serial radionuclide scintigraphy should be reserved for patients who are not eligible for other modalities of monitoring (eg, obese patients) and other variations of thoracic anatomy, such as emphysema, markedly calcified ribs, and narrow intercostal spaces.

The advantages of 2-dimensional echocardiography are the lack of radiation, portability, ability to determine if an effusion is present, evaluation of additional cardiac pathology, and the widespread availability. The limitation of echocardiography is the inherent variability of sequential imaging caused by several factors and, thus, variability in ejection or shortening fraction determination. These challenges include day-to-day physiologic variations (eg, blood pressure), beat-to-beat variation, variable acoustic windows, image acquisition at different parts of the respiratory cycle,

single-photon emission computed tomography (GBPS). Traditionally, serial MUGA has been used to monitor LVEF in adult patients on cardiotoxic chemotherapeutic regimens because of its reliability. However, the utility of MUGA is limited in patients with arrhythmias caused by poor

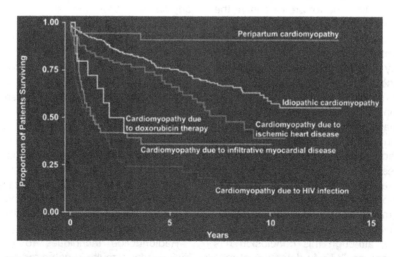

Fig. 1. Adjusted Kaplan-Meier estimates of survival according to the underlying cause of cardiomyopathy. Only idiopathic cardiomyopathy and cardiomyopathy caused by causes for which survival was significantly different from that in patients with idiopathic cardiomyopathy are shown. (*From* Felker GM, Thompson RE, Hare JM, et al. Underlying causes and long-term survival in patients with initially unexplained cardiomyopathy. N Engl J Med 2000;342(15):1077–84; with permission.)

Table 2
Guidelines for monitoring trastuzumab therapy in the National Surgical Adjuvant Breast and Bowel Project B-31

Relationship of LVEF to LLN	Absolute Decrease in LVEF of <10%	Absolute Decrease in LVEF of 10%–15%	Absolute Decrease in LVEF of ≥16%
Within normal limits	Continue	Continue	Hold[a]
1%–5% less than LLN	Continue	Hold[a]	Hold[a]
≥6% less than LLN	Continue	Hold[a]	Hold[a]

Abbreviations: LLN, lower limit of normal; LVEF, left ventricular ejection fraction.
[a] Repeat LVEF assessment after 4 weeks. If the criteria for continuation are met, resume trastuzumab treatment. If 2 consecutive holds or a total of 3 holds occur, discontinue trastuzumab treatment.
Data from Tan-Chiu E, Yothers G, Romond E, et al. Assessment of cardiac dysfunction in a randomized trial comparing doxorubicin and cyclophosphamide followed by paclitaxel, with or without trastuzumab as adjuvant therapy in node-positive, human epidermal growth factor receptor 2-overexpressing breast cancer: NSABP B-31. J Clin Oncol 2005;23(31):7811–9.

obtaining images at an inappropriate depth, artifacts to variable transducer positioning, dependency on gain-dependent edge identification, foreshortening of LV geometry, and variable operator skills. With traditional 2-dimensional echocardiography, the coefficient of variation for LV systolic function can be as high as 15%,[19] making the smallest significant change in ejection fraction that can be detected approximately 11%. Similarly, the test-retest variability of LV volumes varies between 11% for end-diastolic volume and 15% end-systolic volume. Portable echocardiography machines, despite being equipped with software capable of performing tissue Doppler, are limited by similar variation.[20] Sequential imaging using 3-dimensional echocardiography is more reliable because it does

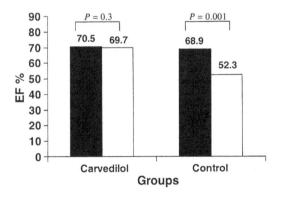

Fig. 2. Carvedilol in anthracycline-induced cardiomyopathy. Left ventricular ejection fraction (EF) at baseline (*black bars*) and after chemotherapy (*white bars*) in carvedilol (N = 25) and control (N = 25) groups. Data expressed as mean values. (*From* Kalay N, Basar E, Ozdogru I, et al. Protective effects of carvedilol against anthracycline-induced cardiomyopathy. J Am Coll Cardiol 2006;48(11):2258–62; with permission.)

not require geometric assumptions like 2-dimensional echocardiography,[21] but it is currently not amenable to sequential imaging in a physician's office.[22]

CMR is the gold standard[23] in the evaluation of LV function because advances in cine assessment (resulting in faster imaging acquisition) and high spatial resolution (making planimetry of interface between the LV cavity and the myocardium accurate) have resulted in easy and reproducible assessment of LV function. The main advantage of CMR is its low intraobserver and interobserver variability.[24] The low interstudy variability and excellent interstudy reproducibility of LV volumes and function means CMR has the highest reproducibility of all imaging techniques. Also, several studies have shown the superiority of CMR over 2-dimensional echocardiography[25]; in a direct comparison of 2-dimensional echocardiography and CMR, considerably lower coefficients of variability were found for end-diastolic volumes (3.7% vs 8.7%, $P = .17$), end-systolic volumes (6.2% vs 17.3%, $P<.001$), and ejection fraction (3.7% vs 11.5%, $P<.001$).[26–28] However, CMR is also not amenable to sequential imaging in a physician's office.

Speckled tracking echocardiography (STE) is a promising newer technique for early detection and monitoring of LV function (**Figs. 3** and **4**),[29] particularly in patients receiving cancer chemotherapy.[30–37] This approach, because it is based on fundamental physiologic principles of myocardial mechanics and obtainable noninvasively, seems particularly suited for monitoring patients on cardiotoxic chemotherapy agents. STE is based on the interference from back-scattered ultrasound waves from neighboring structures that create a speckled pattern that remains stable throughout the cardiac cycle (see **Fig. 3**).[38,39]

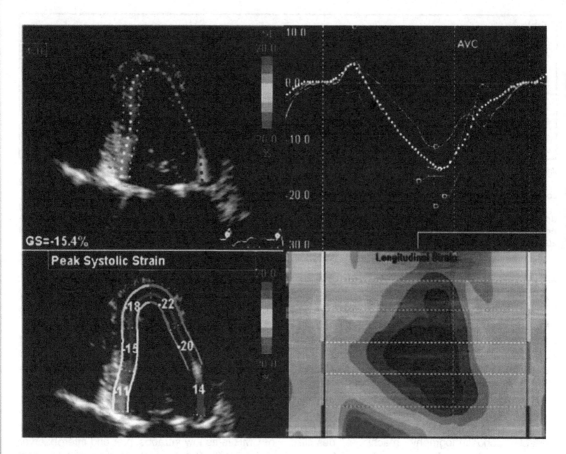

Fig. 3. Peak longitudinal strain obtained using speckle tracking during systolic contraction from 6 regions of interest that are angle independent and occur almost simultaneously in this normal patient. AVC, aortic valve closure; GS, global strain index. (*From* St John Sutton MG, Plappert T, Rahmouni H. Assessment of left ventricular systolic function by echocardiography. Heart Fail Clin 2009;5(2):177–90.)

Strain imaging assesses the deformation of cardiac muscle and is expressed as (1) strain, which is the percentage change of change from the original dimension and measured as the change in myocardial length over resting length[40]: strain $(\varepsilon) = \delta\,L/L_0$, where $\delta\,L$ is $(L_t - L_0)$, L_0 is resting length, and L_t is length at a specific time (t); and (2) strain rate, which is the rate of change of strain over unit time: strain rate $= \delta_\varepsilon/\delta_t$. Strain imaging values have superior reproducibility when compared with LVEF (reproducibility values from strain measurement vary from 5.5%–9.5%[29,41]). STE allows both regional and global assessment of cardiac function. Unlike tissue Doppler imaging, STE is not angle dependent (see **Fig. 3**) and enables assessment of radial and circumferential strain in addition to longitudinal strain (see **Fig. 4**).[38,39] Recent studies report that STE-derived parameters are highly reproducible, with a low interobserver and intraobserver variability,

and are even independent of the type of vendor that is used. It has several additional advantages, including that it is user independent and does not apply complex and error-prone mathematical algorithms to convert tissue velocity into strain parameters, but uses a much simpler principle: the measurement of distances. This technique also allows assessment of circumferential and radial strain components of all myocardial segments.[29] Although STE has not yet been shown to improve clinical outcomes in large studies, because of these advantages, it is increasingly thought that STE will eventually be used in day-to-day clinical cardiology because of its ability to detect subclinical dysfunction before a noticeable change in LVEF.[20,31,42] Indeed, several studies have suggested that STE is able to detect subclinical LV dysfunction before changes in LVEF are noted.[31–34,36] The superiority of STE compared with routine LVEF monitoring in patients undergoing

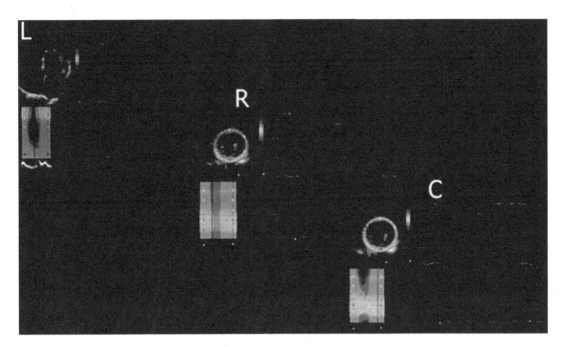

Fig. 4. A plot out of circumferential (C), radial (R), and longitudinal (L) strains from a normal patient in whom there is the usual regional temporal coordination of contraction. (*From* St John Sutton MG, Plappert T, Rahmouni H. Assessment of left ventricular systolic function by echocardiography. Heart Fail Clin 2009;5(2):177–90.)

cancer treatment is because of the fact that chemotherapy-induced cardiotoxicity probably has a regional pattern, and that the function of some myocardial segments may compensate for others, leading to a preserved global LVEF, at least in the early stages.[40] Another possible factor contributing to the higher sensitivity of STE when compared with LVEF may be variability. Strain measurement involves the averaging of the automated measurement of multiple segments (see **Figs. 3** and **4**), whereas LVEF assessment involves a tracing leading to 1 measurement. It has been suggested that the variability (especially in the longitudinal dimension) may, therefore, be lower for strain than for the LVEF,[34] particularly in patients with suboptimal images. Larger study populations are needed to further explore the effect of possible confounding variables in chemotherapy-induced cardiomyopathy, such as prior peripartum cardiomyopathy, accompanying ischemic heart disease, and valvular heart disease.

The availability of these sensitive techniques of detecting and predicting chemotherapy-induced cardiomyopathy suggests that a new approach is required to detect vulnerable myocardium before changes in LVEF or clinical symptoms manifest. A strategy that involves the use of a multi-pronged approach that also includes cardiac biomarkers, such as troponin,[43] and imaging techniques, such as CMR imaging or speckle tracking echocardiography for early detection and prediction will not only allow early initiation of cardioprotective medical therapy or use of less cardiotoxic anticancer drugs and chemotherapeutic regimens but will also allow continuation of treatment in select patients who may have otherwise been deprived of potentially lifesaving anticancer treatment. In our opinion, it is time to change tracks and adopt techniques, such as speckle tracking echocardiography and novel cardiac biomarkers, to detect and monitor chemotherapy-associated cardiotoxicity. To discuss these and other challenges in preventing and treating heart failure in patients with cancer and cancer survivors, Douglas B. Sawyer, MD, PhD and Daniel Lenihan, MD from the Vanderbilt Heart and Vascular Institute have invited an international panel of experts. These articles should not only improve immediate patient care but also form a basis for further research in this rapidly evolving area. With more patients at risk of cardiovascular difficulties developing during cancer treatments and little consensus developed about best monitoring, prevention, and treatments, it is our hope that this excellent compendium will stimulate more attention to this critically important subject.

Ragavendra R. Baliga, MD, MBA
Division of Cardiovascular Medicine
The Ohio State University Medical Center
Columbus, OH, USA

James B. Young, MD
Lerner College of Medicine
Endocrinology & Metabolism Institute
Cleveland Clinic
Cleveland, OH, USA

E-mail addresses:
Ragavendra.baliga@osumc.edu (R.R. Baliga)
youngj@ccf.org (J.B. Young)

REFERENCES

1. Rogers W. Will Rogers speaks: over 1,000 timeless quotations for public speakers (and writers, politicians, comedians, browsers–)/[compiled by] Bryan B. Sterling and Frances N. Sterling. New York: M. Evans and Co; 1996. p. 331.

2. Baliga RR, Pimental DR, Zhao YY, et al. NRG-1-induced cardiomyocyte hypertrophy. Role of PI-3-kinase, p70(S6K), and MEK-MAPK-RSK. Am J Physiol 1999;277(5 Pt 2):H2026–37.

3. Zhao YY, Sawyer DR, Baliga RR, et al. Neuregulins promote survival and growth of cardiac myocytes. Persistence of ErbB2 and ErbB4 expression in neonatal and adult ventricular myocytes. J Biol Chem 1998;273(17):10261–9.

4. Slamon DJ, Leyland-Jones B, Shak S, et al. Use of chemotherapy plus a monoclonal antibody against HER2 for metastatic breast cancer that overexpresses HER2. N Engl J Med 2001;344(11):783–92.

5. Jemal A, Siegel R, Xu J, et al. Cancer statistics. CA Cancer J Clin 2010;60(5):277–300.

6. Shan K, Lincoff AM, Young JB. Anthracycline-induced cardiotoxicity. Ann Intern Med 1996; 125(1):47–58.

7. Felker GM, Thompson RE, Hare JM, et al. Underlying causes and long-term survival in patients with initially unexplained cardiomyopathy. N Engl J Med 2000;342(15):1077–84.

8. Von Hoff DD, Layard MW, Basa P, et al. Risk factors for doxorubicin-induced congestive heart failure. Ann Intern Med 1979;91(5):710–7.

9. Cardinale D, Colombo A, Lamantia G, et al. Anthracycline-induced cardiomyopathy: clinical relevance and response to pharmacologic therapy. J Am Coll Cardiol 2010;55(3):213–20.

10. Telli ML, Hunt SA, Carlson RW, et al. Trastuzumab-related cardiotoxicity: calling into question the concept of reversibility. J Clin Oncol 2007;25(23): 3525–33.

11. Wang TJ, Evans JC, Benjamin EJ, et al. Natural history of asymptomatic left ventricular systolic dysfunction in the community. Circulation 2003; 108(8):977–82.

12. Cardinale D, Colombo A, Sandri MT, et al. Prevention of high-dose chemotherapy-induced cardiotoxicity in high-risk patients by angiotensin-converting enzyme inhibition. Circulation 2006;114(23):2474–81.

13. Kalay N, Basar E, Ozdogru I, et al. Protective effects of carvedilol against anthracycline-induced cardiomyopathy. J Am Coll Cardiol 2006;48(11):2258–62.

14. Zannad F, McMurray JJ, Krum H, et al. Eplerenone in patients with systolic heart failure and mild symptoms. N Engl J Med 2011;364(1):11–21.

15. Baliga RR, Ranganna P, Pitt B, et al. Spironolactone treatment and clinical outcomes in patients with systolic dysfunction and mild heart failure symptoms: a retrospective analysis. J Card Fail 2006; 12(4):250–6.

16. Thorn EM, Mehra MR. Imaging markers of adverse remodeling: from organ to organelle. Heart Fail Clin 2006;2(2):117–27.

17. Bansal S, Vacek JL, Ehler D. Consistency of echocardiographic ejection fraction: variation and 'drift' by interpreter and practice site. Eur J Echocardiogr 2002;3(1):44–6.

18. Einstein AJ, Weiner SD, Bernheim A, et al. Multiple testing, cumulative radiation dose, and clinical indications in patients undergoing myocardial perfusion imaging. JAMA 2010;304(19):2137–44.

19. Otterstad JE, Froeland G, St John Sutton M, et al. Accuracy and reproducibility of biplane two-dimensional echocardiographic measurements of left ventricular dimensions and function. Eur Heart J 1997;18(3):507–13.

20. Hare JL, Brown JK, Marwick TH. Performance of conventional echocardiographic parameters and myocardial measurements in the sequential evaluation of left ventricular function. Am J Cardiol 2008; 101(5):706–11.

21. Takuma S, Ota T, Muro T, et al. Assessment of left ventricular function by real-time 3-dimensional echocardiography compared with conventional noninvasive methods. J Am Soc Echocardiogr 2001;14(4): 275–84.

22. Jenkins C, Bricknell K, Hanekom L, et al. Reproducibility and accuracy of echocardiographic measurements of left ventricular parameters using real-time three-dimensional echocardiography. J Am Coll Cardiol 2004;44(4):878–86.

23. Baliga RR, Young JB. Using a magnet to strike gold. Heart Fail Clin 2009;5(3):ix–x.

24. Grothues F, Braun-Dullaeus R. Serial assessment of ventricular morphology and function. Heart Fail Clin 2009;5(3):301–14, v.

25. Grothues F, Moon JC, Bellenger NG, et al. Interstudy reproducibility of right ventricular volumes, function, and mass with cardiovascular magnetic resonance. Am Heart J 2004;147(2):218–23.

26. Grothues F, Smith GC, Moon JC, et al. Comparison of interstudy reproducibility of cardiovascular magnetic resonance with two-dimensional echocardiography in normal subjects and in patients with heart failure or left ventricular hypertrophy. Am J Cardiol 2002;90(1):29–34.

27. Bellenger NG, Davies LC, Francis JM, et al. Reduction in sample size for studies of remodeling in heart failure by the use of cardiovascular magnetic resonance. J Cardiovasc Magn Reson 2000;2(4):271–8.

28. Bellenger NG, Burgess MI, Ray SG, et al. Comparison of left ventricular ejection fraction and volumes in heart failure by echocardiography, radionuclide ventriculography and cardiovascular magnetic resonance; are they interchangeable? Eur Heart J 2000; 21(16):1387–96.

29. Marwick TH, Leano RL, Brown J, et al. Myocardial strain measurement with 2-dimensional speckle-tracking echocardiography: definition of normal range. JACC Cardiovasc Imaging 2009;2(1):80–4.

30. Cheung YF, Hong WJ, Chan GC, et al. Left ventricular myocardial deformation and mechanical dyssynchrony in children with normal ventricular shortening fraction after anthracycline therapy. Heart 2010; 96(14):1137–41.

31. Hare JL, Brown JK, Leano R, et al. Use of myocardial deformation imaging to detect preclinical myocardial dysfunction before conventional measures in patients undergoing breast cancer treatment with trastuzumab. Am Heart J 2009;158(2):294–301.

32. Ho E, Brown A, Barrett P, et al. Subclinical anthracycline- and trastuzumab-induced cardiotoxicity in the long-term follow-up of asymptomatic breast cancer survivors: a speckle tracking echocardiographic study. Heart 2010;96(9):701–7.

33. Tsai HR, Gjesdal O, Wethal T, et al. Left ventricular function assessed by two-dimensional speckle tracking echocardiography in long-term survivors of Hodgkin's lymphoma treated by mediastinal radiotherapy with or without anthracycline therapy. Am J Cardiol 2011;107(3):472–7.

34. Sawaya H, Sebag IA, Plana JC, et al. Early detection and prediction of cardiotoxicity in chemotherapy-treated patients. Am J Cardiol 2011;107(9):1375–80.

35. Jassal DS, Han SY, Hans C, et al. Utility of tissue Doppler and strain rate imaging in the early detection of trastuzumab and anthracycline mediated cardiomyopathy. J Am Soc Echocardiogr 2009; 22(4):418–24.

36. Ganame J, Claus P, Uyttebroeck A, et al. Myocardial dysfunction late after low-dose anthracycline treatment in asymptomatic pediatric patients. J Am Soc Echocardiogr 2007;20(12):1351–8.

37. Takenaka K, Kuwada Y, Sonoda M, et al. Anthracycline-induced cardiomyopathies evaluated by tissue Doppler tracking system and strain rate imaging. J Cardiol 2001;37(Suppl 1):129–32.

38. Korinek J, Wang J, Sengupta PP, et al. Two-dimensional strain–a Doppler-independent ultrasound method for quantitation of regional deformation: validation in vitro and in vivo. J Am Soc Echocardiogr 2005;18(12):1247–53.

39. Artis NJ, Oxborough DL, Williams G, et al. Two-dimensional strain imaging: a new echocardiographic advance with research and clinical applications. Int J Cardiol 2008;123(3):240–8.

40. St John Sutton MG, Plappert T, Rahmouni H. Assessment of left ventricular systolic function by echocardiography. Heart Fail Clin 2009;5(2):177–90.

41. Sun JP, Popovic ZB, Greenberg NL, et al. Noninvasive quantification of regional myocardial function using Doppler-derived velocity, displacement, strain rate, and strain in healthy volunteers: effects of aging. J Am Soc Echocardiogr 2004;17(2):132–8.

42. Serri K, Reant P, Lafitte M, et al. Global and regional myocardial function quantification by two-dimensional strain: application in hypertrophic cardiomyopathy. J Am Coll Cardiol 2006;47(6):1175–81.

43. Baliga RR, Young JB. Editorial: do biomarkers deserve high marks? Heart Fail Clin 2009;5(4):ix–xii.

Preface

Heart Disease in Cancer Patients: A Burgeoning Field Where Optimizing Patient Care Is Requiring Interdisciplinary Collaborations

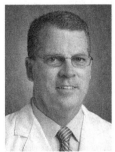 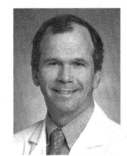

Daniel J. Lenihan, MD   Douglas B. Sawyer, MD, PhD
Guest Editors

In the last decade, it has become increasingly clear that patients who are being cared for by cardiologists are likely to be older and have multiple comorbid conditions and are going to require many more complex decisions that will need full consideration. This is particularly true when it comes to the overall management of heart failure (HF) and left ventricular dysfunction in contemporary medical care. It is no surprise to those practitioners who evaluate and treat patients with HF that the number of recommended tests or medical interventions can be a daunting process and is frequently impossible to fully consider in each patient. Moreover, the primary data or research that forms the basis of each recommendation is typically in a controlled clinical population that may not be completely appropriate for the patient decision at hand.[1] Interestingly, there is no place where these issues are more prominent than in those patients we encounter that have cardiac disease in the setting of cancer.

The concept that a patient who has cancer, either historically or at the current moment, may develop a cardiac issue, specifically HF, is not unusual. In fact, this probably occurs more frequently than typically realized. A large longitudinal study of physicians without established cardiac disease or cancer followed over a decade revealed that the incidence of either condition rose dramatically in the sixth and seventh decade of life and not uncommonly both conditions were coexistent in a substantial number of patients.[2] With this concept in mind, there is a substantial clinical opportunity that now presents itself to the disciplines of cardiology and oncology. There are many areas of clinical overlap, and the patient remains the focal point where the uncertain and challenging decisions occur.

This issue of *Heart Failure Clinics* has a unique presentation of topics aimed at addressing the intersection of heart disease, and specifically HF, in cancer patients. Many of these topics were presented in part at the recent annual meeting of the International CardiOncology Society held in Nashville in October 2010.[3] Although this *Clinics* issue does not include all presentations or important discussions that have been identified by this group of committed cardiology and oncology providers, representative articles explain the complexity and spirit of

Heart Failure Clin 7 (2011) xxi–xxiii
doi:10.1016/j.hfc.2011.04.001

heartfailure.theclinics.com

cooperation that is required to effectively care for these patients.

An impressive group of authors, who have extensive experience in dealing with the dilemmas required by these challenging clinical scenarios, present a wide array of topics. Khakoo and Rees lead off the issue with an excellent basic and clinical overview of the cardiac effects, including hypertension and HF, of anti-angiogenic therapy for cancer. This is followed by a sophisticated discussion from Scherer-Crosbie and colleagues of the latest echocardiographic techniques used to detect cardiotoxicity during chemotherapy. Carver and Ky then further develop the optimal methods for cardiotoxicity detection by carefully summarizing the use of biomarkers for detection of cardiac dysfunction at the earliest potential time and discuss strategies to provide cardioprotection. Witteles and colleagues further this discussion by examining how cardiologists currently respond to the treatment of cardiac toxicities with chemotherapy and explore the practice patterns and how these can be enhanced to improve the provision of care to our patients.

A burgeoning area of research in the treatment of heart failure is stem cell therapy, which has a proven efficacy in certain hematologic malignancies. Naftilan and Schuening summarize the current knowledge of stem cell therapy for cardiac disease and highlight some of the lessons learned from oncology as this treatment option was refined to its present level of efficacy. Chen and Steingart then explore the graduate medical training expectations for the disciplines of both cardiology and oncology and describe the areas for improvement if we are collectively to learn the optimal approaches to patients with cancer and HF.

Ewer and colleagues present an eloquent historical account that covers the development of anthracyclines as a cancer therapy and also how the issues of cardiac damage related to these therapies were detected and managed over the past 30 years. Remick and colleagues then enhance our understanding of how the oncology community ensures adequate patient safety for cardiac conditions in all of their clinical trials by detailing the definitions of cardiac damage in the Common Terminology Criteria. Further, these criteria were recently updated by a multidisciplinary team to be more descriptive and accurate as far as describing cardiac effects of cancer therapy. Next, Seldin and colleagues provide an outstanding overview of the detection and treatment of amyloidosis and areas of direct overlap between oncology and cardiology as it relates to treating this condition. Finally, Porter

and Slosky present important considerations about collaboration among disciplines and use several recent cases as a template for coordinating care in complex clinical decisions.

In reading these contributions, we hope a primary care, oncology, or cardiology provider will gain an increased appreciation for and understanding of the real opportunity that is before us. The significant discoveries in the field of myocardial metabolism and vascular development that have been accelerated because of clinical experience with targeted agents for cancer, the increased appreciation for the overlapping demographics of oncology and cardiology patients, and the finding that therapies developed for one may be a critical adjunct of therapy in the other are but a few of the many exciting developments stimulated by the interaction between cardiology and oncology. It is clearly imperative that we continue to share knowledge and experience across disciplines, as we learn from our patients how to ensure that optimal treatment of both conditions can be achieved. Future directions fertile for exploration include improving our understanding of how stimulatory and inhibitory extracellular and intracellular signaling pathways can be manipulated to treat one disease, without precipitating another. This will require increasing partnership between cardiovascular and oncology investigators at both the bench and the bedside. It is clear our current training programs will need to be adjusted to foster development of future investigators equipped with the knowledge and perspective to lead us forward. If we consider that the overlap between cardiac disease and cancer is a pond, we have figuratively put our toe in to "test the water," but there is certainly momentum, outlined by this issue of *Heart Failure Clinics*, to actually jump in all the way.

Daniel J. Lenihan, MD
Vanderbilt Heart and Vascular Institute
1215 21st Avenue South
Suit 5209
Nashville, TN 37232, USA

Douglas B. Sawyer, MD, PhD
Division of Cardiovascular Medicine
Department of Medicine
Vanderbilt University
2220 Pierce Avenue
Suit 383 Preston Research Building
Nashville, TN 37232, USA

E-mail addresses:
Daniel.lenihan@vanderbilt.edu (D.J. Lenihan)
douglas.b.sawyer@vanderbilt.edu (D.B. Sawyer)

REFERENCES

1. Hunt SA, Abraham WT, Chin MH, et al. 2009 Focused update incorporated into the ACC/AHA 2005 Guidelines for the Diagnosis and Management of Heart Failure in Adults. A Report of the American College of Cardiology Foundation/American Heart Association Task Force on Practice Guidelines Developed in Collaboration With the International Society for Heart and Lung Transplantation. J Am Coll Cardiol 2009; 53:e1–90.

2. Driver JA, Djousse L, Logroscino G, et al. Incidence of cardiovascular disease and cancer in advanced age: prospective cohort study. BMJ 2008;337:a2467.

3. Lenihan DJ, Cardinale D, Cipolla CM. The compelling need for a cardiology and oncology partnership and the birth of the International CardiOncology Society. Prog Cardiovasc Dis 2010;53:88–93.

Molecular Mechanisms of Hypertension and Heart Failure Due to Antiangiogenic Cancer Therapies

Meredith L. Rees, BA[a], Aarif Y. Khakoo, MD, MBA[b],*

KEYWORDS

• Cardiotoxicity • Hypertension • Heart failure • Cancer

In the years since Judah Folkman and colleagues[1] published their discovery of a proangiogenic factor isolated from tumor cells, the field of tumor angiogenesis, along with the development of antiangiogenic cancer therapies, has rapidly evolved. The first milestone was reached in 2004 when the US Food and Drug Administration (FDA) approved bevacizumab, a monoclonal antibody directed against vascular endothelial growth factor (VEGF), which greatly limits tumor angiogenesis and growth. The success of this drug in the treatment of several solid tumor types, including metastatic colorectal cancer (mCRC) and nonsmall cell lung cancer (NSLC), led to the rapid FDA approval of 2 antiangiogenic small molecule tyrosine kinase inhibitors (TKIs): sorafenib in December of 2005 and sunitinib in January of 2006. Both of these agents are approved for use in metastatic renal cell carcinoma (mRCC) among other highly vascularized solid tumors.[2] Recently, 2 other small molecule TKIs have been developed: axitinib and pazopanib. Both are now in different stages of clinical trials.

Small molecule TKIs limit tumor growth by inhibiting proangiogenic growth factors that are typically overexpressed in human cancers. Prominent targets include VEGF receptors 1 through 3 (VEGFR), platelet-derived growth factor receptors α and β (PDGFR), and the stem cell factor receptor CD117 (c-kit).[3,4] The promise of antiangiogenic therapies and other molecularly targeted anticancer agents is that such agents will have a dramatically higher efficacy-to-toxicity ratio than traditional chemotherapy by specifically inhibiting molecules associated with tumor growth. In theory, such agents would be highly effective in treating cancer without adversely affecting normal organs. This is in contrast to traditional chemotherapeutic agents such as anthracyclines, which have been shown to be very effective in the treatment of a number of malignancies yet often result in a cancer survivor with devastating cardiac disease. Although targeted cancer therapies are typically aimed at molecules that are overexpressed in cancer cells, the fact remains that many of these same molecules are expressed in normal tissues, and these molecules may play a role in the normal physiology of many organ systems, including the cardiovascular system. Indeed, over the past decade it has become clear

The authors have nothing to disclose.

[a] Department of Cardiology, University of Texas M.D. Anderson Cancer Center, 1515 Holcombe Boulevard, Unit 1101, Houston, TX 77030, USA

[b] Department of Cardiology, University of Texas M.D. Anderson Cancer Center, 1515 Holcombe Boulevard, Unit 1451, Houston, TX 77030, USA

* Corresponding author.

E-mail address: aykhakoo@mdanderson.org

Heart Failure Clin 7 (2011) 299–311

doi:10.1016/j.hfc.2011.03.004

that there is substantial overlap between biologic systems that are relevant in the pathogenesis of human cancer and cardiovascular disease.[5] For instance, in addition to its well described role in the cardiovascular system, the renin–angiotensin system appears to be a key regulator of human vasculogenesis and tumor angiogenesis.[6] Similarly, cellular bioenergetics, a field that has been studied extensively in the context of cardiac biology, is now being studied by cancer biologists in search of distinct bioenergetic targets in cancer cells.[7]

Further reducing the efficacy-to-toxicity ratio of targeted antiangiogenic therapies are various off-target effects seen with these agents. This is especially true of the small-molecule TKIs, which are designed to competitively inhibit a kinase of interest by interfering with the adenosine triphosphate (ATP) binding pocket of that kinase. Unfortunately, since the ATP binding pocket tends to be structurally conserved across the wide array of human kinases, the specificity of this approach has been limited, even at pharmacologically relevant dosages. Sunitinib malate for example, which has been associated with clinically significant cardiac dysfunction and hypertension (HTN), has been shown to bind to and inhibit a large number of kinases using in vitro assays at clinically relevant dosages.[8]

Thus, while antiangiogenic therapies are effective in prolonging survival, on-target and off-target cardiovascular toxicities including HTN, cardiomyopathies, thromboembolism, and renal dysfunction are major concerns. Although the exact molecular mechanisms by which tyrosine kinase inhibition leads to HTN and cardiotoxicities remain somewhat unclear, recent preclinical and clinical studies have made significant progress.

Table 1 summarizes the relative incidence of HTN and left ventricular (LV) dysfunction that has been reported from clinical studies of antiangiogenic agents in cancer patients. The nature of these toxicities is discussed in more detail throughout this article. It is critically important to note, however, that since cardiovascular toxicities were not primary endpoints of most of these studies and were only reported if clinically manifest, it is likely the true incidence of LV dysfunction and HTN due to antiangiogenic therapies may be higher than currently reported. This article summarizes the incidences of cardiovascular toxicities, namely HTN and heart failure (HF), associated with the most commonly used antiangiogenic therapies, and then presents data from preclinical and clinical studies to provide some insight into the underlying molecular mechanisms.

BEVACIZUMAB

Bevacizumab is a humanized monoclonal antibody directed against VEGF-A and is approved for use in metastatic colorectal cancer (mCRC), nonsmall cell lung cancer, metastatic breast cancer, and metastatic renal cell carcinoma.

Hypertension

In a 1997 phase 1 clinical trial of 25 patients, no common toxicity criteria (CTC) grade 3 or 4 adverse effects were identified.[9] Notably, these criteria have undergone substantial revisions since those applied to this study, and the current grading criteria for HTN, HF, and LV dysfunction, extracted from the Common Terminology Criteria for Adverse Events (CTCAE v 4.0) are presented in **Table 2** for the reader's reference. It was not until a 2003 phase 2 trial of 104 patients with

---

Table 1
Incidence of hypertension and cardiotoxicity with each treatment

Therapy	Type	Targets	Incidence of HTN	Incidence of LV Dysfunction
Bevacizumab (Avastin)	MoAb	VEGF	24%–28%[10,12]	2%–15%[15,17]
Sorafenib (Nexavar)	smTKI	Raf-1, B-Raf, VEGFR2, PDGF, FLt-3, c-Kit	17%–23%[19,20]	10%–21%[20]
Sunitinib (Sutent)	smTKI	VEGFR, PDGFR, c-kit	22%–47%[3,30]	10%–19%[29,31]
Axitinib (AG013736)	smTKI	VEGFR1, 2, and 3; PDGFR; c-Kit	33%–58%[33,35]	3%[33]
Pazopanib (Votrient)	smTKI	VEGFR, PDGFR, c-kit,1, FGF3, IL2	33%–40%[33,36]	Unknown

Abbreviations: HTN, hypertension; IL2, interleukin 2; LV, left ventricular; MoAb, monocolonal antibody; PDGFR, platelet-derived growth factor receptor; smTKI, small molecule tyrosine kinase inhibitor; VEGF, vascular endothelial growth factor.

Table 2
Common terminology criteria for adverse events (CTCAE v 4.0) for cardiovascular events

Adverse Event	Grade				
	1	2	3	4	5
Hypertension	Prehypertension (systolic BP 120–139 mm Hg or diastolic BP 80–89 mm Hg)	Stage 1 hypertension (systolic BP 140–159 mm Hg or diastolic BP 90–99 mm Hg); medical intervention indicated; recurrent or persistent (≥24 h); symptomatic increase by >20 mm Hg (diastolic) or to >140/90 mm Hg if previously within normal limits; monotherapy indicated Pediatric: recurrent or persistent (≥24 hrs) BP >upper limit of normal; monotherapy indicated	Stage 2 hypertension (systolic BP ≥160 mm Hg or diastolic BP ≥100 mm Hg); medical intervention indicated; more than 1 drug or more intensive therapy than previously used indicated Pediatric: same as adult	Life-threatening consequences (eg, malignant hypertension, transient or permanent neurologic deficit, hypertensive crisis); urgent intervention indicated Pediatric: same as adult	Death
Heart Failure	Asymptomatic with laboratory (eg, BNP) or cardiac imaging abnormalities	Symptoms with mild-to-moderate activity or exertion	Severe with symptoms at rest or with minimal activity or exertion; intervention indicated	Life-threatening consequences; urgent intervention indicated (eg, continuous IV therapy or mechanical hemodynamic support)	Death
LV Systolic Dysfunction	N/A	N/A	Symptomatic due to drop in ejection fraction responsive to intervention	Refractory or poorly controlled heart failure due to drop in ejection fraction; intervention such as ventricular assist device, intravenous vasopressor support, or heart transplant indicated	Death

Abbreviations: BNP, B-natriuretic peptide; BP, blood pressure; IV, intravenous; LV, left ventricular.
Adapted from The Common Terminology Criteria for Adverse Events, v 4.0, U.S. Department of Health and Human Services, Published May 28, 2009. Available at: http://evs.nci.nih.gov/ftp1/CTCAE/CTCAE_4.03_2010-06-14_QuickReference_5x7.pdf. Accessed December 23, 2010.

mCRC that significant HTN was first reported.[10] In this trial, 11% of patients treated with 5 mg/kg and 28% of patients treated with 10 mg/kg doses of bevacizumab developed HTN over the course of treatment. HTN was also reported in a 2004 phase 3 trial of 813 patients with previously untreated mCRC.[11] Of the 393 patients treated with irinotecan, bolus fluorouracil, and leucovorin (IFL) plus bevacizumab (5 mg/kg of body weight every 2 weeks), 22.4% developed HTN, while 11% developed CTC grade 3 HTN and were treated with antihypertensive medication. None of the cases resulted in cessation of treatment or death. According to a recent meta-analysis of 12,656 patients with a range of tumors, treatment with bevacizumab results in an incidence of all-grade HTN of 23.6% (95% confidence interval [CI]: 20.5–27.1) and grade 3/4 of 7.9% (95% CI: 6.1–10.2). The calculated RR of developing high-grade HTN was 5.28 (95% CI: 4.15–6.71, $P<.001$).[12]

Cardiotoxicity (LV Dysfunction or HF)

Compared with other antiangiogenic therapies, bevacizumab treatment alone is infrequently associated with LV dysfunction or HF. For example, in a pivotal 2004 study demonstrating benefit of bevacizumab in addition to standard chemotherapy in patients with metastatic colorectal cancer, HF was not reported as an adverse effect, despite a significantly greater incidence of HTN in the bevacizumab treatment arm.[11] Similarly, HF or LV dysfunction was not reported to be significantly increased in a meta-analysis of trials of bevacizumab in metastatic colorectal cancer.[13] As the uses of bevacizumab expand beyond colorectal cancer, the landscape of cardiac toxicity associated with this agent may change. Specifically, previous treatment with known cardiotoxic agents such as anthracyclines may potentiate adverse cardiac effects of bevacizumab.[14] For example, bevacizumab-associated cardiotoxicities have been reported in patients with metastatic breast cancer, most of whom have been pretreated with anthracycline-based regimens and/or trastuzumab.[15,16] In a phase 3 trial of bevacizumab treatment in metastatic breast cancer, 2% (5) of patients treated with a combination of capecitabine and bevacizumab developed CTC grade 3 LV dysfunction.[17] Only 0.5% (1) of the patients in the capecitabine-only group developed grade 4 HF. Data from a number of clinical trials of bevacizumab for early stage breast cancer demonstrate an incidence of LV dysfunction ranging from 2% to 15%.[15] Some of these studies included regimens combining anthracyclines with bevacizumab. These findings suggest that bevacizumab may potentiate clinically significant LV dysfunction in patients simultaneously or previously treated with anthracycline-based regimens, which will need to be formally evaluated in future studies.

SORAFENIB

Sorafenib is an oral small-molecule TKI that was originally developed to inhibit Raf-1 of the MAPK pathways but also blocks B-Raf, VEGFR-2, PDGFR, Flt-3, and c-Kit.[18] It is primarily used in the treatment of mRCC and hepatocellular carcinoma and inhibits angiogenesis by limiting the proliferation of vascular smooth muscle cells. Common systemic adverse effects seen with sorafenib treatment include diarrhea, fatigue, and skin rashes.

Hypertension

Escudier and colleagues[19] performed a comprehensive phase 2 randomized, double-blind, placebo-controlled study of 903 patients with clear cell RCC given 400 mg of sorafenib twice daily. Known as the Treatment Approached in Renal Cancer Global Evaluation Trial (TARGET) and covering 117 centers in 19 different countries, the incidence of all-grade HTN was 17% and 4% for grades 3/4, respectively in the sorafenib group versus 2% for all-grade HTN and <1% for grades 3/4 in the placebo group. Additionally, a meta analysis of 223 studies (4599 patients, 3567 treated with sorafenib alone) indicated that the overall incidence of all-grade HTN was 23.4% (95% CI 16.0–32.9), whereas the incidence of grade 3/4 HTN ranged from 2.1% to 30.7%.[20] This same study looked at the incidence of HTN in mRCC patients regardless of the treatment type with the hypothesis that renal dysfunction would predispose patients to HTN. However, there was no correlation between renal dysfunction/nephrectomy and HTN. In an attempt to understand the mechanisms behind sorafenib-induced HTN, Veronese and colleagues[21] evaluated 20 patients receiving 400 mg sorafenib twice daily for the incidence of HTN and measured serum VEGF, catecholamines, endothelin 1, urotensin 2, renin, and aldosterone levels. Although 75% (15) had at least a 10 mm Hg increase in systolic blood pressure (sBP), and 12 had at least a 20 mm Hg increase in sBP after 3 weeks of therapy, there were no significant changes in the levels of these circulating factors, indicating that sorafenib-induced HTN is not likely due to changes in humoral factors, or at least not those measured in their study. Correspondingly, sorafenib may have a more direct effect on hemodynamics based on the fact that treatment can cause elevation of blood pressure within the first 24 hours.[22] However, this study was careful to note that changes in BP vary widely from patient to patient and that the hypertensive response to sorafenib may be a good clinical indicator of optimal drug dosage.

Cardiotoxicity

Cardiac events in patients treated with sorafenib were first described in a 2008 observational study of patients with RCC treated with either sorafenib or sunitinib.[2,20] Of the sorafenib-treated patients reported in this study, 56% of patients had a cardiac event, defined broadly by an inclusion of electrocardiogram (ECG) changes. In this group, overt LV dysfunction occurred in 21% of patients. Notably, elevations of cardiac biomarkers of injury were seen in a large proportion of patients, accompanied by regional wall motion abnormalities, suggesting an association between sorafenib and regional myocardial ischemia. Isolated case reports further report an association between sorafenib and myocardial ischemia.[23] Additionally, in vitro studies[24] and preclinical in vivo models[25] suggest that sorafenib cardiotoxicity may be an issue of clinical concern, but the true incidence of myocardial ischemia or HF due to sorafenib is not clearly defined.

SUNITINIB

Sunitinib is a small-molecule TKI whose targets include VEGFR, PDGFR and c-kit. Sunitinib has demonstrated significant antitumor effect when used for the treatment of mRCC and imatinib-resistant gastrointestinal stromal tumors (GIST). Although VEGFR and PDGFR are the dominant targets of sunitinib and may account for a significant portion of its observed antitumor effects, sunitinib is an extremely promiscuous TKI. In a study of its in vitro activity, sunitinib exerted significant inhibition of close to 20% of all kinases tested,[26,27] suggesting that off-target effects of sunitinib may play a role in both its antitumor effect and cardiovascular toxicities.

HTN

HTN associated with sunitinib treatment was first observed in a 2006 randomized, double-blind phase 3 trial of sunitinib for the second-line treatment of imatinib-resistant GIST.[28] Grade 3/4 HTN was observed in 3% (6) of patients in the sunitinib group versus none in the placebo-treated group. A similar phase 3 trial found that 24% of patients develop HTN, with 8% developing grade 3 or higher.[29] Two other single-arm multicenter trails also indicated hypertension as an adverse

effect.[22] In 2007, Chu and colleagues[3] analyzed a phase 1/2 study of 75 patients with imatinib-resistant GIST for the presence of adverse cardiac effects and found that 47% (35 patients) developed HTN (>150/100 mm Hg). The incidences of HTN associated with sunitinib treatment seem to vary widely, and in an attempt to broadly define the incidence of HTN with sunitinib treatment, Zhu and colleagues[30] performed a meta analysis of 13 clinical trials in which patients with RCC, GIST, or other malignancies received either 37.5 mg of sunitinib daily (continuous daily dosing or 50 mg of sunitinib daily for 4 weeks followed by 2 weeks off, for a 6 week cycle. Out of the 4999 patients analyzed, the incidence of all-grade HTN was 21.6%, with 6.8% developing grade 3/4 HTN. This puts the incidence of hypertension with sunitinib treatment in line with the other antiangiogenic therapies.

Cardiotoxicity

Concern about cardiotoxicity due to sunitinib first arose from early phase clinical trials. In a 2007 study of patients with GIST, 10% of sunitinib-treated patients experienced LV dysfunction compared with 3% in the placebo-treated arm.[26] In addition, in an early phase trial of sunitinib for metastatic RCC, 15% of patients developed objective LV dysfunction.[26] The Chu and colleagues study found that of the 75 sunitinib-treated patients with no prior history of LV dysfunction or HF, 19% experienced a 15% or greater decline in LV ejection fraction (LVEF), with 8% of patients developing high-grade cardiac dysfunction and HF.[3] In a retrospective analysis of 175 patients with mRCC at 8 different Italian institutions treated with sunitinib, DiLorenzo and colleagues[31] found that 19% of patients had objective declines in cardiac function, including 7% who experienced HF. After noting a high incidence of HF in patients receiving sunitinib for RCC or GIST, Telli and colleagues[32] at Stanford University conducted a retrospective analysis of patients treated with sunitinib between July 1, 2004, and July 1, 2007. Of the 48 patients who received therapy, 15% (7 patients) presented with grade 3/4 LV dysfunction. All 7 patients presented with symptomatic HF; 5 patients required hospitalization, and 3 patients continued to experience cardiac dysfunction after cessation of treatment and initiation of therapy for HF. In a referral-based study, the authors reported that 6 sunitinib-treated patients (3% of the total sunitinib-treated population over the time period in question) developed LV dysfunction and HF associated with profound morbidity and mortality.[4]

In each of these studies, cardiac dysfunction occurred within the first several cycles of treatment and was often associated with the development of significant systemic HTN. Importantly, in contrast to the studies described, a randomized, double-blind phase 3 trial by Rock and colleagues[26] recorded grade 3/4 decreases in LVEF in 1% (2) of patients versus none in the placebo-treated group. Similarly, a multicenter phase 2 trial by Motzer and colleagues[29] of 750 patients with previously untreated mRCC found a decline in LVEF in 10% of patients, though only 2% were classified as grade 3 or higher. Discrepancies in the event rate of cardiac dysfunction associated with sunitinib may relate to differences in definitions or to the extent of cardiac monitoring. Nevertheless, the sum of all of the data suggests that sunitinib may have the most associated cardiac toxicity when compared with other antiangiogenic agents currently used in clinical practice.

AXITINIB AND PAZOPANIB

Axitinib and pazopanib are both new-generation small-molecule TKIs used in the treatment of mRCC and colorectal cancer.[18,33] Pazopanib has also been beneficial in treating ovarian cancer, breast cancer, nonsmall cell lung cancer, soft tissue sarcoma, and multiple myeloma.[34] Shared targets include VEGFR1, VEGFR2, VEFGR3, PDGFR, and c-kit, although pazopanib has been shown to inhibit other targets such as the fibroblast growth factors 1 and 3 and the interleukin-(IL)2 receptor. Common adverse effects for both include nausea, fatigue, vomiting, and diarrhea.

Hypertension

Although there are not nearly as many clinical trials with these drugs as there are for the three already discussed, HTN has been shown to be a notable adverse effect in early phase clinical trials with both of these agents. In a 2007 phase 1 trial of axitinib in 52 patients with mRCC who had progressive diseases despite previous treatment with cytokine-based therapy, 58% (30) of patients developed some level of HTN with 8 patients developing grade 3/4 HTN.[33] One patient each developed cardiomyopathy, myocardial infarction (MI), and LV dysfunction. Antihypertensive treatment was used by 36 of the patients in the study; however 23 had a history of HTN. In a similar phase 1 trial, 63 patients with advanced-stage refractory solid tumors were treated with pazopanib on a dose-escalation or dose-expansion protocol.[35] Thirty-three percent (21) developed HTN, with 25% (16) developing grade 3/4 toxicity. In this case, the incidence of HTN was similar in patients

with and without and history of HTN. The average time to elevation of BP by greater than 15 mmHg was 7.5 days. In a larger randomized, double-blind phase 3 trial of pazopanib in 435 patients with previously untreated (233 patients, 54%) or cytokine pretreated (202 patients, 46%) advanced RCC, the incidence of HTN was 40%.[36] In this same study, MI or ischemia occurred in 3% of patients. Similarly, a phase 2 trial of pazopanib for use in recurrent glioblastoma found an incidence of HTN of 37% (13 patients).

MOLECULAR MECHANISMS OF HYPERTENSION AND CARDIOTOXICITY DUE TO ANTIANGIOGENIC AGENTS

Recent research has begun to reveal the mechanisms underlying TKI-induced HTN and cardiotoxicity and has implicated processes from mitochondrial dysfunction and apoptosis to vessel refraction and decreased nitric oxide bioavailability. None of the TKIs are truly specific, and the level of cardiotoxicity may be correlated with lack of target specificity.[37] In some cases, previously unidentified roles for certain tyrosine kinases in the heart have been discovered.[38] Mechanistically, it appears that HTN and cardiac dysfunction may be coupled, and may relate to effects of these agents on the vasculature or result from direct effects on cardiomyocytes. Putative mechanisms of cardiotoxicity of antiangiogenic TKIs will be discussed, with an overview of known vascular and cardiac effects of VEGFR and PDGFR, the dominant targets of the currently used antiangiogenic therapies. **Fig. 1** illustrates putative mechanisms by which inhibition of VEGFR or PDGFR may result in clinically significant HTN. Aspects of this figure are discussed in more detail.

VASCULAR EFFECTS
VEGF/VEGFR

VEGFR signaling is a key target of most antiangiogenic cancer therapy. VEGFRs play an important role in tumor angiogenesis but also regulate normal vascular permeability and endothelial cell survival. The VEGF family includes 7 members: VEGF-A, VEGF-B, VEGF-C, VEGF-D, VEGF-E, VEGF-F, and placenta growth factor, PIGF. Most of the common proangiogenic functions (endothelial cell proliferation and migration) of VEGF family members have been attributed to VEGF-A (commonly and herein referred to as simply VEGF).[39] VEGF-B is thought to mainly function in embryonic angiogenesis, but recent evidence has suggested that VEGF-B may be the predominant form in the adult heart and may be

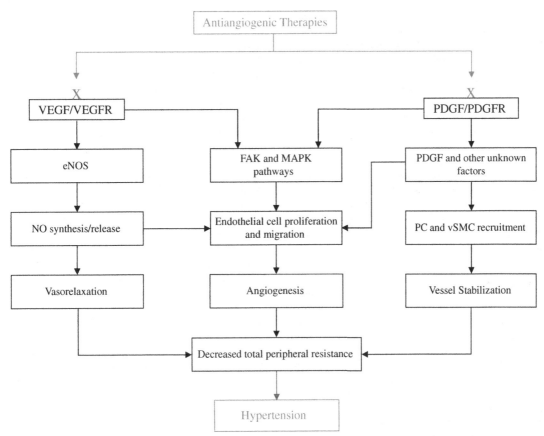

Fig. 1. Mechanisms for blood pressure changes with antiangiogenic therapies. Antiangiogenic therapies cause hypertension through the inactivation of both the vascular endothelial growth factor and platelet-derived growth factor receptors. Disruption of normal signaling results in a loss of angiogenesis and vasoconstriction. This leads to an increase in total peripheral resistance and thus a rise in blood pressure.

cardioprotective. VEGF-C and VEGF-D are involved in lymphangiogenesis, whereas VEGF-E and VEGF-F have been found in viruses and snake venom, respectively.

Alternative splicing of the 8 exons of the VEGF-A gene results in 4 different isoforms: $VEGF_{121}$, $VEGF_{165}$, $VEGF_{189}$, and $VEGF_{206}$. $VEGF_{165}$ is the most common isoform and can either be secreted or bound by a heparin-binding domain to the extracellular matrix (ECM). $VEGF_{121}$ lacks the binding domain and is freely diffusible. $VEGF_{189}$ and $VEGF_{206}$ have high heparin binding affinity and are found predominately in the ECM. ECM-bound forms of VEGF can be cleaved to the enzyme plasmin and then become freely diffusible.[39]

The main transcription factor driving VEGF expression is hypoxia-inducible factor 1α (HIF-1α), whose activity is tightly coupled to oxygen tension. Under normal oxygen tension conditions, HIF-1α is sequestered in the cytoplasm by the product of the von Hippel-Lindau (VHL) gene. When oxygen levels drop, VHL is degraded, and HIF1-α translocates to the nucleus, where it induces transcription of several proangiogenic and prosurvival genes. It is also thought that VEGF can be released in response to physical forces such a shear stress and stretch. This mode of release of VEGF may be important in HTN and may be central to bevacizumab-associated HTN.

There are 2 main VEGF receptors: VEGFR1 (also known as Flt-1) and VEGFR2 (KDR or Flk-1). The function of VEGFR1 is less well understood compared with VEGFR2. Activation of VEGFR1 does not seem to induce angiogenesis, and therefore some have argued that endothelial VEGFR1 acts as a decoy receptor and regulates angiogenesis by preventing VEGF from binding to VEGFR2[39] Importantly, VEGF-B and PlGF only bind to VEGFR1,[40] and therefore it seems likely that VEGFR1 has yet-to-be-defined vascular functions. In vessels, VEGFR2 mediates cell proliferation through MAPK pathways, migration via focal adhesion kinase (FAK), and survival through Akt[41] as well as stimulating endothelial nitric oxide synthase (eNOS) and the consequent production of nitric oxide (NO). The role of NO in vascular biology is well characterized, having profound vasorelaxation capabilities; thus NO plays an essential role in the regulation of BP and consequentially the development of HTN.[42] Interestingly, VEGF levels are elevated in hypertensive patients, much like insulin in type 2 diabetics. However, levels decrease with aggressive antihypertensive therapies, implying that changes in VEGF levels and signaling may be secondary to the development of HTN. Nonetheless, the high incidence of HTN induced by agents that block VEGFR signaling suggests that this pathway may play a more important role than previously appreciated in the regulation of systemic vascular resistance.

PDGF/PDGFR

PDGFR plays an important paracrine role in embryonic angiogenesis, vessel maturation, and stabilization and wound healing by stimulating the growth and recruitment of a variety of cells including vascular smooth muscle cells, pericytes, fibroblasts, endothelial and glial cells.[43–45] PDGF is stored, and was originally discovered, in the alpha granules of platelets. However, it can also be synthesized by a variety of cell types including endothelial cells and cardiomyocytes. Various stimuli can induce synthesis of PDGF including low oxygen tension (via HIF1α), thrombin and other growth factors such as FGF. The PDGF ligand is found as either a homodimer or heterodimer of 2 PDGF chains, alpha and beta. Both chains are synthesized as precursor molecules that spontaneously form dimers upon cleavage in an apparently random fashion.[43] Because the molecule is a dimer, it binds 2 receptors at once, causing autophosphorylation of the receptors. PDGF works through 2 structurally related receptor tyrosine kinases, alpha and beta. The two receptors have similar but independent functions. For instance, PDGFR-β activation induces chemotaxis in vitro, whereas activation of PDGFR-α inhibits it.[43] Downstream effectors include, but are not limited to, GRB2/SOS, PI3K, Akt, and members of the MAPK pathways. After activation, the receptor can be internalized and degraded via a lysosomal-dependent process. Antiangiogenic drugs that target the PDGF receptors almost exclusively inactivate the ATP-binding domain.

Healthy vasculature is mainly comprised of endothelial cells surrounded by vascular smooth muscle cells (vSMC) or pericytes (PC), depending on vessel diameter and tissue location. Pericytes cover the smallest of vessels, sharing a basement membrane with endothelial cells in capillaries. Communication between endothelial cells and vascular smooth muscle cells or pericytes appears to be essential for normal vessel development.[45] For instance, loss of the Tie2 receptor in endothelial cells results in loss of pericytes. And, loss of the PDGFR-β in the developing vasculature not only leads to pericyte loss but also endothelial dysfunction.[45] Although PDGF is known to induce angiogenesis on its own, it functions mainly to enhance vSMC and PC recruitment for maturation and stabilization of new vessels. In vivo experiments showed that blood vessels that had not recruited vSMC/PC required VEGF for survival, but the same was not true for vessels that had recruited these support cells.[46] Similarly, ectopic injection of PDGF-BB selectively disrupted endothelial–pericyte interactions in a neonatal rat model of retinal remodeling.[47] The only pericytes affected were those expressing PDGFR-B, which is commonly thought to only be expressed on migrating pericytes. PDGF-BB injection had no effect on mature vessels.

It is extremely well established that the cardiomyocyte hypertrophies in response to pressure overload stress. In compensatory cardiac hypertrophy, this increase in cardiomyocyte size or number is tightly coupled to an increase in angiogenesis. It is thought that an imbalance between hypertrophy and angiogenesis leads to decompensated cardiac remodeling and ultimately to HF. Therefore, cardiotoxicity and HF due to PDGF receptor inhibition may be due in part to the inability to stabilize new vessels in the myocardium in the setting of vascular stress such as HTN.

CARDIOMYOCYTE EFFECTS
VEGF

Both VEGF receptors are found on cardiomyocytes. However, they seem to have separate functions in maintaining cardiovascular function. The cardioprotective effects of VEGF have almost exclusively been studied in the setting of ischemia–reperfusion injury. Exogenous delivery of VEGF (via adenoviral or cDNA injection) has been found to reduce infarct size, promote angiogenesis, preserve cardiac function, and reduce cardiomyocyte apoptosis in rodent,[48] canine[49] and porcine,[50] models of ischemic injury. VEGF seems to be upregulated by exercise after the induction of MI in mice.[51] An interesting study by Zhou and colleagues[52] looked at the roles of each VEGF receptor in mediating cardiomyocyte response to copper-induced regression of phenylephrine-induced hypertrophy.

The administration of copper did not affect media levels of VEGF but increased the ratio of VEGFR1 to VEGFR2 twofold. Additionally, gene silencing of VEGFR1 prevented copper-induced regression of hypertrophy, whereas silencing of VEGFR2 prevented phenylephrine-induced hypertrophy, suggesting that VEGFR1 and VEGFR2 signaling have opposite effects on cardiomyocyte hypertrophy. Cardiac-specific knockout of VEGFR2 results in a loss of microvascular density and depressed contractile function.[53] The importance of VEGFR1 signaling in the heart was further highlighted by a study by Huusko and colleagues Adenoviral constructs of VEGFA$_{165}$, VEGFB$_{186}$ (VEGFR1-specific), and VEGFE were delivered to the anterior wall of the left ventricle of mice. Although VEGF-A induced the strongest angiogenic effect, it also caused large dilation of capillaries, tissue damage, and edema. VEGFA and VEGF-E caused proliferation mostly in endothelial cells, whereas VEGFB mostly stimulated cardiomyocyte proliferation. The authors therefore concluded that VEGFB, which is specific for VEGFR1, has a more direct effect on cardiomyocytes, whereas VEGF-A plays a more important role in the vasculature. A similar study by Zentillin and colleagues[54] found that post-MI VEGFB treatment resulted in decreased fibrosis and increased cardiac function despite the absence of significant angiogenesis. The investigators also found VEGFB to be antiapoptotic and induced expression of genes most commonly associated with compensatory cardiac hypertrophy such as increased α-MHC and repression of β-MHC, as well as skeletal α-actin in both isolated cardiomyocytes and infarcted hearts. Lastly, overexpression of VEGFB in the heart (driven by the α-MHC promoter) induced significant cardiomyocyte hypertrophy and increases in capillary lumen diameter, but not vessel density, without any obvious affects on cardiac function. Ultimately, the cardiotoxic effects of anti-VEGF therapies may be due in part to specific inhibition of VEGFR1 signaling compared with VEGFR2. However, not all VEGF inhibitors are cardiotoxic; therefore the cardiotoxic effects of these specific antiangiogenic drugs must also be due to effects on other kinases such as PDGFR.

PDGFR

The role of PDGFR in the heart is poorly understood. However, emerging evidence indicates that there is significant crosstalk between cardiomyocytes, endothelial cells, and pericytes, and that PDGFR in the heart may play a critical role in promoting this crosstalk. Edelberg and colleagues[55] found that cardiac microvascular endothelial cells constitutively express PDGF-A in culture but can be induced to express PDGF-B when cocultured with cardiomyocytes. The presence of cardiomyocytes in the culture also increased expression of VEGF and VEGFR2 on endothelial cells. Like VEGF, PDGF, has been shown to be cardioprotective from ischemic injury. Pretreatment with PDGF before acute ligation of the left anterior descending coronary artery in rats promoted angiogenesis, reduced infarct size, and preserved cardiac function.[56] Hsieh and colleagues[57] saw a similar result with delivery of PDGF-BB by self-assembling nanofibers after induction of MI. It should be noted that this was seen with exogenous administration of PDGF and may not correspond with the actions of endogenous PDGF. Nonetheless, stem cell overexpression of both VEGF and PDGF also improved cardiac function after MI.[58]

Recent work by the authors' group has demonstrated that cardiomyocyte PDGFR plays an essential role in the heart's ability to respond to pressure overload stress by promoting myocardial angiogenesis and preserving of microvascular density.[59] PDGFR-β expression and activation are significantly increased in response to pressure overload stress induced by transaortic constriction. Correspondingly, the authors constructed a cardiomyocyte-specific, inducible knockout of the PDGFR-β and exposed these mice to pressure overload stress. Knockout of the receptor resulted in significant cardiac dysfunction and failure. Hearts from PDGFR-β cardiac-specific knockout mice also displayed reduced coronary flow reserve and marked reductions in microvessel density (vessels per myocyte). This resulted in increased subendocardial fibrosis and hypoxia. The exact mechanism of PDGFR activation in response to pressure overload stress is not known. It has been demonstrated that angiotensin 2 can activate the receptor on cardiomyocytes but in a way that is different from PBGF-BB treatment. This activation seems to be dependent on crosstalk between the receptor and the angiotensin 2 receptor, AT1R.[44,60] Stretch also activates PDGFR-β in pulmonary artery tissue and smooth muscle cells.[61] As mentioned previously, cardiotoxicity due to PDGF receptor inhibition may result from the heart's inability to stabilize new vessel formation in response to pressure overload stress.

PRECLINICAL STUDIES OF ANTIANGIOGENIC DRUGS

Many studies have looked at the direct effects of drug treatment in animal models. French and colleagues[25] treated rats with sunitinib, sorafenib, or pazopanib concurrently with the cardiac stressor dobutamine. Analysis via echocardiography revealed modest cardiac dysfunction with sorafenib but not sunitinib or pazopanib, including premature ventricular contractions and decreased heart rate. Evaluation by transmission electron microscopy revealed mitochondrial swelling and structural abnormalities with sunitinib and sorafenib but not pazopanib. Mitochondrial dysfunction was seen in rats treated with sunitinib and sorafenib but not pazopanib, including depletion of intracellular ATP. Along that same line, treatment of H9c2 cells with sunitinib substantially increased cellular autophagy.[62] Mitochondrial structural abnormalities have also been seen in patients, possibly due to inhibition of AMPK activity.[63] While mitochondrial dysfunction seems to be significant in TKI-associated cardiotoxicity, others have implicated the endothelin-1 system.[64] It is clear that different TKIs do not have the same toxicities. The molecular mechanisms of tyrosine kinase inhibition leading to cardiotoxicity are extremely complex and most likely are the result of multiple on-target and off-target kinase inhibition, reviewed in greater detail by Force and colleagues.[65–67]

HTN AND ANTITUMOR RESPONSE

Interestingly, a growing body of mostly unpublished data seems to indicate that antiangiogenic therapies have a stronger antitumor effect in patients who develop HTN while on the drug, including time of progression-free survival (PFS) and overall survival (OS). This is suggestive of an underlying connection between the host vasculature and antiangiogenic therapies. In a retrospective review of 131 patients with mRCC of clear cell histology who received antiangiogenic therapy (sunitinib, sorafenib, and bevacizumab), Wilhelm and colleagues[68] found that PFS at 12 months was 37% for patients who developed HTN (63% of all patients) versus 56% in patients who did not. Correspondingly, the mortality rate was 8% in hypertensive patients versus 27% in normotensive patients. However, adverse cardiovascular events occurred in 10% of patients and were exclusive to the HTN group, including 2 MIs. A similar study by Scartozzi and colleagues[69] found a significant correlation between PFS and the development of HTN in patients with mCRC treated with bevacizumab. Median PFS was 14.5 months in patients who developed HTN versus 3.1 months in those who did not ($P = .04$). However, a similar study in mRCC did not find an association between the development of HTN and time to tumor progression.[70] Nonetheless, Rini and colleagues[71] performed a retrospective

analysis of 4 clinical trails in which patients with mRCC received 50 mg of sunitinib and found that all indicators of drug efficacy (eg, PFS) favored patients who developed HTN on sunitinib. Additionally, antihypertensive medication did not have an effect on PFS. After a multivariate analysis, the development of HTN was found to be an independent predictor of PFS in patients with mRCC who were treated with sunitinib.

Possibly there are certain qualities inherent to the patient's vasculature that not only aid in the efficacy of the drugs in treating the cancer but may also predispose them to the development of clinically relevant cardiotoxicities. For instance, this may be preexisting endothelial dysfunction or a higher reliance on growth factors such as VEGF and PDGF for normal vascular homeostasis. VEGF single-nucleotide polymorphisms (SNPs) have already been associated with coronary heart disease.[72] In an insightful single-arm phase 2 clinical trail of 46 patients with nonclear cell RCC treated with sunitinib, Ilias-Khan and colleagues[73] not only stratified PFS by the development of HTN but also by the presence of established coronary artery disease (CAD) risk factors. Overall, 33% of patients developed grade 2 or higher HTN while on treatment. However, none (0/12) of the patients without established CAD risk factors developed HTN, whereas 74% (13/17) of patients with established CAD risk factors developed HTN. Treatment decreased circulating VEGFR2 levels in all patients, but, and as a possible insight into the molecular mechanism of patient vasculature–drug interaction, circulating VEGFR2 levels were 2 times lower in patients who developed HTN and were reduced at baseline in patients who developed HTN.

SUMMARY

HTN and cardiotoxicities associated with anticancer TKIs are a major concern, and careful cardiovascular monitoring of cancer patients on TKI therapy is necessary. Further research into the underlying mechanisms as well as efforts to identify patients specifically predisposed to cardiovascular complications will not only limit the severity of HTN and associated LV dysfunction during TKI therapy but also may lead to novel discoveries about cardiac physiology and pathophysiology.

REFERENCES

1. Folkman J, Merler E, Abernathy C, et al. Isolation of a tumor factor responsible for angiogenesis. J Exp Med 1971;133(2):275–88.

2. Schmidinger M, Zielinski CC, Vogl UM, et al. Cardiac toxicity of sunitinib and sorafenib in patients with metastatic renal cell carcinoma. J Clin Oncol 2008; 26(32):5204–12.

3. Chu TF, Rupnick MA, Kerkela R, et al. Cardiotoxicity associated with tyrosine kinase inhibitor sunitinib. Lancet 2007;370(9604):2011–9.

4. Khakoo AY, Kassiotis CM, Tannir N, et al. Heart failure associated with sunitinib malate. Cancer 2008;112(11):2500–8.

5. Dorn GW. Myocardial angiogenesis: its absence makes the growing heart founder. Cell Metab 2007;5(5):326–7.

6. Khakoo AY, Sidman RL, Pasqualini R, et al. Does the renin–angiotensin system participate in regulation of human vasculogenesis and angiogenesis? Cancer Res 2008;68(22):9112–5.

7. Gogvadze V, Orrenius S, Zhivotovsky B. Mitochondria in cancer cells: what is so special about them? Trends Cell Biol 2008;18(4):165–73.

8. Fabian MA, Biggs WJ 3rd, Treiber DK, et al. A small molecule-kinase interaction map for clinical kinase inhibitors. Nat Biotechnol 2005;23(3):329–36.

9. Gordon MS, Margolin K, Talpaz M, et al. Phase I safety and pharmacokinetic study of recombinant human antivascular endothelial growth factor in patients with advanced cancer. J Clin Oncol 2001; 19(3):843–50.

10. Kabbinavar F, Hurwitz HI, Fehrenbacher L, et al. Phase II, randomized trial comparing bevacizumab plus fluorouracil (FU)/leucovorin (LV) with FU/LV alone in patients with metastatic colorectal cancer. J Clin Oncol 2003;21(1):60–5.

11. Hurwitz H, Fehrenbacjer L, Novotny W, et al. Bevacizumab plus irinotecan, fluorouracil, and leucovorin for metastatic colorectal cancer. N Engl J Med 2004;350(23):2335–42.

12. Ranpura V, Pulipati B, Chu D, et al. Increased risk of high-grade hypertension with bevacizumab in cancer patients: a meta-analysis. Am J Hypertens 2010;23(5):460–8.

13. Wagner AD, Arnold D, Grothey AA, et al. Antiangiogenic therapies for metastatic colorectal cancer. Cochrane Database Syst Rev 2009;3:CD005392.

14. Vaklavas C, Lenihan D, Kurzrock R, et al. Antivascular endothelial growth factor therapies and cardiovascular toxicity: what are the important clinical markers to target? Cancer Biology. Oncologist 2010;15:130–41.

15. Yardley DA. Integrating bevacizumab into the treatment of patients with early stage breast cancer: focus on cardiac safety. Clin Breast Cancer 2010; 10(2):119–29.

16. Miller K, Wang M, Gralow J, et al. Paclitaxel plus bevacizumab versus paclitaxel alone for metastatic breast cancer. N Engl J Med 2007;357(26): 2666–76.

17. Miller KD, Chap LI, Holmes FA, et al. Randomized phase III trial of capecitabine compared with bevacizumab plus capecitabine in patients with previously treated metastatic breast cancer. J Clin Oncol 2005;23:792–9.

18. Ratain MJ, Eisen T, Stadler WM, et al. Phase II placebo-controlled randomized discontinuation trial of sorafenib in patients with metastatic renal cell carcinoma. J Clin Oncol 2006;24:2505–12.

19. Escudier B, Eisen T, Stadler WM, et al. Sorafenib in advanced clear-cell renal-cell carcinoma. N Engl J Med 2007;356(2):125–34.

20. Wu S, Chen JJ, Kudelka A, et al. Incidence and risk of hypertension with sorafenib in patients with cancer: a systematic review and meta-analysis. Lancet Oncol 2008;9(2):117–23.

21. Veronese ML, Mosenkis A, Flaherty KT, et al. Mechanisms of hypertension associated with BAY 43-9006. J Clin Oncol 2006;24:1363–9.

22. Maitland ML, Kasza KE, Karrison T, et al. Ambulatory monitoring detects sorafenib-induced blood pressure elevations on the first day of treatment. Clin Cancer Res 2009;15:6250–7.

23. Arima Y, Oshima S, Noda K, et al. Sorafenib-induced acute myocardial infarction due to coronary artery spasm. J Cardiol 2009;54(3):512–5.

24. Hasinoff BB, Patel D. Mechanisms of myocyte cytotoxicity induced by the multikinase inhibitor sorafenib. Cardiovasc Toxicol 2010;10(1):1–8.

25. French KJ, Coatney RW, Renninger JP, et al. Differences in effects on myocardium and mitochondria by angiogenic inhibitors suggest separate mechanisms of cardiotoxicity. Toxicol Pathol 2010;38(5): 691–702.

26. Rock EP, Goodman V, Jiang JX, et al. Food and Drug Administration drug approval summary: sunitinib malate for the treatment of gastrointestinal stromal tumor and advanced renal cell carcinoma. Oncologist 2007;12(1):107–13.

27. Hasinoff BB, Patel D, O'Hara KA. Mechanisms of myocyte cytotoxicity induced by the multiple receptor tyrosine kinase inhibitor sunitinib. Mol Pharmacol 2008;74(6):1722–8.

28. Demetri GD, van Oosterom AT, Garrett CR, et al. Efficacy and safety of sunitinib in patients with advanced gastrointestinal stromal tumour after failure of imatinib: a randomised controlled trial. Lancet 2006;368(9544):1329–38.

29. Motzer RJ, Hutson TE, Tomczak P, et al. Sunitinib versus interferon alfa in metastatic renal-cell carcinoma. N Engl J Med 2007;356(2):115–24.

30. Zhu X, Stergiopoulos K, Wu S. Risk of hypertension and renal dysfunction with an angiogenesis inhibitor sunitinib: systematic review and meta-analysis. Acta Oncol 2009;48(1):9–17.

31. Di Lorenzo G, Autorino R, Bruni G, et al. Cardiovascular toxicity following sunitinib therapy in metastatic

renal cell carcinoma: a multicenter analysis. Ann Oncol 2009;20(9):1535–42.

32. Telli ML, Witteles RM, Fisher GA, et al. Cardiotoxicity associated with the cancer therapeutic agent sunitinib malate. Ann Oncol 2008;19(9):1613–8.

33. Rixe O, Bukowski RM, Michaelson MD, et al. Axitinib treatment in patients with cytokine-refractory metastatic renal cell cancer: a phase II study. Lancet Oncol 2007;8(11):975–84.

34. LaPlant KD, Louzon PD. Pazopanib: an oral multitargeted tyrosine kinase inhibitor for use in renal cell carcinoma. Ann Pharmacother 2010;44:1054–60.

35. Hurwitz HI, Dowlati A, Saini S, et al. Phase I trial of pazopanib in patients with advanced cancer. Clin Cancer Res 2009;15(12):4220–7.

36. Sternberg CN, Davis ID, Mardiak J, et al. Pazopanib in locally advanced or metastatic renal cell carcinoma: results of a randomized phase III trial. J Clin Oncol 2010;28(6):1061–8.

37. Hasinoff BB. The cardiotoxicity and myocyte damage caused by small molecule anticancer tyrosine kinase inhibitors is correlated with lack of target specificity. Toxicol Appl Pharmacol 2010;244(2):190–5.

38. Force T, Krause DS, Van Etten RA. Molecular mechanisms of cardiotoxicity of tyrosine kinase inhibition. Nat Rev Cancer 2007;7(5):332–44.

39. Ferrara N, Gerber HP, LeCouter J. The biology of VEGF and its receptors. Nat Med 2003;9: 669–76.

40. Madonna R, De Caterina R. VEGF receptor switching in heart development and disease. Cardiovasc Res 2009;84(1):4–6.

41. Yogi AA, O'Connor SE, Callera GE, et al. Receptor and nonreceptor tyrosine kinases in vascular biology of hypertension. Curr Opin Nephrol Hypertens 2010;19(2):169–76.

42. Cooke JP, Dzau VJ, et al. Nitric oxide synthase: role in the genesis of vascular disease. Annu Rev Med 1997;48(1):489–509.

43. Heldin CH, Westermark B. Mechanism of action and in vivo role of platelet-derived growth factor. Physiol Rev 1999;79(4):1283–316.

44. Wang C, Wu LL, Liu J, et al. Crosstalk between angiotensin II and platelet derived growth factor receptor BB mediated signal pathways in cardiomyocytes. Chin Med J (Engl) 2008;121(3):236–40.

45. Hellstrom M, Kalen M, Lindahl P, et al. Role of PDGF-B and PDGFR-beta in recruitment of vascular smooth muscle cells and pericytes during embryonic blood vessel formation in the mouse. Development 1999;126:3047–55.

46. Benjamin LE, Golijanin D, Itin A, et al. Selective ablation of immature blood vessels in established human tumors follows vascular endothelial growth factor withdrawal. J Clin Invest 1999;103(2):159–65.

47. Benjamin LE, Hemo I, Keshet E. A plasticity window for blood vessel remodeling is defined by pericyte

coverage of the preformed endothelial network and is regulated by PDGF-B and VEGF. Development 1998;125(9):1591–8.

48. Ruixing Y, Dezhai Y, Hai W, et al. Intramyocardial injection of vascular endothelial growth factor gene improves cardiac performance and inhibits cardiomyocyte apoptosis. Eur J Heart Fail 2007;9(4):343–51.

49. Ferrarini M, Arsic N, Recchia FA, et al. Adeno-associated virus-mediated transduction of VEGF165 improves cardiac tissue viability and functional recovery after permanent coronary occlusion in conscious dogs. Circ Res 2006;98(7):954–61.

50. Wang X, Hu Q, Mansoor A, et al. Bioenergetic and functional consequences of stem cell-based VEGF delivery in pressure-overloaded swine hearts. Am J Physiol Heart Circ Physiol 2006;290(4):H1393–405.

51. Wu G, Rana JS, Wykrzykowska J, et al. Exercise-induced expression of VEGF and salvation of myocardium in the early stage of myocardial infarction. Am J Physiol Heart Circ Physiol 2009;296(2): H389–95.

52. Zhou Y, Bourcy K, Kang YJ. Copper-induced regression of cardiomyocyte hypertrophy is associated with enhanced vascular endothelial growth factor receptor-1 signaling pathway. Cardiovasc Res 2009;84(1):54–63.

53. Giordano FJ, Gerber HP, Williams SP, et al. A cardiac myocyte vascular endothelial growth factor paracrine pathway is required to maintain cardiac function. Proc Natl Acad Sci U S A 2001; 98:5780–5.

54. Zentilin L, Puligadda U, Lionetti V, et al. Cardiomyocyte VEGFR-1 activation by VEGF-B induces compensatory hypertrophy and preserves cardiac function after myocardial infarction. FASEB J 2010; 24(5):1467–78.

55. Edelberg JM, Aird WC, Wu W, et al. PDGF mediates cardiac microvascular communication. J Clin Invest 1998;102(4):837–43.

56. Zheng J, Shin JH, Xaymardan M, et al. Platelet-derived growth factor improves cardiac function in a rodent myocardial infarction model. Coron Artery Dis 2004;15(1):59–64.

57. Hsieh PC, Davis ME, Gannon J, et al. Controlled delivery of PDGF-BB for myocardial protection using injectable self-assembling peptide nanofibers. J Clin Invest 2006;116(1):237–48.

58. Das H, Geroge JC, Joseph M, et al. Stem cell therapy with overexpressed VEGF and PDGF genes improves cardiac function in a rat infarct model. PLoS One 2009;4(10):e7325.

59. Chintalgattu V, Patel SS, Khakoo AY. Cardiovascular effects of tyrosine kinase inhibitors used for gastrointestinal stromal tumors. Hematol Oncol Clin North Am 2009;23(1):97–107.

60. Heeneman S, Haendeler J, Saito Y, et al. Angiotensin II induces transactivation of two different

populations of the platelet-derived growth factor $\hat{I}^2$ receptor. J Biol Chem 2000;275(21):15926–32.

61. Tanabe Y, Saito M, Ueno A, et al. Mechanical stretch augments PDGF receptor β expression and protein tyrosine phosphorylation in pulmonary artery tissue and smooth muscle cells. Mol Cell Biochem 2000;215:103–13.

62. Zhao Y, Xue T, Yang X, et al. Autophagy plays an important role in sunitinib-mediated cell death in H9c2 cardiac muscle cells. Toxicol Appl Pharmacol 2010;248(1):20–7.

63. Kerkela R, Woulfe KC, Durand JB, et al. Sunitinib-induced cardiotoxicity is mediated by off-target inhibition of AMP-activated protein kinase. Clin Transl Sci 2009;2(1):15–25.

64. Kappers MH, van Esch JH, Sluiter W, et al. Hypertension induced by the tyrosine kinase inhibitor sunitinib is associated with increased circulating endothelin-1 levels. Hypertension 2010;56(4):675–81.

65. Cheng H, Force T. Molecular mechanisms of cardiovascular toxicity of targeted cancer therapeutics. Circ Res 2010;106(1):21–34.

66. De Keulenaer GW, Doggen K, Lemmens K. The vulnerability of the heart as a pluricellular paracrine organ: lessons from unexpected triggers of heart failure in targeted ErbB2 anticancer therapy. Circ Res 2010;106(1):35–46.

67. Force T. Introduction to cardiotoxicity review series. Circ Res 2010;106(1):19–20.

68. Wilhelm KL, Atkinson BJ, Khakoo AY, et al. A retrospective evaluation of antiangiogenic therapy induced hypertension in metastatic renal cell carcinoma [meeting abstracts]. J Clin Oncol 2010; 28(Suppl 15):e15047.

69. Scartozzi M, Galizia E, Chiorrini S, et al. Arterial hypertension correlates with clinical outcome in colorectal cancer patients treated with first-line bevacizumab. Ann Oncol 2009;20(2):227–30.

70. Bono P, Elfving H, Utriainen T, et al. Hypertension and clinical benefit of bevacizumab in the treatment of advanced renal cell carcinoma. Ann Oncol 2009; 20:393–4.

71. Rini B, Cohen DP, Lu D, et al. Hypertension (HTN) as a biomarker of efficacy in patients (pts) with metastatic renal cell carcinoma (mRCC) treated with sunitinib. Presented at: ASCO 2010 Genitourinary Cancers Symposium, San Francisco (CA), March 5–7, 2010.

72. Wang Y, Zheng Y, Zhang W, et al. Polymorphisms of KDR gene are associated with coronary heart disease. J Am Coll Cardiol 2007;50(8):760–7.

73. Ilias-Khan NA, Khakoo AY, Tannir NM. A clinical and biological profile to predict risk of development of hypertension in patients with non-clear cell renal cell carcinoma treated with sunitinib [meeting abstracts]. J Clin Oncol 2010;28(Suppl 15):4601.

Newest Echocardiographic Techniques for the Detection of Cardiotoxicity and Heart Failure During Chemotherapy

Heloisa Sawaya, MD, PhD[a], Juan Carlos Plana, MD[b],
Marielle Scherrer-Crosbie, MD, PhD[a],*

KEYWORDS

- Echocardiography • Cardiotoxicity • Chemotherapy

Therapy for cancer has progressed tremendously over the last decade and chemotherapy-induced cardiotoxicity has been increasingly recognized as a major health threat. Although the overall rate of cancer incidence has declined since the early 2000s (National Cancer Institute, Cancer Trends Progress Report –2009/2010 Update),[1] cancers necessitating aggressive chemotherapy, including melanoma, non-Hodgkin lymphoma, leukemia, pancreas, and esophagus, among others, have been on the rise. Accompanying this trend, the length of cancer survival has increased for all cancers combined. In 2001, 68.3% of patients with cancer were alive 5 years after their diagnosis, allowing for the potential cardiac side effects of chemotherapeutic agents to manifest. As the cancer survivors become older, their risk of cardiovascular disease increases significantly. For individuals free of cardiovascular disease at 50 years of age, more than half of men and nearly 40% of women will develop cardiovascular disease during their remaining lifespan.[2,3] In addition, some patients with cancer may be at a higher risk for cardiovascular complications as compared with the general population.[2,4] Finally, multiple classes of potentially cardiotoxic anticancer agents are currently being developed.[5] In summary, the combination of increased use of chemotherapy, overall increased survival, and development of newer agents have led to the emergence of chemotherapy-induced cardiotoxicity as a major public health issue.

DEFINITION OF CARDIOTOXICITY

The therapeutic agents used in the treatment of cancer can cause a wide array of toxic effects in the cardiovascular system. The acute or subacute cardiotoxicity can be characterized by the presence of abnormalities in ventricular repolarization and the

This work was supported by an investigator-initiated grant from Susan G. Komen for the Cure Foundation and Caflin Distinguished Scholar Award and a Clinical Innovation Award.
The authors have nothing to disclose.
[a] Cardiac Ultrasound Laboratory, Division of Cardiology, Massachusetts General Hospital, Harvard Medical School, 55 Fruit Street, Boston, MA 02114, USA
[b] Section of Imaging, Department of Cardiovascular Medicine, The Cleveland Clinic Foundation, Cleveland Clinic Main Campus, Mail Code J1-5, 9500 Euclid Avenue, Cleveland, OH 44195, USA
* Corresponding author.
E-mail address: marielle@crosbie.com

Heart Failure Clin 7 (2011) 313–321
doi:10.1016/j.hfc.2011.03.003

QT-interval (supraventricular and ventricular arrhythmias), acute coronary syndromes, and pericarditis or myocarditislike syndromes, which can occur at the initiation of chemotherapy or up to 2 weeks after its termination. Other toxic cardiac side effects include sinus bradycardia, atrioventricular block, hypotension or hypertension, and mild functional mitral regurgitation.[6–10] Chronic cardiotoxicity is characterized by asymptomatic systolic or diastolic left ventricular dysfunction leading to severe congestive cardiomyopathy.[11] The present review focuses on the detection of chemotherapy-induced left ventricular dysfunction.

A consensus regarding the definition of cardiotoxicity still needs to be clarified as clinical trials present with different definitions of cardiomyopathy (**Table 1**).

DETECTION OF CARDIOTOXICITY BY LEFT VENTRICULAR EJECTION FRACTION

The regular monitoring of heart function during chemotherapy is of major importance so that cardiac dysfunction can be detected. Currently, there are guidelines for monitoring the chemotherapy-induced cardiotoxicity in children treated with anthracyclines.[19] For the adult population, the American Heart Association recommends close monitoring of cardiac function during anthracycline therapy, however, it does not specify how often these patients need to be followed, which methods should be used, and what thresholds should be used.[20] For patients treated with anthracyclines,

the evaluation of left ventricular ejection fraction (LVEF) has been the traditionally preferred method for assessing cardiac function,[21–25] although no clear consensus has been reached on the percentage of change, which represents a clinically relevant decline in myocardial contractile function, requiring intervention.

ROUTINE METHODS OF EVALUATING LVEF

Left ventricular ejection fraction is the most common method of monitoring cardiac function during cancer treatment. Evaluation of left ventricular ejection fraction is commonly assessed through echocardiography or multiple gated acquisition (MUGA) scan.[26] The measurement of LVEF using MUGA scan has the advantage of low interobserver variability (<5%[27]) and the lack of use of geometric modeling. Disadvantages of MUGA include the exposure to radioactivity and the limited information than can be obtained on cardiac structure and diastolic function. Echocardiography is noninvasive and does not involve the use of radiation. It also provides more information on cardiac morphology valvular and diastolic function.[28] However, the interobserver and intraobserver variability may be slightly higher than in MUGA scan (8.8% vs 6.8% for 2-dimensional [2-D] echocardiography[29]), magnetic resonance imaging (MRI) is another method used to evaluate myocardial function. Its spatial resolution is higher than that of echocardiography, but its temporal resolution is lower. MRI may be used as an

---

Table 1
Definition of cardiotoxicity for anthracyclines and trastuzumab

Author	Definition of Cardiotoxicity	Drug
Tan-Chiu et al,[12] 2005	Decline LVEF by 10% to <55%	Trastuzumab
Perez et al,[13] 2004	Asymptomatic LVEF decline ≥10% but <20% compared with baseline (toxicity grade 1) or asymptomatic decline ≥20% to below the LLN (toxicity grade 2)	Doxorubicin and cyclophosphamide
Suter et al,[14] 2004	Decline of LVEF ≥15 points to <50%	Trastuzumab
O'Brien et al,[15] 2004	Decline in LVEF of 20 points to >50% or at least 10 points to <50% or clinical CHF	Doxorubicin
Smith et al,[16] 2007	Decline in LVEF of ≥10 points from baseline to <50%	Trastuzumab after adjuvant or neoadjuvant chemotherapy
Romond et al,[17] 2005	Decline of LVEF ≥16 points or <LLN	Doxorubicin and cyclophosphamide followed by trastuzumab
Ryberg et al,[18] 2008	Decline of LVEF <45% or 15 points from baseline	Epirubicin

Abbreviations: CHF, congestive heart failure; LLN, lower limit of normal; LVEF, left ventricular ejection fraction.

important tool to assess myocardial function and damage after chemotherapy, however, its high costs and limited availability limits its routine use.[28]

USEFULNESS OF LVEF

Although LVEF is the most commonly used parameter to monitor chemotherapy-induced cardiotoxicity, its prognostic value is controversial. In an initial study Alexander and colleagues[32] demonstrated the usefulness of sequential evaluation of LVEF in patients with chemotherapy for the detection of heart failure. Nousiainen and colleagues[30] in a study of 28 patients with non-Hodgkin lymphoma receiving doxorubicin, reported a significant decline of LVEF at low cumulative doses, which was predictive of later development of cardiotoxicity. In contrast, in a study of 120 patients with breast cancer followed before, during, and 3 years after treatment with epirubicin, monitoring of LVEF did not seem to correlate with later development of cardiotoxicity.[31] It is crucial that baseline measurements be obtained for comparison with follow-ups during the course of any chemotherapy implemented.

IMPROVING THE MEASURED LVEF

Novel methods have been developed to access cardiotoxicity. One approach is to improve the acquisition and measurement of the LVEF.

CONTRAST ECHO AND CARDIOTOXICITY

Several multicenter and single-center trials have demonstrated the usefulness of contrast echocardiography in clinical practice. Ultrasound contrast agents are approved for opacification of heart chambers, improving the endocardial border definition (see example on **Fig. 1**), and as a result reducing the intraobserver and interobserver variability of the studies.[32] They are especially useful when a precise measurement of left ventricular (LV) function is necessary, as is the case for selection of treatment and monitoring of patients undergoing chemotherapy with cardiotoxic drugs.[33] Although the indication for the use of contrast is not specified in the chemotherapy guidelines, it is reasonable to apply general American Society of Echocardiography and European Association of Echocardiography guidelines, which recommend contrast echocardiography in those patients in whom the endocardium is not well visualized in 2 or more segments.[33]

THREE-DIMENSIONAL ECHOCARDIOGRAPHY AND CARDIOTOXICITY

The assessments of LV systolic function by M-mode and 2-D images rely on geometric assumptions and visual extrapolations. Three-dimensional (3-D) echocardiography overcomes these limitations and allows a more accurate assessment of LV volume and ejection fraction (**Fig. 2**), with good correlation with computed tomography and magnetic resonance imaging.[34–36] Several studies have demonstrated 3-D–echocardiography to be superior to the more routinely used 2-D images. The advantages of this new technique include higher reproducibility and lower interobserver variability.[37,38] Furthermore, analysis time was

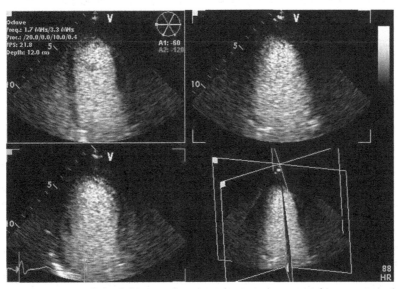

Fig. 1. Triplane reconstruction of the left ventricle using ultrasound contrast for accurate calculation of left ventricular ejection fraction.

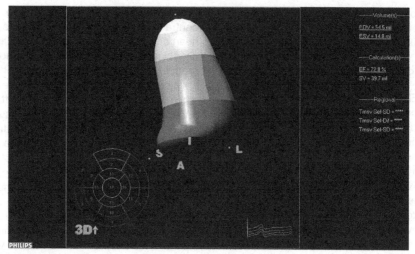

Fig. 2. A 3-D echocardiogram for accurate calculation of end diastolic and systolic volumes and left ventricular ejection fraction.

considerably reduced. However, these studies included a small number of patients.[37] In the study of Hare and colleagues,[39] 3-D echocardiography was used to measure LVEF in women undergoing treatment with trastuzumab for breast cancer with measurements performed every 3 months between baseline and 12 months. The investigators did not detect any changes in 3-D LVEF before and after trastuzumab.

DIASTOLE AND CARDIOTOXICITY

In chemotherapy-induced cardiotoxicity as in other cardiac diseases, (such as ischemia for example,[40–43]) alterations in diastole may occur before systolic dysfunction. The impairment of Doppler-derived diastolic indexes seems to represent an sign of subtle LV dysfunction in patients treated with chemotherapy.[44] More than 50% of patients treated with anthracyclines presented with impaired early peak flow velocity to atrial peak flow velocity (E/A) ratio, deceleration time (DT), and isovolumetric relaxation time (IVRT) when evaluated approximately 27 months after discontinuation of anthracycline.[45] Alterations of the LV diastolic performance (significant reductions in peak E velocity, increase in the peak A velocity, prolongation of the pressure half time of E wave and in the IVRT) was also documented in a study group of subjects treated with epirubicin who had different malignancies when compared with a sex- and age-matched control group of subjects with malignancies who did not receive cardiotoxic agents. Neither the treated nor the untreated group presented with significant variations in the LVEF.[46] In another study of 26 patients with acute leukemia treated with 2 to 6 cycles of conventional chemotherapy containing anthracycline, the changes in diastolic LV function developed very early on after the initiation of chemotherapy with significant reduction in the E/A ratio, prolongation of DT, and in the IVRT before LVEF decreased.[47] These findings were also reproduced in another study as well.[48] Stoddard and colleagues[49] prospectively evaluated 26 patients before receiving chemotherapy (doxorubicin) and 3 weeks after cumulative doses. These investigators observed prolongation of isovolumetric relaxation time preceding a significant decrease in LVEF. The studies previously mentioned reinforce the possible value of the diastolic indices in the detection of early cardiotoxicity, however larger studies would be needed to confirm the value of diastolic measurements in cardiotoxicity.

STRESS ECHO AND CARDIOTOXICITY

Exercise and pharmacologic stress testing has been studied as a way to unmask subclinical abnormalities of LV function induced by chemotherapeutic agents. Low doses of dobutamine do not seem to unmask systolic dysfunction limiting its usefulness.[50,51] Subtle changes in diastolic parameters have been reported. In contrast, high dose dobutamine used in 26 patients treated with high-dose anthracycline and without symptoms of cardiac dysfunction, revealed an alteration of the fractional shortening and the transmitral E/A ratio.[52] Exercise echocardiography can unmask subclinical cardiac dysfunction as demonstrated by Jarfelt and colleagues[53] in 23 young adults. These patients were acute lymphoblastic leukemia survivors who had received anthracyclines before the onset of puberty and were followed for a median of 21 years after remission. Ten out of the 23 patients presented with reduced LVEF at stress, whereas such a reduced LVEF was not observed in any of the controls. Although these results are promising, stress echo involves an additional procedure, still strictly in the research perspective.

STRAIN AND STRAIN RATE

Novel echocardiographic techniques, including myocardial velocity, strain, and strain rate imaging, have been used to evaluate global and regional myocardial dysfunction in a variety of cardiac pathologies. The recently developed 2-D strain based on speckle tracking provides a multidimensional evaluation of myocardial mechanics (longitudinal, radial, and circumferential strain).[54] Several studies have shown that strain and strain rate may be more sensitive in the detection of LV dysfunction than LVEF.[55–58] The analysis of regional myocardial function appears to be more sensitive to detect myocardial dysfunction after anthracycline therapy when compared with conventional echocardiographic parameters of systolic and diastolic function[59] (see example on Figs. 3 and 4). More than 80% of pediatric patients who received low to moderate cumulative dose of anthracyclines presented with regional LV free wall motion abnormality 6 months after the end of the treatment. No changes were observed in fractional shortening in these patients. In a study employing pulsed tissue Doppler imaging to evaluate the short- and long-term effects of anthracycline chemotherapy in adults, Tassan-Magina and colleagues[60] demonstrated that mitral annular diastolic velocities decreased rapidly after initiation of anthracycline therapy even though normal systolic function was still present.

Significant decreases in longitudinal and radial LV myocardial strain and strain rate were observed after the first dose of anthracycline was administered to 13 children receiving 3 successive cycles of chemotherapy. In this study, decreased LV shortening fraction and ejection fraction were only evident after the second cycle of anthracycline treatment. The reduction in strain and strain rate persisted after subsequent doses of anthracyclines.[61] The same investigators demonstrated that strain and strain rate were able to detect the long-term effects of anthracyclines. Fifty-six pediatric patients who had previously received anthracycline treatment for acute lymphoblastic leukemia, lymphoma, solid tumors, or acute myeloblastic leukemia were studied at a median of 5.2 years after the last dose of anthracycline. A significant decrease in both radial and longitudinal peak systolic strain rate and strain in the lateral wall and LV diastolic abnormalities were observed.[62]

Recently, Jurcut and colleagues[63] demonstrated that myocardial deformation parameters, which included longitudinal and radial strain and strain rate, allowed detecting subtle alterations in longitudinal and radial LV function following 6 cycles of pegylated liposomal doxorubicin in 16 elderly women with breast cancer. The LV dimensions,

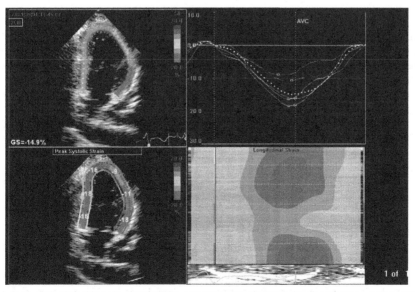

Fig. 3. A 2-D–based peak global longitudinal strain assessment in the apical 2-chamber view in a patient receiving anthracyclines. Note the abnormal strain values at the mid and apical segments of the anterior wall, suggestive of anthracycline toxicity.

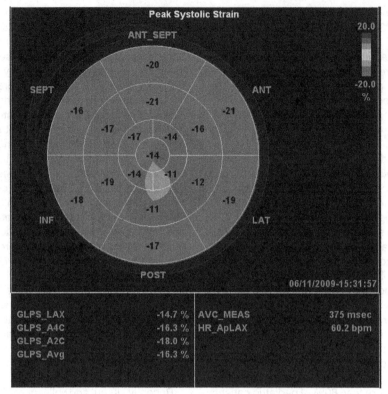

Fig. 4. Bull's eye display peak global longitudinal strain of the patient described in **Fig. 3**. The peak global longitudinal strain is reduced (<18.6). Note the abnormal peak strain values (>−14%) in several of the segments.

ejection fraction, and systolic myocardial velocity did not change during the follow-up.

The analysis of myocardial deformation parameters has also been demonstrated to be a more sensitive mean to detecting early LV dysfunction in patients treated with anthracyclines and trastuzumab. Significant reduction in 2-D longitudinal strain was observed in 51% of women receiving trastuzumab for HER2 positive breast cancer and significant reduction in 2-D radial strain rate was observed in 37% of these women.[39]

Finally, in a recent study of 43 breast cancer patients treated with anthracyclines followed by trastuzumab and taxol, a drop in peak global longitudinal strain from baseline to 3 months could predict later development of cardiotoxicity at 6 months while LVEF and parameters of diastolic function did not.[64]

SUMMARY

The improvements in detection and therapy of cancer have created a new cohort of patients who will live with sufficient survival to develop the cardiac complications of the cancer therapy. Three-dimensional echocardiography has been validated as the ultrasound modality with the best accuracy for the calculation of ejection

fraction when compared with MRI, the current gold standard, making it the tool of choice, when available, for the initial evaluation and follow-up of patients receiving chemotherapy.

If 3-D echocardiography is not available, or the quality of the images is challenging, the use of ultrasound contrast can be useful for the definition of the endocardial border and the identification of the true apex of the heart, enhancing the ability of the interpreter to accurately calculate volumes and ejection fraction.

2-D–based strain appears promising as a tool to identify abnormalities in myocardial mechanics early on during cardiotoxicity, allowing the prediction of later overt systolic dysfunction. These parameters may be useful in the detection of patients treated with chemotherapy who could benefit from alternate therapies, thereby decreasing the incidence of cardiotoxicity and its associated morbidity and mortality.

REFERENCES

1. Cancer Trends Progress Report - 2009/2010 Update. Available at: http://progressreport.cancer.gov/. 2010.
2. Clarke CA, Purdie DM, Glase SL. Population attributable risk of breast cancer in white women

associated with immediately modifiable risk factors. BMC Cancer 2006;6:170.

3. Lloyd-Jones DM, Dyer AR, Wang R, et al. Risk factor burden in middle age and lifetime risks for cardiovascular and non-cardiovascular death (Chicago Heart Association Detection Project in Industry). Am J Cardiol 2007;99:535.

4. Lloyd-Jones DM, Leip EP, Larson MG, et al. Prediction of lifetime risk for cardiovascular disease by risk factor burden at 50 years of age. Circulation 2006; 113:791.

5. Cheng H, Force T. Molecular mechanisms of cardiovascular toxicity of targeted cancer therapeutics. Circ Res 2010;106:21.

6. Chu TF, Rupnick MA, Kerkela R, et al. Cardiotoxicity associated with tyrosine kinase inhibitor sunitinib. Lancet 2007;370:2011.

7. Schmidinger M, Zielinski CC, Vogl UM, et al. Cardiac toxicity of sunitinib and sorafenib in patients with metastatic renal cell carcinoma. J Clin Oncol 2008; 26:5204.

8. Sereno M, Brunello A, Chiappori A, et al. Cardiac toxicity: old and new issues in anti-cancer drugs. Clin Transl Oncol 2008;10:35.

9. Yeh ET, Tong AT, Lenihan DJ, et al. Cardiovascular complications of cancer therapy: diagnosis, pathogenesis, and management. Circulation 2004;109: 3122.

10. Zver S, Zadnik V, Bunc M, et al. Cardiac toxicity of high-dose cyclophosphamide in patients with multiple myeloma undergoing autologous hematopoietic stem cell transplantation. Int J Hematol 2007;85:408.

11. Pai VB, Nahata MC. Cardiotoxicity of chemotherapeutic agents: incidence, treatment and prevention. Drug Saf 2000;22:263.

12. Tan-Chiu E, Yothers G, Romond E, et al. Assessment of cardiac dysfunction in a randomized trial comparing doxorubicin and cyclophosphamide followed by paclitaxel, with or without trastuzumab as adjuvant therapy in node-positive, human epidermal growth factor receptor 2-overexpressing breast cancer: NSABP B-31. J Clin Oncol 2005;23:7811.

13. Perez EA, Suman VJ, Davidson NE, et al. Effect of doxorubicin plus cyclophosphamide on left ventricular ejection fraction in patients with breast cancer in the North Central Cancer Treatment Group N9831 Intergroup Adjuvant Trial. J Clin Oncol 2004;22:3700.

14. Suter TM, Cook-Bruns N, Barton C. Cardiotoxicity associated with trastuzumab (Herceptin) therapy in the treatment of metastatic breast cancer. Breast 2004;13:173.

15. O'Brien ME, Wigler N, Inbar M, et al. Reduced cardiotoxicity and comparable efficacy in a phase III trial of pegylated liposomal doxorubicin HCl (CAELYX/Doxil) versus conventional doxorubicin for first-line treatment of metastatic breast cancer. Ann Oncol 2004;15:440.

16. Smith I, Procter M, Gelber RD, et al. 2-year follow-up of trastuzumab after adjuvant chemotherapy in HER2-positive breast cancer: a randomised controlled trial. Lancet 2007;369:29.

17. Romond EH, Perez EA, Bryant J, et al. Trastuzumab plus adjuvant chemotherapy for operable HER2-positive breast cancer. N Engl J Med 2005;353:1673.

18. Ryberg M, Nielsen D, Cortese G, et al. New insight into epirubicin cardiac toxicity: competing risks analysis of 1097 breast cancer patients. J Natl Cancer Inst 2008;100:1058.

19. Steinherz LJ, Graham T, Hurwitz R, et al. Guidelines for cardiac monitoring of children during and after anthracycline therapy: report of the Cardiology Committee of the Childrens Cancer Study Group. Pediatrics 1992;89:942.

20. Hunt SA, Abraham WT, Chin MH, et al. ACC/AHA 2005 Guideline Update for the Diagnosis and Management of Chronic Heart Failure in the Adult: a report of the American College of Cardiology/American Heart Association Task Force on Practice Guidelines (Writing Committee to Update the 2001 Guidelines for the Evaluation and Management of Heart Failure): developed in collaboration with the American College of Chest Physicians and the International Society for Heart and Lung Transplantation: endorsed by the Heart Rhythm Society. Circulation 2005;112:e154.

21. Batist G, Ramakrishnan G, Rao CS, et al. Reduced cardiotoxicity and preserved antitumor efficacy of liposome-encapsulated doxorubicin and cyclophosphamide compared with conventional doxorubicin and cyclophosphamide in a randomized, multicenter trial of metastatic breast cancer. J Clin Oncol 2001;19:1444.

22. Harris L, Batist G, Belt R, et al. Liposome-encapsulated doxorubicin compared with conventional doxorubicin in a randomized multicenter trial as first-line therapy of metastatic breast carcinoma. Cancer 2002;94:25.

23. Ng R, Better N, Green MD. Anticancer agents and cardiotoxicity. Semin Oncol 2006;33:2.

24. Schwartz RG, McKenzie WB, Alexander J, et al. Congestive heart failure and left ventricular dysfunction complicating doxorubicin therapy. Seven-year experience using serial radionuclide angiocardiography. Am J Med 1987;82:1109.

25. Swain SM, Whaley FS, Gerber MC, et al. Cardioprotection with dexrazoxane for doxorubicin-containing therapy in advanced breast cancer. J Clin Oncol 1997;15:1318.

26. Jannazzo A, Hoffman J, Lutz M. Monitoring of anthracycline-induced cardiotoxicity. Ann Pharmacother 2008;42:99.

27. Skrypniuk JV, Bailey D, Cosgriff PS, et al. UK audit of left ventricular ejection fraction estimation from equilibrium ECG gated blood pool images. Nucl Med Commun 2005;26:205.

28. Jurcut R, Pappas CJ, Masci PG, et al. Detection of regional myocardial dysfunction in patients with acute myocardial infarction using velocity vector imaging. J Am Soc Echocardiogr 2008;21:879.

29. Chuang ML, Hibberd MG, Salton CJ, et al. Importance of imaging method over imaging modality in noninvasive determination of left ventricular volumes and ejection fraction: assessment by two- and three-dimensional echocardiography and magnetic resonance imaging. J Am Coll Cardiol 2000;35:477.

30. Nousiainen T, Jantunen E, Vanninen E, et al. Early decline in left ventricular ejection fraction predicts doxorubicin cardiotoxicity in lymphoma patients. Br J Cancer 2002;86:1697.

31. Jensen BV, Skovsgaard T, Nielsen SL. Functional monitoring of anthracycline cardiotoxicity: a prospective, blinded, long-term observational study of outcome in 120 patients. Ann Oncol 2002;13:699.

32. Hoffmann R, von Bardeleben S, ten Cate F, et al. Assessment of systolic left ventricular function: a multi-centre comparison of cineventriculography, cardiac magnetic resonance imaging, unenhanced and contrast-enhanced echocardiography. Eur Heart J 2005;26:607.

33. Olszewski R, Timperley J, Szmigielski C, et al. The clinical applications of contrast echocardiography. Eur J Echocardiogr 2007;8:S13.

34. Jenkins C, Bricknell K, Chan J, et al. Comparison of two- and three-dimensional echocardiography with sequential magnetic resonance imaging for evaluating left ventricular volume and ejection fraction over time in patients with healed myocardial infarction. Am J Cardiol 2007;99:300.

35. Qi X, Cogar B, Hsiung MC, et al. Live/real time three-dimensional transthoracic echocardiographic assessment of left ventricular volumes, ejection fraction, and mass compared with magnetic resonance imaging. Echocardiography 2007;24:166.

36. Sugeng L, Mor-Avi V, Weinert L, et al. Quantitative assessment of left ventricular size and function: side-by-side comparison of real-time three-dimensional echocardiography and computed tomography with magnetic resonance reference. Circulation 2006; 114:654.

37. Jacobs LD, Salgo IS, Goonewardena S, et al. Rapid online quantification of left ventricular volume from real-time three-dimensional echocardiographic data. Eur Heart J 2006;27:460.

38. Takuma S, Ota T, Muro T, et al. Assessment of left ventricular function by real-time 3-dimensional echocardiography compared with conventional noninvasive methods. J Am Soc Echocardiogr 2001;14:275.

39. Hare JL, Brown JK, Leano R, et al. Use of myocardial deformation imaging to detect preclinical myocardial dysfunction before conventional measures in patients undergoing breast cancer treatment with trastuzumab. Am Heart J 2009;158:294.

40. Moller JE, Pellikka PA, Hillis GS, et al. Prognostic importance of diastolic function and filling pressure in patients with acute myocardial infarction. Circulation 2006;114:438.

41. Moller JE, Sondergaard E, Poulsen SH, et al. Pseudonormal and restrictive filling patterns predict left ventricular dilation and cardiac death after a first myocardial infarction: a serial color M-mode Doppler echocardiographic study. J Am Coll Cardiol 2000; 36:1841.

42. Moller JE, Whalley GA, Dini FL, et al. Independent prognostic importance of a restrictive left ventricular filling pattern after myocardial infarction: an individual patient meta-analysis: Meta-Analysis Research Group in Echocardiography acute myocardial infarction. Circulation 2008;117:2591.

43. Nijland F, Kamp O, Karreman AJ, et al. Prognostic implications of restrictive left ventricular filling in acute myocardial infarction: a serial Doppler echocardiographic study. J Am Coll Cardiol 1997;30:1618.

44. Marchandise B, Schroeder E, Bosly A, et al. Early detection of doxorubicin cardiotoxicity: interest of Doppler echocardiographic analysis of left ventricular filling dynamics. Am Heart J 1989;118:92.

45. Tjeerdsma G, Meinardi MT, van Der Graaf WT, et al. Early detection of anthracycline induced cardiotoxicity in asymptomatic patients with normal left ventricular systolic function: autonomic versus echocardiographic variables. Heart 1999;81:419.

46. Radulescu D, Pripon S, Parv A, et al. Altered left ventricular diastolic performance in oncologic patients treated with epirubicin. Congest Heart Fail 2007;13:215.

47. Pudil R, Horacek JM, Strasova A, et al. Monitoring of the very early changes of left ventricular diastolic function in patients with acute leukemia treated with anthracyclines. Exp Oncol 2008;30:160.

48. Nagy AC, Tolnay E, Nagykalnai T, et al. Cardiotoxicity of anthracycline in young breast cancer female patients: the possibility of detection of early cardiotoxicity by TDI. Neoplasma 2006;53:511.

49. Stoddard MF, Seeger J, Liddell NE, et al. Prolongation of isovolumetric relaxation time as assessed by Doppler echocardiography predicts doxorubicin-induced systolic dysfunction in humans. J Am Coll Cardiol 1992;20:62.

50. Bountioukos M, Doorduijn JK, Roelandt JR, et al. Repetitive dobutamine stress echocardiography for the prediction of anthracycline cardiotoxicity. Eur J Echocardiogr 2003;4:300.

51. Cottin Y, L'Huillier I, Casasnovas O, et al. Dobutamine stress echocardiography identifies anthracycline cardiotoxicity. Eur J Echocardiogr 2000;1:180.

52. Hamada H, Ohkubo T, Maeda M, et al. Evaluation of cardiac reserved function by high-dose dobutamine-stress echocardiography in asymptomatic

anthracycline-treated survivors of childhood cancer. Pediatr Int 2006;48:313.

53. Jarfelt M, Kujacic V, Holmgren D, et al. Exercise echocardiography reveals subclinical cardiac dysfunction in young adult survivors of childhood acute lymphoblastic leukemia. Pediatr Blood Cancer 2007;49:835.

54. Cho GY, Marwick TH, Kim HS, et al. Global 2-dimensional strain as a new prognosticator in patients with heart failure. J Am Coll Cardiol 2009;54:618.

55. Chetboul V, Escriou C, Tessier D, et al. Tissue Doppler imaging detects early asymptomatic myocardial abnormalities in a dog model of Duchenne's cardiomyopathy. Eur Heart J 2004;25:1934.

56. Nagueh SF, Bachinski LL, Meyer D, et al. Tissue Doppler imaging consistently detects myocardial abnormalities in patients with hypertrophic cardiomyopathy and provides a novel means for an early diagnosis before and independently of hypertrophy. Circulation 2001;104:128.

57. Neilan TG, Jassal DS, Perez-Sanz TM, et al. Tissue Doppler imaging predicts left ventricular dysfunction and mortality in a murine model of cardiac injury. Eur Heart J 2006;27:1868.

58. Sebag IA, Handschumacher MD, Ichinose F, et al. Quantitative assessment of regional myocardial function in mice by tissue Doppler imaging: comparison with hemodynamics and sonomicrometry. Circulation 2005;111:2611.

59. Kapusta L, Groot-Loonen J, Thijssen JM, et al. Regional cardiac wall motion abnormalities during and shortly after anthracyclines therapy. Med Pediatr Oncol 2003;41:426.

60. Tassan-Mangina S, Codorean D, Metivier M, et al. Tissue Doppler imaging and conventional echocardiography after anthracycline treatment in adults: early and late alterations of left ventricular function during a prospective study. Eur J Echocardiogr 2006;7:141.

61. Ganame J, Claus P, Eyskens B, et al. Acute cardiac functional and morphological changes after Anthracycline infusions in children. Am J Cardiol 2007;99:974.

62. Ganame J, Claus P, Uyttebroeck A, et al. Myocardial dysfunction late after low-dose anthracycline treatment in asymptomatic pediatric patients. J Am Soc Echocardiogr 2007;20:1351.

63. Jurcut R, Wildiers H, Ganame J, et al. Strain rate imaging detects early cardiac effects of pegylated liposomal Doxorubicin as adjuvant therapy in elderly patients with breast cancer. J Am Soc Echocardiogr 2008;21:1283.

64. Sawaya H, Sebag I, Plana JC, et al. Early detection and prediction of cardiotoxicity in chemotherapy-treated patients. Am J Cardiol 2011;107(9):1375–80.

Biomarker Approach to the Detection and Cardioprotective Strategies During Anthracycline Chemotherapy

Bonnie Ky, MD, MSCE[a,b,c,*], Joseph R. Carver, MD[a,c]

KEYWORDS

- Anthracyclines • Biomarker • Chemotherapy cardiotoxicity
- Cardioprotective agents

Chemotherapeutics used in the treatment of malignancies are widely effective but have potential devastating effects on specific organs, with cardiac toxicity of considerable concern.[1,2] Anthracyclines, commonly used in the treatment of pediatric and adult cancers, are associated with an important long-term risk of cardiac dysfunction and poor prognosis once symptomatic heart failure ensues.[3,4] Over the past decade, the number of patients at risk for adverse cardiac events has risen, secondary to both the increasing incidence of cancer and improved survival rates of treated patients. In breast cancer alone, for example, current estimates predict that more than 2 million survivors are at risk for cardiotoxicity.[5,6] A key strategy to decreasing the risk of cardiovascular complications associated with chemotherapy is the early identification of patients at high risk for heart failure and cardiac dysfunction.

Current standards for screening patients and for monitoring cardiac function during chemotherapy rely primarily on the measurement of left ventricular ejection fraction (LVEF) by echocardiography or multigated acquisition scanning. Assessment of ejection fraction (EF), however, is limited by an inability to detect early changes or predict late declines in function with chemotherapy exposure and can be highly variable secondary to dynamic changes in preload and afterload.[3] The application of new metrics, such as circulating biomarkers, that are reproducible, sensitive, and cost effective, is critical to identifying vulnerable patients at a preclinical stage. Biomarkers aimed at the early detection of cardiotoxicity could lead to an enhanced ability of clinicians to manage high-risk patients through the initiation of early cardioprotective measures and the development of a personalized, tailored chemotherapeutics regimen to decrease cardiotoxicity risk.

The purpose of this review is to first briefly discuss the effects of anthracyclines on the myocardium and then review in detail the current data on biomarker prediction of anthracycline-induced cardiac dysfunction as well as describe

[a] Division of Cardiovascular Medicine, University of Pennsylvania School of Medicine, 3400 Spruce Street, Philadelphia, PA 19104, USA
[b] Center for Clinical Epidemiology and Biostatistics, University of Pennsylvania School of Medicine, Blockley Hall, 423 Guardian Drive, Philadelphia, PA 19104, USA
[c] Abramson Cancer Center, University of Pennsylvania School of Medicine, 1600 Penn Tower, Philadelphia, PA 19104, USA
* Corresponding author. Division of Cardiovascular Medicine, University of Pennsylvania School of Medicine, 3400 Spruce Street, 9054 West Gates, Philadelphia, PA 19104.
E-mail address: bonnie.ky@uphs.upenn.edu

Heart Failure Clin 7 (2011) 323–331
doi:10.1016/j.hfc.2011.03.002
1551-7136/11/$ – see front matter © 2011 Elsevier Inc. All rights reserved.

current prophylactic cardioprotective strategies in the pediatric and adult populations.

MECHANISMS OF ANTHRACYCLINE CARDIOTOXICITY: OVERVIEW

The mechanisms of anthracycline-induced cardiac dysfunction are under active investigation, and several pathways have been implicated. Structurally, anthracycline-associated abnormalities include mitochondrial and cytoplasmic vacuolization and myofibrillar and sarcomeric disarray.[7] Chemotoxin-exposed human cardiac tissue demonstrates mitochondrial swelling and chromatin contraction.[4,8]

Oxidative stress is hypothesized to be one mechanism of myocyte apoptosis and necrosis. Free radical formation results in oxidation of myocyte proteins, nucleic acids, and cell membranes that lead to a reduction in sarco/endoplasmic reticulum Ca^{2+}-ATPase (SERCA2), intracellular calcium overload, and mitochondrial dysfunction, which altogether accelerate titin degradation and sarcomeric disarray.[8,9] Additional mechanisms potentially related to the cardiotoxicity of anthracyclines include a decline in energy reserves via changes in excitation-contraction coupling, mitochondrial respiratory function, and fatty acid metabolism.[7,10]

Several antiapoptotic pathways are also affected with anthracyclines, including Phosphatidylinositol 3-kinase, with an overall disruption in the cardioprotective mechanisms involving glutathione reductase, metallothionein, cyclooxygenase, nitric oxide, glycoprotein 130, and neuregulin/ErbB signaling.[4,8] This latter pathway is particularly interesting because ErbB2-targeted therapy with trastuzumab seems to sensitize the heart to anthracyclines.[11] More recently, there are data that suggest anthracycline cardiotoxicity may be associated with a depletion of cardiac progenitor cells that are important in cellular differentiation, vascular development, and DNA repair.[12,13] An improved understanding of the mechanisms of anthracycline toxicity is central to further advancing the field of biomarkers and cardioprotective therapeutics.

BIOMARKERS: OVERVIEW

There has been an important interest in the application of circulating biomarkers to improve the management of patients receiving cardiotoxic agents.[14] Biomarkers can fulfill several roles, including the identification of patients at an elevated risk of developing incident disease; screening for the early presence of subclinical disease; as an adjunctive diagnostic tool in cases where conventional metrics, such as EF, are

equivocal; and as a prognostic marker of adverse outcomes in patients who have developed cardiovascular disease.[15] Overall, biomarkers are attractive tools given their relative ease of use, predictive ability, precision, and accuracy.

In order for biomarkers to be useful, however, several criteria must be met. A biomarker must be easy to measure and implement clinically, be accurate and reproducible in independent populations, and demonstrate a strong, consistent association with the outcome. The information should add to existing tests, and biomarker-guided triage should improve care, for example, by leading to an earlier intervention with significant impact.[16] Ideally, a biomarker should also be reflective of the underlying mechanism of cardiac dysfunction. Current biomarkers in anthracycline-induced cardiac dysfunction, although they show excellent promise, have not yet fulfilled all these criteria (**Box 1**).

Box 1
Current state and future goals for biomarker assessment of anthracycline-induced cardiac dysfunction. Panel A highlights the current state of biomarker assessment in anthracycline-induced cardiac dysfunction, whereas Panel B identifies future goals

- Panel A: Current State
  - Strengths
    - Potential utility of troponin I (TnI) and brain natriuretic peptide (BNP)
    - Ability of TnI testing to identify patients that benefit from early cardioprotective measures
  - Weaknesses
    - Timing of specimen collection
    - Duration of follow-up in clinical studies
    - Definition of cardiac endpoints
    - Patient heterogeneity without adjustment for confounding in clinical studies
    - Limited sample size in clinical studies
- Panel B: Future Goals
  - Standardized, practical approach to biomarker assessment
  - Longer follow-up time
  - Consensus definition of cardiotoxicity
  - Control for confounding variables
  - Larger sample size
  - Rigorous reporting methods
  - Novel, mechanistic markers and use of a multimarker strategy
  - Cooperative working groups

BIOMARKERS FOR PREDICTION OF ANTHRACYCLINE CARDIOTOXICITY IN CHILDREN

Most of the current cardiac biomarker data in the pediatric population are related to troponin release, which is directly reflective of cardiomyocyte membrane integrity, and natriuretic peptides, which are released from the heart in response to volume expansion and increased wall stress.[17] The UK National Health Service Health Technology Program recently commissioned a group of investigators to objectively assess the utility of biomarkers in pediatric anthracycline cardiotoxicity.[18] This analysis highlighted 6 cohort studies and 1 randomized controlled trial that met the inclusion criteria of having a control or comparison group.[19–25] The studies presented included measurements of atrial natriuretic peptide (ANP), BNP, troponinT (TnT), lipid peroxide levels, or carnitine. Of these, no study demonstrated an improvement in cardiovascular outcomes with biomarker knowledge. The overall conclusion of the panel was that the evidence for use of cardiac markers for quantifying cardiac damage with chemotherapy exposure was too limited in quantity and quality to make substantive recommendations.

One of the largest studies worth noting was of 206 pediatric acute lymphocytic leukemia patients, where TnT was used as an outcome measure, but not predictor, of subclinical cardiac damage.[19] In this study, 101 children with acute lymphocytic leukemia were randomized to receive doxorubicin alone and 105 children were randomized to receive dexrazoxane followed immediately by doxorubicin. Serial measures of cardiac TnT were made, with a median of 15.1 measures per patient. Elevations of TnT occurred in 35% of the patients and more commonly in those who received doxorubicin alone. Although this study demonstrated that dexrazoxane was associated with less-frequent TnT elevations compared with placebo, the relationship between TnT and cardiac function by echocardiography was not determined. Additional smaller studies in children have failed to show changes in TnT or TnI with doxorubicin or a strong correlation with echocardiographic measures of cardiac function.[22,26–30]

With respect to natriuretic peptide assessment, the majority of the studies have been even less definitive.[20,22,24,26,31–33] One cross-sectional study of 34 patients in remission who had previously been treated with anthracyclines compared ANP and BNP levels to cardiac function by echocardiography. Cardiac dysfunction was defined as LVEF less than 60% or by the presence of regional wall motion abnormalities. BNP levels were significantly different in 8 children with cardiac dysfunction versus those who did not experience toxicity ($P<.05$).[20] There was wide variability in BNP measurements, however, with the mean 29.0 (31.2) pg/mL in the cardiac dysfunction group and 9.0 (14.8) pg/mL in the normal group. Other studies have corroborated this finding—that although there may be some degree of correlation between natriuretic peptides and cardiac function by echo, there is wide interindividual variability in natriuretic peptide levels and considerable overlap between groups of patients with and without cardiac dysfunction.[31] Such variability has thus far limited its utility as a screening marker for subclinical cardiotoxicity in children.

BIOMARKERS FOR PREDICTION OF ANTHRACYCLINE CARDIOTOXICITY IN ADULTS

Several studies in adults have further defined the distribution of circulating TnT and TnI with exposure to high-dose chemotherapy (HDC).[34–44] The highest-impact studies include a detailed investigation in 204 patients, which defined the relationship between longitudinal assessments of repeated measures of TnI and LVEF with HDC exposure.[42] This study demonstrated that elevated TnI is a risk marker for the development of incident cardiac dysfunction. Biomarker measurements were made before, immediately after, and then 12, 24, 36, and 72 hours after each cycle of chemotherapy, with the average number of cycles per patient 3.2. Again, similar to the pediatric studies, there were nearly 18 biomarker measures per patient. Of the 204 patients, 65 had a positive TnI in 112 of the 661 chemotherapy cycles. Approximately half of the elevations were observed at less than 12 hours, but the other half occurred 12 to 72 hours postexposure. Overall, 29% of the 65 patients with TnI positivity had a significant decline in EF to less than 50% during 9 to 10 months of follow-up. Patients with TnI negativity had a transient decrease in LVEF after 3 months but recovered to an LVEF greater than 50% by 4 to 7 months. This highly important study demonstrated a predictive role for TnI in the identification of patients at high risk for cardiac dysfunction.

Subsequently, these same investigators expanded their findings to a significantly larger group of 703 patients with various malignancies undergoing HDC.[40] In this cohort, more than two-thirds had received prior anthracyclines and one-third prior mediastinal radiation. Again, plasma TnI was measured over various time points (baseline; immediately after; 12, 24, 36, and 72 hours after drug infusion; and 1 month after chemotherapy completion). Echocardiography was performed at baseline; 1, 3, 6, and 12 months after the end of each cycle; and every 6 months thereafter or whenever required clinically. Clinical endpoints included not only LVEF decline but also the combined outcome of death, overt heart failure, acute pulmonary edema, asymptomatic LVEF reduction ($\geq$25% reduction from baseline), life-threatening arrhythmias, and conduction disturbances. Patients were followed over an extended period of time (mean 20 (13) months) and classified into 3 subgroups based on the combined presence of any detectable TnI either within 72 hours (early) or 1 month after the last administration of chemotherapy (late). In 208 patients, early low levels of TnI were detected at levels greater than or equal to 0.08 ng/mL, and in 63 of these patients there were also persistent late elevations. The majority of the patients (495) had no elevations. There were 111 adverse cardiovascular events, with all but 5 occurring in the 2 subgroups with TnI elevations. The correlation between TnI positivity and LVEF maximal reduction was 0.78 to 0.92, with positive and negative predictive values of 84% and 99%, respectively.

As demonstrated by these 2 studies, TnI positivity seems highly predictive of chemotherapy-induced cardiac dysfunction. Questions remain, however, regarding the optimal timing of TnI assessment; the cost-effectiveness of multiple, repeated TnI measures; the independent predictive value of biomarker assessment after adjustment for potential confounders; and replication of these findings in multiple external cohorts.

Serum concentrations of natriuretic peptides, such as ANP, BNP, and N-terminal proBNP (NT-proBNP), have also been measured in adults undergoing HDC, but these findings are less consistent. One study of 100 patients demonstrated transient increases in NT-proBNP in 13 patients, but no association with diastolic or systolic function.[36] Other small studies have also demonstrated a lack of association[34,45,46] or only cross-sectional associations between BNP and diastolic function.[47]

Early point-of-care testing and serial assessment of certain natriuretic peptides, however, may have predictive utility and both need to be more fully examined. A pilot study of 109 patients undergoing anthracycline-based therapy demonstrated that BNP elevation by point-of-care testing was predictive of subsequent cardiac events. Patients with a BNP elevation greater than 200 pg/mL had a significantly increased risk of subsequent cardiotoxicity, as observed in 11 patients in the cohort.[48]

In another retrospective study, 52 patients had serial assessments of NT-proBNP before the initiation of, immediately after the completion of, and 12, 24, 36, and 72 hours of high-dose chemotherapy.[49] Patients were divided into groups based on (1) persistent elevation, (2) transient elevation, or (3) decrease/no change in biomarker level. Serial echocardiograms were performed during 1 year of follow-up. In 17 patients with a persistent BNP increase, there was a worsening of diastolic and systolic function indices from baseline to 12 months. The mean LVEF decreased from 62.8 (3.4)% to 45.6 (11.5)%. No patients in the other 2 groups had a decline in LVEF to less than 55%.

Thus, repeated measures of biomarkers, such as troponins or natriuretic peptides, show excellent promise in their predictive ability of chemotherapy-induced cardiac dysfunction. Although many of these studies demonstrate important findings, altogether there remain important methodological issues. These include a need to clarify the optimal timing of biomarker assessment and specimen collection; variable definition of the outcome cardiac dysfunction; need for consideration of the independent predictive value of biomarkers and control for confounding variables; the inclusion of patients with pre-existing cardiovascular disease within these cohorts given that they are commonly treated in everyday clinical practice; need for extended follow-up time; and validation of these findings in multiple independent cohorts.[50]

CARDIOPROTECTIVE STRATEGIES: OVERVIEW

There are several prophylactic, cardioprotective strategies that have been studied in the hopes of minimizing toxicity (**Box 2**), but currently there are no well-established or highly effective therapies that are commonly used in everyday clinical practice.[51,52] Current measures include limiting the cumulative anthracycline dose, altering anthracycline administration timing and duration, and using liposomal anthracycline derivatives.[53] Various cardioprotectants that are believed to have antioxidant effects, such as probucol, amifostine, and N-acetylcysteine, have been studied in small human trials. The 3 most promising and commonly used agents are dexrazoxane, angiotensin-converting enzyme inhibitors (ACE-Is), and β-blockers.

CARDIOPROTECTIVE STRATEGIES IN CHILDREN

Dexrazoxane is the major agent that has been studied in the pediatric anthracycline-treated population.[19,53–57] Dexrazoxane is a derivative of

---

Box 2
Current state and future goals for cardioprotective strategies in anthracycline-induced cardiac dysfunction. Panel A highlights the current state of cardioprotective strategies in anthracycline-induced cardiac dysfunction whereas Panel B identifies future goals

- Panel A: Current State
  - Strengths
    - Utility of dexrazoxane, ACE-Is, angiotensin receptor blockers, and carvedilol
    - Potential utility of biomarkers to identify high-risk patients
  - Weaknesses
    - Small number of double-blind, placebo-controlled randomized trials
    - Potential for worse oncologic response rate with dexrazoxane
- Panel B: Future Goals
  - Novel, mechanistically relevant agents for cardioprotection
  - Established method for identifying patients who may benefit from early cardioprotective strategies
  - Randomized, double-blind, placebo-controlled trials

EDTA that acts as an intracellular chelating agent against iron, which may act by decreasing anthracycline-induced free radical generation. Animal studies have demonstrated an important cardioprotective effect of dexrazoxane and, to date, 6 human clinical studies corroborate this.

An early study of pediatric sarcoma patients undergoing doxorubicin chemotherapy randomized 38 subjects to dexrazoxane versus placebo.[54] There was a statistically significant albeit small difference in EF decline in the control versus dexrazoxane group (2.7% vs 1%, $P = .02$). Of the 15 patients who received the full-intended dose of doxorubicin (410 mg/m^2), the mean EF in the control group (n = 5) was 44 (2.8)% versus 53.9 (2.2)% in the dexrazoxane group (n = 10). As discussed previously, a larger randomized placebo-controlled study compared all patients who received doxorubicin alone (30 mg/m^2 every 3 weeks for 10 doses) with those who received dexrazoxane and doxorubicin.[19] Both TnT and echocardiographic assessment of cardiac function were used to access differential responses to therapy. Serial measurements of TnT were made in a majority of the subjects before, during (on the same day and then 7 days after induction therapy), and on completion of treatment with doxorubicin, the dexrazoxane group had significantly fewer elevations in TnT compared with the control group (21% vs 50% of the population having any TnT abnormality, $P<.001$), but there was no difference in cardiac function by echocardiography at time of therapy completion. Based on these available data, the American Society of Clinical Oncology states that there is insufficient evidence to make a guideline recommendation supporting the use of dexrazoxane in pediatric malignancies.[58,59]

In addition, although there have been encouraging results in adults treated with ACE-I therapy, the benefits in children are still largely unproven.[60,61] In the only randomized, placebo-controlled trial of ACE-I therapy in children previously exposed to chemotherapy, 135 long-term survivors of pediatric malignancies who had at least one cardiac abnormality after anthracycline exposure were randomized to enalapril versus placebo. Enalapril was initiated at a dose of 0.05 mg/kg per day and scaled to 0.15 mg/kg per day. Over a median follow-up of 2.8 years, there was no difference in exercise performance, fractional shortening, stroke velocity index, or overall rate of change in maximal cardiac index on exercise testing. In the first year of therapy, there was a significant difference in end-systolic wall stress largely related to differences in end systolic pressure. Among the 135 patients in the study, 7 had significant declines in cardiac performance and were taken off randomly assigned medications. Six of these 7 patients had been randomized to placebo therapy ($P = .11$). Currently, prophylactic use of ACE-Is in pediatric patients without clinical evidence of cardiac dysfunction is not a practice standard.

CARDIOPROTECTIVE STRATEGIES IN ADULTS

In adults, however, ACE-Is are a cornerstone in the treatment of heart failure and systolic dysfunction and are believed to be effective as a prophylactic strategy in adult anthracycline-treated patients at high risk for cardiotoxicity.[62] ACE-Is decrease left ventricular (LV) size and vascular resistance through effects on the renin-angiotensin system and may also act to scavenge free radicals.[63] In a randomized, placebo-controlled trial of patients undergoing HDC, those with any evidence of cardiac damage by TnI positivity were selected for prophylactic ACE-I therapy.[51] TnI was measured at 6 time points surrounding each chemotherapy cycle. In 58 of 114 patients with early TnI positivity, enalapril was initiated and titrated as tolerated. In this group, dramatic reductions in cardiotoxicity were observed without any decline in LVEF during the 12-month follow-up duration. Conversely, 25 of 58 patients in the placebo control group had an LVEF decline of greater than 10%. Although this study demonstrates the benefits of ACE-I therapy in cardiotoxicity prevention and the use of TnI to help identify patients who may benefit from such therapy, the incremental utility of biomarker-guided therapies in this setting is not yet entirely clear. As discussed later, similar treatment benefits have been observed when other agents were administered in a randomized fashion.

Several smaller studies have also looked at the cardioprotective effects of the angiotensin receptor blocker, valsartan, and β-blocker, carvedilol. In a randomized study of 40 patients with treatment-naïve non-Hodgkin lymphoma, 20 were randomized to valsartan therapy (80 mg once daily). Although not clearly blinded or placebo-controlled, the investigators determined that during 7 days of monitoring, patients not treated with valsartan had significant increases in BNP, ANP, and LV end-diastolic diameter as measured by echocardiography. valsartan therapy was associated with statistically significant smaller LV end-diastolic diameters and BNP levels in repeated measures over 7 days.[64]

In a single-blind, placebo-controlled trial of 50 patients undergoing 6 cycles of doxorubicin-containing or epirubicin-containing chemotherapy, those treated with oral carvedilol (with 12.5 mg once daily) had no significant change in LVEF after 5.2 (1.2) months. Conversely, patients in the control group had notable EF reductions compared with baseline (mean 68.9% to 52.3%, $P<.001$) and changes in LV end-diastolic and end-systolic chamber size ($P<.01$).[65] Although these findings need to be validated in larger populations, there is some mechanistic basis for these observations. It is believed that carvedilol may exert cardioprotective effects via antioxidant effects and reduction of free oxygen radicals, restoration of SERCA2 activity in cardiomyocytes, and potentially the inhibition of apoptotic signaling pathways.[65]

There have also been several studies in the adult population with dexrazoxane. A recent meta-analysis by the Cochrane Collaboration determined that there is significant efficacy of dexrazoxane in preventing cardiotoxicity (hazard ratio [HR] 0.29; 95% CI, 0.20–0.41); however, the majority of the patients included in the studies were adults with advanced breast cancer.[66] Although there was no clear difference in tumor response rate (HR 0.89; 95% CI, 0.78–1.02) or progression-free survival (HR 1.01; 95% CI, 0.86–1.18), one individual study did detect a significantly worse response rate in the dexrazoxane

group, which may have been related to an anomalously high response rate in the control group.[57] In terms of other side effects, the Cochrane meta-analysis did determine that there was significant myelosuppression in the dexrazoxane-treated group (relative risk 1.16; 95% CI, 1.05–1.29; $P = .005$ favoring control).

Currently, the American Society of Clinical Oncology has recommended that the use of dexrazoxane can be considered for breast cancer patients who have received more than 300 mg/m^2 of doxorubicin in the metastatic setting and who may benefit from continued doxorubicin-containing therapy.[58,59] The use of dexrazoxane is still not recommended for patients in the adjuvant setting or with epirubicin therapy. For those patients previously treated with more than 300 mg/m^2 in the adjuvant setting but with recurrent metastatic disease, the guidelines state that the decision to treat with dexrazoxane should be individualized with the "consideration given to the potential for dexrazoxane to decrease response rates as well as decreasing the risk of cardiotoxicity."[58] Clinically, dexrazoxane has not yet achieved widespread use, however.

FUTURE RESEARCH—BIOMARKERS AND CARDIOPROTECTIVE STRATEGIES

Strategies reflective of the underlying biology and pathophysiologic derangements would be ideal for biomarker and therapeutics development. The authors propose that specifically focusing on biomarkers and therapeutics involved in cardiomyocyte metabolism and survival reflective of the alterations in cardiac homeostasis during anthracycline therapy can provide a major advance in the early detection and cardioprotection of anthracycline toxicity. In addition, a multimarker strategy may be particularly useful in capturing various mechanisms of the disease process.[17] There is a growing need to expand the use of biomarkers, such as troponins or natriuretic peptides, to the population of patients that are treated with cancer therapies that are also associated with an increased risk of cardiotoxicity, such as trastuzumab and sunitinib. There are few published data to date regarding the effectiveness of biomarkers regarding these newer agents.[67]

SUMMARY

Significant advances have been made over the past 10 years regarding the biomarker assessment of cardiotoxicity due to chemotherapy and in prophylactic cardioprotective strategies. There is promise that certain biomarkers, mainly troponins and natriuretic peptides, may represent a future, fundamental strategy for risk prediction and cardiotoxicity detection. There are many important considerations that still remain a barrier to implementing such an approach, however. There needs to be greater emphasis on the development of common definitions of cardiac outcomes, larger sample sizes with longer follow-up time, standardization of the timing of biomarker measurements, and validation in additional populations. Biomarkers specific to cardiomyocyte metabolism and survival and the use of a multimarker strategy are also necessary to advance this field, as is the continued application of knowledge in basic and translational research to develop novel therapeutic strategies. In addition, this research needs to expand outside of anthracyclines alone, to include commonly used agents that are also associated with significant cardiotoxic effects, such as trastuzumab and sunitinib. Finally, more research needs to be performed in the validation of promising cardioprotective strategies, including randomized controlled trials in both adults and children.

REFERENCES

1. Felker GM, Thompson RE, Hare JM, et al. Underlying causes and long-term survival in patients with initially unexplained cardiomyopathy. N Engl J Med 2000;342(15):1077–84.

2. Yeh ET, Tong AT, Lenihan DJ, et al. Cardiovascular complications of cancer therapy: diagnosis, pathogenesis, and management. Circulation 2004; 109(25):3122–31.

3. Altena R, Perik PJ, van Veldhuisen DJ, et al. Cardiovascular toxicity caused by cancer treatment: strategies for early detection. Lancet Oncol 2009;10(4): 391–9.

4. Chen B, Peng X, Pentassuglia L, et al. Molecular and cellular mechanisms of anthracycline cardiotoxicity. Cardiovasc Toxicol 2007;7(2):114–21.

5. Jones LW, Haykowsky MJ, Swartz JJ, et al. Early breast cancer therapy and cardiovascular injury. J Am Coll Cardiol 2007;50(15):1435–41.

6. Gianni L, Herman EH, Lipshultz SE, et al. Anthracycline cardiotoxicity: from bench to bedside. J Clin Oncol 2008;26(22):3777–84.

7. Tokarska-Schlattner M, Zaugg M, Zuppinger C, et al. New insights into doxorubicin-induced cardiotoxicity: the critical role of cellular energetics. J Mol Cell Cardiol 2006;41(3):389–405.

8. Zuppinger C, Timolati F, Suter TM. Pathophysiology and diagnosis of cancer drug induced cardiomyopathy. Cardiovasc Toxicol 2007;7(2):61–6.

9. Lim CC, Zuppinger C, Guo X, et al. Anthracyclines induce calpain-dependent titin proteolysis and

10. Jeyaseelan R, Poizat C, Wu HY, et al. Molecular mechanisms of doxorubicin-induced cardiomyopathy. Selective suppression of Reiske iron-sulfur protein, ADP/ATP translocase, and phosphofructokinase genes is associated with ATP depletion in rat cardiomyocytes. J Biol Chem 1997;272(9): 5828–32.

11. Slamon DJ, Leyland-Jones B, Shak S, et al. Use of chemotherapy plus a monoclonal antibody against HER2 for metastatic breast cancer that overexpresses HER2. N Engl J Med 2001;344(11):783–92.

12. De Angelis A, Piegari E, Cappetta D, et al. Anthracycline cardiomyopathy is mediated by depletion of the cardiac stem cell pool and is rescued by restoration of progenitor cell function. Circulation 2010; 121(2):276–92.

13. Huang C, Zhang X, Ramil JM, et al. Juvenile exposure to anthracyclines impairs cardiac progenitor cell function and vascularization resulting in greater susceptibility to stress-induced myocardial injury in adult mice. Circulation 2010;121(5):675–83.

14. Cardinale D, Colombo A, Cipolla CM. Prevention and treatment of cardiomyopathy and heart failure in patients receiving cancer chemotherapy. Curr Treat Options Cardiovasc Med 2008;10(6):486–95.

15. Vasan RS. Biomarkers of cardiovascular disease: molecular basis and practical considerations. Circulation 2006;113(19):2335–62.

16. Morrow DA, de Lemos JA. Benchmarks for the assessment of novel cardiovascular biomarkers. Circulation 2007;115(8):949–52.

17. Braunwald E. Biomarkers in heart failure. N Engl J Med 2008;358(20):2148–59.

18. Bryant J, Picot J, Baxter L, et al. Use of cardiac markers to assess the toxic effects of anthracyclines given to children with cancer: a systematic review. Eur J Cancer 2007;43(13):1959–66.

19. Lipshultz SE, Rifai N, Dalton VM, et al. The effect of dexrazoxane on myocardial injury in doxorubicin-treated children with acute lymphoblastic leukemia. N Engl J Med 2004;351(2):145–53.

20. Hayakawa H, Komada Y, Hirayama M, et al. Plasma levels of natriuretic peptides in relation to doxorubicin-induced cardiotoxicity and cardiac function in children with cancer. Med Pediatr Oncol 2001;37(1):4–9.

21. Pinarli FG, Oguz A, Tunaoglu FS, et al. Late cardiac evaluation of children with solid tumors after anthracycline chemotherapy. Pediatr Blood Cancer 2005; 44(4):370–7.

22. Soker M, Kervancioglu M. Plasma concentrations of NT-pro-BNP and cardiac troponin-I in relation to doxorubicin-induced cardiomyopathy and cardiac function in childhood malignancy. Saudi Med J 2005;26(8):1197–202.

23. Yaris N, Ceviz N, Coskun T, et al. Serum carnitine levels during the doxorubicin therapy. Its role in cardiotoxicity. J Exp Clin Cancer Res 2002;21(2): 165–70.

24. Bauch M, Ester A, Kimura B, et al. Atrial natriuretic peptide as a marker for doxorubicin-induced cardiotoxic effects. Cancer 1992;69(6):1492–7.

25. Horino N, Kobayashi Y, Usui T. Elevation of lipid peroxide in children treated with a combination of chemotherapeutic agents including doxorubicin. Acta Paediatr Scand 1983;72(4):549–51.

26. Germanakis I, Anagnostatou N, Kalmanti M. Troponins and natriuretic peptides in the monitoring of anthracycline cardiotoxicity. Pediatr Blood Cancer 2008;51(3):327–33.

27. Fink FM, Genser N, Fink C, et al. Cardiac troponin T and creatine kinase MB mass concentrations in children receiving anthracycline chemotherapy. Med Pediatr Oncol 1995;25(3):185–9.

28. Kismet E, Varan A, Ayabakan C, et al. Serum troponin T levels and echocardiographic evaluation in children treated with doxorubicin. Pediatr Blood Cancer 2004;42(3):220–4.

29. Kremer LC, Bastiaansen BA, Offringa M, et al. Troponin T in the first 24 hours after the administration of chemotherapy and the detection of myocardial damage in children. Eur J Cancer 2002;38(5): 686–9.

30. Mathew P, Suarez W, Kip K, et al. Is there a potential role for serum cardiac troponin I as a marker for myocardial dysfunction in pediatric patients receiving anthracycline-based therapy? A pilot study. Cancer Invest 2001;19(4):352–9.

31. Aggarwal S, Pettersen MD, Bhambhani K, et al. B-type natriuretic peptide as a marker for cardiac dysfunction in anthracycline-treated children. Pediatr Blood Cancer 2007;49(6):812–6.

32. Tikanoja T, Riikonen P, Perkkio M, et al. Serum N-terminal atrial natriuretic peptide (NT-ANP) in the cardiac follow-up in children with cancer. Med Pediatr Oncol 1998;31(2):73–8.

33. Ekstein S, Nir A, Rein AJ, et al. N-terminal-proB-type natriuretic peptide as a marker for acute anthracycline cardiotoxicity in children. J Pediatr Hematol Oncol 2007;29(7):440–4.

34. Horacek JM, Pudil R, Jebavy L, et al. Assessment of anthracycline-induced cardiotoxicity with biochemical markers. Exp Oncol 2007;29(4):309–13.

35. Horacek JM, Pudil R, Tichy M, et al. Cardiac troponin I seems to be superior to cardiac troponin T in the early detection of cardiac injury associated with anthracycline treatment. Onkologie 2008; 31(10):559–60.

36. Dodos F, Halbsguth T, Erdmann E, et al. Usefulness of myocardial performance index and biochemical markers for early detection of anthracycline-induced cardiotoxicity in adults. Clin Res Cardiol 2008;97(5): 318–26.

37. Auner HW, Tinchon C, Brezinschek RI, et al. Monitoring of cardiac function by serum cardiac troponin T levels, ventricular repolarisation indices, and echocardiography after conditioning with fractionated total body irradiation and high-dose cyclophosphamide. Eur J Haematol 2002;69(1):1–6.

38. Morandi P, Ruffini PA, Benvenuto GM, et al. Serum cardiac troponin I levels and ECG/Echo monitoring in breast cancer patients undergoing high-dose (7 g/m(2)) cyclophosphamide. Bone Marrow Transplant 2001;28(3):277–82.

39. Kilickap S, Barista I, Akgul E, et al. cTnT can be a useful marker for early detection of anthracycline cardiotoxicity. Ann Oncol 2005;16(5):798–804.

40. Cardinale D, Sandri MT, Colombo A, et al. Prognostic value of troponin I in cardiac risk stratification of cancer patients undergoing high-dose chemotherapy. Circulation 2004;109(22):2749–54.

41. Cardinale D, Sandri MT, Martinoni A, et al. Myocardial injury revealed by plasma troponin I in breast cancer treated with high-dose chemotherapy. Ann Oncol 2002;13(5):710–5.

42. Cardinale D, Sandri MT, Martinoni A, et al. Left ventricular dysfunction predicted by early troponin I release after high-dose chemotherapy. J Am Coll Cardiol 2000;36(2):517–22.

43. Suzuki T, Hayashi D, Yamazaki T, et al. Elevated B-type natriuretic peptide levels after anthracycline administration. Am Heart J 1998;136(2):362–3.

44. Sandri MT, Cardinale D, Zorzino L, et al. Minor increases in plasma troponin I predict decreased left ventricular ejection fraction after high-dose chemotherapy. Clin Chem 2003;49(2):248–52.

45. Knobloch K, Tepe J, Lichtinghagen R, et al. Monitoring of cardiotoxicity during immunotherapy with Herceptin using simultaneous continuous wave Doppler depending on N-terminal pro-brain natriuretic peptide. Clin Med 2007;7(1):88–9 [author reply: 89].

46. Knobloch K, Tepe J, Rossner D, et al. Combined NT-pro-BNP and CW-Doppler ultrasound cardiac output monitoring (USCOM) in epirubicin and liposomal doxorubicin therapy. Int J Cardiol 2008; 128(3):316–25.

47. Nousiainen T, Jantunen E, Vanninen E, et al. Natriuretic peptides as markers of cardiotoxicity during doxorubicin treatment for non-Hodgkin's lymphoma. Eur J Haematol 1999;62(2):135–41.

48. Lenihan DJ, Massey MR, Baysinger KB, et al. Superior detection of cardiotoxicity during chemotherapy using biomarkers. J Card Fail 2007;13(Suppl 2): S151.

49. Sandri MT, Salvatici M, Cardinale D, et al. N-terminal pro-B-type natriuretic peptide after high-dose

chemotherapy: a marker predictive of cardiac dysfunction? Clin Chem 2005;51(8):1405–10.

50. Maruvada P, Srivastava S. Joint National Cancer Institute-Food and Drug Administration workshop on research strategies, study designs, and statistical approaches to biomarker validation for cancer diagnosis and detection. Cancer Epidemiol Biomarkers Prev 2006;15(6):1078–82.

51. Cardinale D, Colombo A, Sandri MT, et al. Prevention of high-dose chemotherapy-induced cardiotoxicity in high-risk patients by angiotensin-converting enzyme inhibition. Circulation 2006;114(23):2474–81.

52. Albini A, Pennesi G, Donatelli F, et al. Cardiotoxicity of anticancer drugs: the need for cardio-oncology and cardio-oncological prevention. J Natl Cancer Inst 2010;102(1):14–25.

53. Wouters KA, Kremer LC, Miller TL, et al. Protecting against anthracycline-induced myocardial damage: a review of the most promising strategies. Br J Haematol 2005;131(5):561–78.

54. Wexler LH, Andrich MP, Venzon D, et al. Randomized trial of the cardioprotective agent ICRF-187 in pediatric sarcoma patients treated with doxorubicin. J Clin Oncol 1996;14(2):362–72.

55. Swain SM, Vici P. The current and future role of dexrazoxane as a cardioprotectant in anthracycline treatment: expert panel review. J Cancer Res Clin Oncol 2004;130(1):1–7.

56. Swain SM, Whaley FS, Gerber MC, et al. Delayed administration of dexrazoxane provides cardioprotection for patients with advanced breast cancer treated with doxorubicin-containing therapy. J Clin Oncol 1997;15(4):1333–40.

57. Swain SM, Whaley FS, Gerber MC, et al. Cardioprotection with dexrazoxane for doxorubicin-containing therapy in advanced breast cancer. J Clin Oncol 1997;15(4):1318–32.

58. Hensley ML, Hagerty KL, Kewalramani T, et al. American Society of Clinical Oncology 2008 clinical practice guideline update: use of chemotherapy and radiation therapy protectants. J Clin Oncol 2009; 27(1):127–45.

59. Schuchter LM, Hensley ML, Meropol NJ, et al. 2002 Update of recommendations for the use of chemotherapy and radiotherapy protectants: clinical practice guidelines of the American Society of Clinical Oncology. J Clin Oncol 2002;20(12):2895–903.

60. Lipshultz SE, Lipsitz SR, Sallan SE, et al. Long-term enalapril therapy for left ventricular dysfunction in doxorubicin-treated survivors of childhood cancer. J Clin Oncol 2002;20(23):4517–22.

61. Silber JH, Cnaan A, Clark BJ, et al. Enalapril to prevent cardiac function decline in long-term survivors of pediatric cancer exposed to anthracyclines. J Clin Oncol 2004;22(5):820–8.

62. Jessup M, Abraham WT, Casey DE, et al. 2009 focused update: ACCF/AHA Guidelines for the diagnosis and management of heart failure in adults: a report of the American College of Cardiology Foundation/American Heart Association Task Force on Practice Guidelines: developed in collaboration with the International Society for Heart and Lung Transplantation. Circulation 2009;119(14):1977–2016.

63. Vaynblat M, Shah HR, Bhaskaran D, et al. Simultaneous angiotensin converting enzyme inhibition moderates ventricular dysfunction caused by doxorubicin. Eur J Heart Fail 2002;4(5):583–6.

64. Nakamae H, Tsumura K, Terada Y, et al. Notable effects of angiotensin II receptor blocker, valsartan, on acute cardiotoxic changes after standard chemotherapy with cyclophosphamide, doxorubicin, vincristine, and prednisolone. Cancer 2005;104(11): 2492–8.

65. Kalay N, Basar E, Ozdogru I, et al. Protective effects of carvedilol against anthracycline-induced cardiomyopathy. J Am Coll Cardiol 2006;48(11):2258–62.

66. van Dalen EC, Caron HN, Dickinson HO, et al. Cardioprotective interventions for cancer patients receiving anthracyclines. Cochrane Database Syst Rev 2008;2:CD003917.

67. Morris PG, Hudis CA. Trastuzumab-related cardiotoxicity following anthracycline-based adjuvant chemotherapy: how worried should we be? J Clin Oncol 2010;28(21):3407–10.

Chemotherapy-Associated Cardiotoxicity: How Often Does it Really Occur and How Can it Be Prevented?

Ronald M. Witteles, MD[a,*], Michael B. Fowler, MB, FRCP[a],
Melinda L. Telli, MD[b]

KEYWORDS

- Cardiotoxicity • Chemotherapy • Cancer • Malignancy
- Heart failure

Since the earliest days of chemotherapy, treatment-related cardiotoxicity has remained an "Achilles heel" for the medical treatment of malignancy. This problem, which has only grown with time because of the introduction of new cardiotoxic agents, more sensitive methods of screening for cardiotoxicity, and increased survival times for patients with malignancy, has manifested itself in two forms:

1. Morbidity and mortality associated with cardiotoxicity
2. Inability for patients to receive optimal treatment of cancer, resulting in morbidity and mortality from their malignancies.

Unfortunately, the semantics of what constitutes cardiotoxicity, and specifically heart failure, has resulted in substantial and persistent confusion. In fact, it is important to understand that cardiovascular toxicity might include a spectrum of problems, including arrhythmias, pericardial disease, alterations of blood pressure, arterial and venous thromboembolism, and, of course, left ventricular dysfunction. Hence, the true rates of cardiotoxicity, and the clinical relevance when it occurs, are often misunderstood. This article outlines the current clinical evidence for left ventricular dysfunction and heart failure for the two most important classes of cardiotoxic chemotherapeutic agents (anthracyclines and anti-HER2–directed therapies, including trastuzumab). The potential pitfalls that have led to underestimated rates of left ventricular dysfunction and strategies for screening for and prophylaxing against chemotherapy-associated left ventricular dysfunction are discussed.

ANTHRACYCLINES

Anthracyclines are among the most commonly used chemotherapeutic agents, with antineoplastic activity against a wide variety of tumors. In particular, they represent a cornerstone of chemotherapy for lymphomas, hematologic malignancies, breast carcinomas, and sarcomas.

Almost since the time that anthracycline use began, the presence of a dose-dependent rate of cardiotoxicity has been recognized.[1–5] Early reports examined the levels of clinical cardiotoxicity, usually manifesting as overt heart failure and symptoms of vascular congestion.

[a] Division of Cardiovascular Medicine, Stanford University School of Medicine, 300 Pasteur Drive, Falk CVRC, Stanford, CA 94305, USA
[b] Division of Medical Oncology, Stanford University School of Medicine, 300 Pasteur Drive, Stanford, CA 94305, USA
* Corresponding author.
E-mail address: witteles@stanford.edu

Heart Failure Clin 7 (2011) 333–344
doi:10.1016/j.hfc.2011.03.005

Specifically, two influential studies in the 1970s recommended a cutoff for doxorubicin at a cumulative dose of 550 mg/m^2, based on a perceived relatively low incidence of heart failure (0.3%–7%) in doses up to that level.[2,4] In an often-quoted study by Von Hoff and colleagues[4] in 1979, an inflection point in the cardiotoxicity curve seemed to occur at a cumulative doxorubicin dose of 550 mg/m^2.

Over the past 3 decades, it has become increasingly evident that these predicted rates vastly underestimated the true incidence of left ventricular dysfunction and heart failure. The explanation for the difference lies in the definitions used for cardiotoxicity. "Severe congestive heart failure"[2] or "clinical signs and symptoms of congestive heart failure believed to be secondary to doxorubicin by the clinical investigator"[4] were standard definitions in the 1970s.

More modern analyses concur with current American College of Cardiology (ACC)/American Heart Association (AHA) guidelines[6] in which development of left ventricular systolic dysfunction, either symptomatic or asymptomatic, is considered to represent major cardiotoxicity and represents a class I indication for instituting heart failure therapy (**Box 1**). Therefore, more recent

---

Box 1
2005 ACC/AHA heart failure guidelines[a]

- Stage A: Risk for heart failure but without structural heart disease or symptoms of heart failure
- Stage B: Structural heart disease without symptoms of heart failure
- Stage C: Structural heart disease with current or prior symptoms of heart failure
- Stage D: Refractory heart failure

[a] All patients receiving potentially cardiotoxic chemotherapy (eg, anthracyclines, trastuzumab, tyrosine kinase inhibitors) are stage A. Patients with left ventricular dysfunction (even if asymptomatic) are at least stage B. Note that therapy with ß-blockers and either angiotensin-converting enzyme inhibitors or angiotensin II receptor blockers is a class I indication for all patients with stage B or C heart failure.

Data from Hunt SA, Abraham WT, Chin MH, et al. ACC/AHA 2005 Guideline Update for the Diagnosis and Management of Chronic Heart Failure in the Adult: a report of the American College of Cardiology/American Heart Association Task Force on Practice Guidelines (Writing Committee to Update the 2001 Guidelines for the Evaluation and Management of Heart Failure): developed in collaboration with the American College of Chest Physicians and the International Society for Heart and Lung Transplantation: endorsed by the Heart Rhythm Society. Circulation 2005;112:e154–235.

---

studies have focused on screening for left ventricular dysfunction, either symptomatic or asymptomatic.

A 2003 study by Swain and colleagues[7] analyzed three anthracycline trials, and found a dramatically higher incidence of cardiotoxicity than had previously been recognized. Specifically, the incidence of significant left ventricular dysfunction (mostly representing a reduction in left ventricular ejection fraction [LVEF] of $\geq$10 absolute percentage points to a level below normal) was 16.2%, 32.4%, and 65.4% at cumulative doxorubicin doses of 300, 400, and 550 mg/m^2, respectively. Even at relatively low doses of anthracyclines (cumulative doses, 200–250 mg/m^2), a significant risk of cardiotoxicity was estimated at 7.8% to 8.8%, which is similar to that observed in recent large trials with prospective cardiac screening.[8]

Multiple strategies have been used to counteract the left ventricular dysfunction associated with anthracyclines. One approach has been structural modification of anthracyclines. The most prominent example has been with epirubicin, which has evidence for less cardiotoxicity on a milligram-for-milligram basis compared with doxorubicin.[9] Despite early optimism, subsequent analyses have found a similar incidence of cardiotoxicity with functionally equivalent doses of the less-potent epirubicin, particularly at cumulative doses greater than 800 to 900 mg/m^2.[10,11] A recent Cochrane meta-analysis found a strong trend favoring epirubicin for minimizing cardiotoxicity, although a smaller trend favored doxorubicin for tumor responsiveness, suggesting the possibility that the anthracycline doses in the trials were not equivalent.[12] Less left ventricular dysfunction (clinical and subclinical) has been observed with the administration of liposomal-encapsulated doxorubicin compared with conventional doxorubicin, with similar antineoplastic efficacy, but a trend has been seen toward worsened overall survival.[12]

Another strategy has been the use of continuous infusions of anthracyclines (rather than boluses) to decrease peak levels and possibly decrease resultant left ventricular dysfunction. Although some evidence shows a cardioprotective effect with this strategy, it is hampered by the cost and inconvenience of continuous infusion regimens and some evidence of decreased antineoplastic efficacy.[13,14]

The strategy with the greatest evidence for decreasing anthracycline cardiotoxicity involves the coadministration of dexrazoxane, an EDTA-like chelator that likely prevents cardiotoxicity through preventing oxidative injury. Dexrazoxane not only has prevented deterioration in cardiac function but also has been shown to prevent rises in cardiac biomarkers (troponin T) associated with cardiac injury.[15] Unfortunately, meta-analyses have suggested a decrease in antineoplastic efficacy, greater myelosuppression and a higher rate of secondary leukemia, and trends toward worsened survival with dexrazoxane, and therefore its widespread use has been limited.[16]

Defining the Injury: Acute Versus Early Versus Late Toxicity

Anthracycline cardiotoxicity is largely described in terms of causing acute, early, and late cardiotoxicity. According to the usual description, acute toxicity is believed to be relatively rare, and is manifested by electrocardiogram changes, reductions in LVEF, left ventricular dilatation, elevated B-type natriuretic peptide (BNP), and is self-limited in nature, usually resolving in 1 week. Early cardiotoxicity is defined as occurring within the first year after anthracycline exposure (peaking at 3 months after exposure) and is the main focus of most studies. Late toxicity is described as left ventricular dysfunction and heart failure, which comes to clinical attention years after anthracycline administration, and is best described in studies of survivors of childhood leukemia.

Implicit in these classifications is the notion that the early and late anthracycline injuries are occurring months or years after the administration of the agent. If looked for closely, subtle signs of cardiac injury (acute toxicity) can be discovered during most anthracycline administration, including QT prolongation, increased left ventricular size, mild reductions in LVEF, and elevated BNP.[17] The cardiac response to injury at this point is likely similar to the response to other forms of injury (eg, myocardial infarction or myocarditis). In these cases, if the injury is small enough and the patient has no risk factors for left ventricular dysfunction (eg, advanced age, diabetes), the cardiac function will often recover without development of overt heart failure. If the injury is large enough or enough other concomitant risk factors are present, symptomatic heart failure can immediately occur, likely representing the relatively uncommon syndrome of acute anthracycline cardiomyopathy. Finally, if the injury is of moderate size (or repetitive, as occurs with multiple cycles of anthracycline administration or when anthracyclines are coadministered with other cardiotoxic therapies), the left ventricle gradually remodels because of upregulation of neurohormonal systems (eg, catecholamines, renin-angiotensin-aldosterone system), and the

patient will have a delayed presentation with symptomatic heart failure, either months or years later.

Almost identical risk factors to those defining susceptibility to other cardiac insults predict the development of left ventricular dysfunction from chemotherapy: hypertension, advanced age, obesity, diabetes mellitus, coronary artery disease, radiation, prior cardiotoxin exposure, and prior heart failure.[7,18–20] This fact helps explain the observed cardiotoxicity curves seen with anthracyclines: at low-level exposure (eg, 200–250 mg/m^2 doxorubicin), left ventricular dysfunction will usually only become apparent in a particularly susceptible patient. At high-level exposure (eg, 600 mg/m^2 doxorubicin), the anthracycline cardiotoxicity alone is enough to develop symptomatic left ventricular dysfunction in many individuals, even without prior susceptibility.

Limited studies of late toxicity show the magnitude of the problem of left ventricular dysfunction, particularly when anthracyclines are used to treat curable tumors and patients live many years or decades thereafter. In one study of 201 survivors of anthracycline-treated pediatric malignancies, 23% of the cohort had abnormal cardiac function on noninvasive imaging; this figure increased to 38% for those with more than 10 years of follow-up (mean dose, 495 mg/m^2 of doxorubicin), and to a staggering 63% in those who had been exposed to more than 500 mg/m^2 of doxorubicin.[21] In a study of 229 adult survivors who had received doxorubicin as children for solid tumors at least 15 years prior (mean, 18 years), 10% had symptomatic heart failure, and an additional 6% were asymptomatic but had marked or severe systolic dysfunction on cardiac imaging; the only independent risk factors were the cumulative dose of doxorubicin received and the average radiation dose to the heart.[22] In a recent study of the Surveillance, Epidemiology, and End Results (SEER) Medicare database examining women aged 66 to 80 years with newly diagnosed stages I through III breast cancer, patients were divided into three groups: those who received no adjuvant chemotherapy, those who received adjuvant anthracycline chemotherapy, and those who received adjuvant chemotherapy without an anthracycline. The investigators queried the database for the frequency of a new diagnosis code for heart failure (ICD-9 code 428), which clearly underestimates the true risk of cardiotoxicity, particularly asymptomatic left ventricular dysfunction. Nevertheless, the frequency for heart failure diagnoses was much higher in the anthracycline group (38.4% by 120 months in the anthracycline cohort), and screening was infrequent, with only one-third of patients receiving anthracyclines ever undergoing cardiac imaging.[23]

Controversy remains regarding the importance of transient left ventricular dysfunction if the dysfunction resolves after discontinuing chemotherapy.[24–26] However, the fact that prior heart failure/left ventricular dysfunction of any cause remains the strongest risk factor for the subsequent development of left ventricular dysfunction illustrates the point that any myocardial injury leaves individuals more susceptible to future insults (eg, coronary artery disease, administration of another cardiotoxic agent), even if the overall left ventricular function returns to normal.

ANTI-HER2 TARGETED THERAPY: TRASTUZUMAB AND LAPATINIB

Besides the anthracycline drugs, no other cancer medication has been studied in more detail for left ventricular dysfunction than trastuzumab. Trastuzumab is a monoclonal antibody against HER2, an epidermal growth factor receptor family member overexpressed in 20% to 25% of breast cancers.[27] HER2 overexpression/amplification connotes a more aggressive tumor with increased rates of metastasis and mortality.[27]

In addition to its role in breast cancer, HER2 is an important growth factor receptor in human development. Animal experiments have established that HER2 is vital to normal cardiac development and myocardial trabeculation.[28,29]

In 2001, the pivotal phase III trial was published examining trastuzumab therapy for patients with metastatic breast cancer. Cardiac monitoring consisted of clinical assessments at prespecified timepoints, and heart failure was graded according to the New York Heart Association (NYHA) Classification system.[30] Unexpectedly, patients in the trastuzumab arm had significantly higher rates of left ventricular dysfunction. An independent review showed that 27% of patients receiving anthracyclines/trastuzumab and 13% of those receiving paclitaxel/trastuzumab developed cardiac dysfunction, compared with 8% receiving anthracyclines alone and 1% receiving paclitaxel alone.[30] Symptomatic NYHA class III and IV heart failure developed in 16% of the anthracycline/trastuzumab group, compared with 3% or less in the other three groups.[30] Proving the fact that even in the 21st century confusion remains regarding differing definitions of toxicity, the authors referred to the 1979 Von Hoff and colleagues[4] data on symptomatic cardiotoxicity while comparing their results including asymptomatic cardiotoxicity when noting, "The 27% incidence of cardiac

dysfunction among patients who were given AC+H (anthracycline/cyclophosphamide/trastuzumab) and the 13% incidence among those given T+H (taxane/trastuzumab) exceeded the expected incidence of <7% associated with cumulative doses of doxorubicin of up to 550 mg/m^2."[30]

Combined results of two large adjuvant trials (NSABP B-31 and NCCTG N9831) in patients with operable, high-risk early-stage breast cancer were published in 2005.[8] These trials, comprising more than 3600 combined patients, randomized subjects to receive either anthracycline-based chemotherapy alone or anthracycline-based chemotherapy followed by 52 weeks of trastuzumab. Cardiac monitoring was prospectively built into the trials at baseline, after the anthracycline portion of therapy was completed, and at months 6, 9, and 18. If the LVEF fell from normal to abnormal (or if cardiac symptoms developed) during the anthracycline portion, patients did not receive trastuzumab regardless of their randomization. Asymptomatic reductions in LVEF were considered significant if they fell 10% or more in absolute terms from baseline to below the lower limit of normal, or 16% or more from baseline but remained in the normal range. If patients met these end points, trastuzumab was held for 4 weeks and LVEF reassessed; if LVEF recovered beyond these criteria, then trastuzumab was resumed.[8] Trastuzumab was permanently discontinued when cardiotoxicity was symptomatic or if the hold criteria were again met at the 4-week reassessment for patients who were asymptomatic.

Besides providing data on trastuzumab cardiotoxicity, these trials also provide some of the best available data on anthracycline cardiotoxicity at commonly used doses in patients with breast cancer. The standard 240 mg/m^2 cumulative doxorubicin dose used in these trials resulted in a 6.7% to 7.5% incidence of significant reduction in LVEF (before any trastuzumab therapy); these patients were unable to proceed to the trastuzumab arm per the study protocol.[8,31] This estimate is consistent with the data from the retrospective review by Swain and colleagues,[7] and is notable because current screening guidelines do not recommend routine cardiac imaging for anthracycline exposure until a cumulative doxorubicin dose of 250 mg/m^2.[32]

Of 1159 patients who received trastuzumab, 19% discontinued the medication before the indicated 52 weeks because of cardiotoxicity; 14% for asymptomatic declines in LVEF, and 5% for symptomatic heart failure or other adverse cardiac events.[8,33] NYHA class III and IV heart failure occurred in 4.1% of subjects randomized to trastuzumab in B-31 versus 0.6% of control subjects, and in 2.9% of subjects randomized to trastuzumab in N9831 versus 0% of control subjects. In absolute numbers in the joint analysis, 51 subjects developed NYHA class III and IV heart failure in the trastuzumab arm compared with 4 in the control arm.[8] A follow-up of 27 of the 31 patients in the B-31 trial who developed trastuzumab-associated cardiotoxicity painted a mixed picture: although 96% remained free of clinical heart failure symptoms, 67% remained on cardiac medications and 71% had an LVEF that remained below their baseline.[33]

If asymptomatic reductions in LVEF associated with trastuzumab are considered, cardiotoxicity rates are significantly higher. In B-31, trastuzumab was held or permanently stopped in 31% of patients; 24% for asymptomatic reduction in LVEF, and 7% for symptomatic heart failure.[33] The incidence of a significant LVEF drop during the 52 weeks of trastuzumab therapy was 34% in the trastuzumab arm compared with 17% in the control arm, although all patients had also received baseline anthracyclines.[33] The timing of trastuzumab-associated reductions in LVEF was difficult to predict, but nearly three-quarters of the patients discontinued trastuzumab therapy because of cardiotoxicity in the 3- to 9-month interval of therapy, versus only one-quarter in the first or last 3 months.[33] Risk-factors for trastuzumab-associated reductions in LVEF in this series included age older than 50 years, requirement for antihypertensive medication, and postanthracycline LVEF values of 50% to 55%, which was the strongest risk factor of all, and emphasizing the synergistic nature of anthracycline/trastuzumab cardiotoxicity.[31]

The Herceptin Adjuvant (HERA) trial studied the administration of 0, 1, or 2 years of trastuzumab after the completion of neoadjuvant or adjuvant chemotherapy for early-stage HER2-positive breast cancer.[34] This trial reported a substantially lower incidence of trastuzumab-related cardiotoxicity than prior studies, with a "confirmed significant LVEF drop" of 3.04% in the trastuzumab cohort and 0.53% in the cohort who did not receive trastuzumab.[35] Only 4.3% of patients discontinued trastuzumab because of cardiac adverse events.[35] However, many important differences exist that likely explain the lower reported incidence of cardiotoxicity. Prior chemotherapy regimens varied from doxorubicin-containing protocols to epirubicin-containing protocols to nonanthracycline protocols; in addition, there was a much longer interval between completion of prior chemotherapy and starting trastuzumab: a median of 89 days.[35] Patients could only be included if their post-(neo)adjuvant chemotherapy

LVEF was 55% or more, representing a significantly stricter criterion than most other studies. In HERA, reductions in LVEF were only counted in the end point if they were confirmed on a second assessment approximately 3 weeks after the initial assessment; this is the only trial that used this criterion, potentially allowing transitory trastuzumab-associated LVEF drops to be missed. If the confirmatory LVEF assessment was not required, the cardiotoxicity rate more than doubled to 7% (vs 2% among patients not receiving trastuzumab).[35] Finally, median follow-up in HERA was relatively short at 12 months.[35]

Because of cardiotoxicity concerns, some protocols for HER2-positive patients have been designed to be anthracycline-sparing. In the BCIRG 006 trial, 3222 patients with early-stage breast cancer were randomized to one of three arms: an anthracycline-containing arm without trastuzumab, a trastuzumab-containing arm without anthracycline, or an arm containing both anthracycline and trastuzumab.[36,37] At the second interim analysis, the rates of significant (>10%) LVEF decline were approximately twice as high in the anthracycline/trastuzumab cohort (18%) as in either the anthracycline/no trastuzumab cohort (10%) or the trastuzumab/no anthracycline cohort (8.6%).

A recent mechanistic study has offered insights into the synergistic nature of anthracycline and trastuzumab toxicity, and may help explain the lower apparent rate of cardiotoxicity observed in HERA versus other studies. Ten HER2-negative patients were scanned with radiolabeled trastuzumab 3 weeks after completing treatment with four to six cycles of anthracycline; radiolabeled trastuzumab was also administered to 10 patients with chronic heart failure without anthracycline exposure. Five of the patients treated with anthracycline had significant myocardial uptake of radiolabeled trastuzumab, compared with none of the patients with chronic heart failure.[38] When this scanning was previously performed in 15 patients treated after a median of 11 months post-anthracycline exposure, uptake was only observed in one patient.[39] This finding suggests that myocardial HER2 may be unregulated early in response to anthracycline injury, leaving the myocardium particularly vulnerable to trastuzumab exposure in this period.

Lapatinib is a small molecule tyrosine kinase inhibitor that inhibits HER2 in addition to epidermal growth factor receptor 1 (HER1); it is predominantly used in patients with advanced HER2-positive breast cancer with trastuzumab resistance. In the pivotal phase III trial published in 2006, patients for whom prior therapy with anthracyclines, taxanes, and trastuzumab failed and who still had normal LVEF were randomized to receive capecitabine alone or in combination with lapatinib.[40] Cardiac events were defined as either symptomatic heart failure or reductions in LVEF of 20% or more. Although more patients in the lapatinib arm had a cardiac event, rates were low in both groups (2.45% vs 0.62%). Reasons for the low rates could be a lower incidence of left ventricular dysfunction with lapatinib than with trastuzumab, the fact that the patients had already shown that they did not have LVEF drops with trastuzumab to get into the trial, and the fact that the 20% or more percentage point reduction of LVEF criterion was higher than was used in any other major trial.[40] Subsequent studies (with similar caveats) seem to confirm a genuinely lower risk of left ventricular dysfunction with lapatinib compared with trastuzumab.[41,42]

Second second-generation anti-HER2 therapies are currently in clinical development. Neratinib is a small molecule tyrosine kinase inhibitor that, like lapatinib, is a dual HER2 and HER1 inhibitor. Trastuzumab-DM1 (T-DM1) is an antibody–drug conjugate that combines the biologic activity of trastuzumab with the targeted delivery of a highly potent antimicrotubule agent called DM1. Pertuzumab is a recombinant humanized monoclonal antibody that binds to the extracellular domain of the HER2 receptor and blocks its ability to dimerize with other HER receptors. Careful attention to cardiotoxicity signals in ongoing clinical trials of these novel agents is a high priority.

PREVENTING CARDIOTOXICITY WITH COADMINISTRATION OF CARDIAC MEDICATIONS

Standard medical treatment for heart failure uses similar strategies regardless of the underlying cause of the cardiomyopathy. Although older treatments (digoxin, diuretics) were focused on treating the symptoms of heart failure, therapy over the past 3 decades has increasingly focused on neurohormonal antagonism (eg, β-blockers, angiotensin-converting enzyme inhibitors [ACE-Is], angiotensin II receptor blockers [ARBs], aldosterone antagonists).[6] The neurohormonal antagonist strategy focuses on reversing the maladaptive remodeling process in heart failure, in which the left ventricle gradually grows larger and more spherical.[6]

One potential treatment strategy for preventing cancer therapy–associated left ventricular dysfunction is the coadministration of standard heart failure medications. Although most evidence collected so far is for anthracycline cardiac injury, the strategy (which uses agents directed at general cardioprotection rather than agents specifically aimed at mitigating injury mediated through anthracycline effects) has great potential for being effective with other cardiotoxic cancer therapy agents.

One study has evaluated ameliorating acute effects of anthracycline toxicity through coadministering the angiotensin-receptor blocker valsartan with standard anthracycline-based chemotherapy (cyclophosphamide, vincristine, doxorubicin, and prednisone [CHOP]) for non-Hodgkin's lymphoma. Although the study was small (n = 40), significant improvements were seen in left ventricular size, QT interval, and BNP levels, all signs of preventing acute injury. The improvements were largest at day 3 after chemotherapy administration, largely reverting to baseline in both cohorts by day 7.[17] An animal study with a knockout of angiotensin II offered further support for this model, in which the angiotensin II receptor knockout mice (and wild-type mice given ARBs) were protected from doxorubicin injury compared with wild-type mice.[43]

An intriguing method to monitor for chemotherapy-related left ventricular dysfunction is the use of cardiac biomarkers, such as BNP or cardiac troponins. BNP is a hormone secreted by the atria/ventricles in response to increased wall-stretch,[44] and therefore is a relatively sensitive marker for heart failure. Cardiac troponins (troponin I and troponin T) are part of the contractile apparatus, and their expression is limited to the myocardium; because no plasma level of cardiac troponins should be detectable, their presence, even in small quantities, is very sensitive and specific for cardiac injury.[45]

One important study which validated the utility of using troponin monitoring to detect chemotherapy-associated cardiac injury examined the relative rates of troponin rises when anthracyclines were administered with or without the cardioprotective agent dexrazoxane. In this study (testing troponin T values in children being treated for acute lymphocytic leukemia), dexrazoxane was extremely effective at preventing troponin elevations, with detectable troponin values in nearly half of the patients in the standard therapy arm by 181 to 240 days, compared with less than 10% in the dexrazoxane arm.[15]

This strategy was taken one step further in a study of patients undergoing high-dose chemotherapy, through linking development of a detectable troponin level with clinical outcomes. In this study, 703 patients who had normal baseline cardiac function underwent high-dose chemotherapy for a variety of tumor types and with a variety of treatment protocols. All patients had either been previously exposed to anthracyclines or were being exposed to anthracyclines as part of the high-dose chemotherapy protocol. Troponin I levels were measured at baseline and at five additional times within the first 3 days of receiving chemotherapy, and were then remeasured 1 month after high-dose chemotherapy. The cutoff level for a positive troponin was 0.08 ng/mL, the threshold of detectability for the assay. The investigators found that 70% of patients had undetectable troponins at all time points, 21% of patients had a detectable troponin value within the first 3 days but had undetectable values at 1 month, and 9% of patients had detectable troponin values after both 3 days and 1 month.[46] No patient developed a reverse pattern of detectability in which troponin was negative during the first 3 days but positive at 1 month, supporting the concept that toxicity is apparent early if it is going to happen at all. Troponin I positivity was almost always at low levels, typically 0.1 to 0.4 ng/mL, and the likelihood of troponin positivity correlated with whether the high-dose chemotherapy regimen contained anthracycline or not.[46]

The primary end point, which was a composite of cardiac death, acute pulmonary edema, overt heart failure, large asymptomatic LVEF reduction (≥25% absolute drop from baseline), and life-threatening tachyarrhythmias, was highly correlated with troponin positivity. Specifically, it occurred in 1% of the troponin-negative cohort, 37% of the early-troponin–positive but late-troponin–negative cohort, and 84% of the early- and late-troponin–positive cohort.[46] Reductions in LVEF showed similarly impressive results; significant ejection fraction drops (>15% absolute ejection fraction drop from baseline) occurred in 2% of the troponin-negative cohort, 65% of the early-troponin–positive but late-troponin–negative cohort, and 84% of the early- and late-troponin–positive cohort.[46]

Building on these results, the same group published a study examining a similar (though new) population of 114 patients undergoing high-dose chemotherapy. In this cohort, all 114 patients had early troponin positivity (a detectable troponin value within the first 3 days) and were randomized to receive or not receive the ACE-I enalapril, starting one month after the end of chemotherapy and continuing throughout the study.[47] Troponin positivity was present at month 1 (just before initiation of the enalapril) in 45% of the enalapril-randomized cohort and 43% of the control cohort. By month two, 4% of the enalapril cohort, compared with 41% of the control cohort, still

had troponin positivity; by month three, 0% of the enalapril cohort and 21% of the control cohort were positive.[47] Even more impressively, the primary end point (drop in LVEF by >10% to an absolute level <50%) occurred in 0% of the enalapril group, compared with 43% of the control group.[47] Although these findings are clearly of enormous importance, it is vital that they be duplicated in other centers, and that they be shown in patients receiving other cancer therapy besides high-dose chemotherapy.

A smaller study examined the use of the β-blocker carvedilol as prophylaxis against anthracycline-mediated reductions in LVEF in a population receiving de novo anthracycline treatment. In this trial, average LVEF stayed constant at 70% in the carvedilol group, whereas it fell from 69% to 52% in the control group.[48] However, the trial was limited by several factors, including its small size (n = 50), once-daily dosing of short-acting carvedilol, and inconsistencies regarding the number of cycles received (six) and the cumulative anthracycline doses reported (approximately 520 mg/m^2 of doxorubicin).[48]

How to Monitor: Symptoms Versus MUGA Versus Echocardiography Versus MRI Versus Biomarkers

The original method of monitoring for cardiotoxicity relied entirely on the development of heart failure symptoms.[4,5] Although the presence of new symptomatic heart failure is undoubtedly specific for cardiotoxicity, the sensitivity is extremely low.[7] Therefore, newer techniques using imaging and cardiac biomarkers are now available, with varying degrees of evidence supporting them. Given that treatment with ACE-Is/ARBs/β-blockers is considered a class I indication for the treatment of asymptomatic left ventricular dysfunction,[6] left ventricular dysfunction is important to detect as early as possible.

Multiple-gated acquisition scans and echocardiography

The primary method of monitoring for cancer therapy–associated left ventricular dysfunction, besides screening for heart failure symptoms, is to monitor the LVEF. This monitoring is accomplished most frequently through the use of echocardiography or nuclear imaging, usually in the form of a multiple-gated acquisition (MUGA) scan.

Both techniques yield reliable measurements of LVEF for most patients. Historically, MUGA scans have been the most commonly used modality for monitoring LVEF in patients with cancer. The reasons for this are likely multiple:

1. Low intertest and interobserver variability,
2. Generation of an exact LVEF value, as opposed to a range, which is often reported on echocardiography studies, and
3. The fact that MUGA once was a superior imaging modality, before echocardiography technology improved in the 1990s and 2000s.

MUGA, however, is now largely an outdated test. With vast imaging improvements over the past 2 decades, high-quality echocardiographic images can be obtained for most patients. The main advantages for echocardiography are the lack of any ionizing radiation, and a more complete cardiac assessment (beyond LVEF measurement), including chamber sizes for all cardiac chambers, valvular assessments, pericardial assessments, and diastolic function assessments.

One fundamental problem with MUGA imaging is the fact that it only yields data for LVEF and left ventricular size. Besides cardiotoxicity, many other factors can have profound effects on LVEF, including states of adrenergic stimulation, volume status/preload, systemic vascular resistance/afterload, valvular regurgitation, and adrenal insufficiency. Patients undergoing chemotherapy are particularly at risk for many of these changes, such as hypovolemia from nausea/diarrhea, sympathetic hyperstimulation from anxiety/infection/anemia, and direct effects on systemic vascular resistance of the chemotherapy itself (eg, tyrosine kinase inhibitors). Furthermore, focusing only on LVEF misses the potential for detecting other cardiotoxic effects of chemotherapy, such as the development of diastolic dysfunction or pericardial disease.

In addition, some authors have questioned whether MUGA scans provide results with truly lower interobserver variability, or if this is simply a consequence of the fact that in most cases a computer is generating the LVEF value. A recent study examining variability across multiple centers found a surprisingly high variability rate.[49]

For these reasons, the authors' group recommends using echocardiography as the primary imaging modality to screen for left ventricular dysfunction, except when echocardiography is not readily available or if echocardiographic images are unsuitable.

MRI

Cardiac MRI has several unique advantages, along with important disadvantages, for monitoring for cancer therapy–induced left ventricular dysfunction. On the positive side, cardiac MRI offers the most accurate/reproducible assessment of LVEF, exposes the patient to no ionizing radiation, and provides outstanding structural information. In addition, if gadolinium contrast is administered, the presence of regions of delayed enhancement may represent the earliest sign of myocardial injury, and allow interventions to be performed before reductions in LVEF are apparent.[50] On the negative side, cardiac MRI requires expensive equipment and technical expertise not readily available to most practitioners; it cannot be performed in patients with metal devices/hardware; and the gadolinium contrast cannot be safely administered to patients with significant renal dysfunction. Hence, MRI likely has great usefulness in the research setting, but decidedly less of a role in clinical practice.

Biomarkers

Waiting for the LVEF to be substantially reduced to detect cardiotoxicity is not ideal, because this implies that damage has already occurred; detecting significant cardiotoxicity before it is profound enough to cause a drop in LVEF is far preferable. Serum biomarker screening (particularly using cardiac troponins) is an attractive method for detecting early injury, and impressive early evidence exists for its use.[15,46,51–53] However, further study is needed before routine biomarker screening is used in clinical practice.

Is Appropriate Monitoring and Treatment Occurring?

Despite the accumulation of evidence for cardiac monitoring and treatment, rates of appropriate screening/treatment remain low. Even when screening shows a diagnosis of left ventricular dysfunction, action is often not undertaken. In a recent analysis, a cohort of patients with cancer who had reductions in LVEF observed during echocardiographic screening, only 40% received ACE-I or ARB therapy, 51% received β-blocker therapy, and 54% were referred to cardiologists. In the group with asymptomatic reductions in LVEF, the rates of therapy were even lower; 31% received ACE-Is or ARBs, 35% received β-blockers, and 42% were referred to cardiologists. Therapy with these agents is considered a class I indication by consensus ACC/AHA guidelines, even in the setting of asymptomatic left ventricular dysfunction.[6] Clearly, much work must be done to better understand these practice patterns, and to foster a closer collaboration between oncologists and cardiologists in the treatment of this unique patient group.

DEFINITIONS OF LEFT VENTRICULAR DYSFUNCTION AND HEART FAILURE

Much of the confusion regarding how to classify cardiotoxicity manifesting as either asymptomatic drops in LVEF or as symptomatic heart failure is attributable to internal confusion in the consensus criteria. In the current "Common Terminology Criteria for Adverse Events (CTCAE) version 4.0," the same toxicity is listed under three separate headings, and the definition contradicts each another.[54] For example, an individual who experienced an asymptomatic treatment-emergent drop in LVEF from 60% to 35% would be considered as having grade 0 "left ventricular dysfunction," grade 1 "heart failure," and grade 3 "ejection fraction decrease" for the same event (**Table 1**).

Table 1
Common terminology criteria for adverse events v4.0 and recommended changes from Stanford cardiology

Current CTCAE 4.0 Criteria

Adverse Event	Grade 1	Grade 2	Grade 3	Grade 4
Heart failure	Asymptomatic with laboratory (eg, BNP) or cardiac imaging abnormalities	Symptoms with mild to moderate activity or exertion	Severe with symptoms at rest or with minimal activity or exertion; intervention indicated	Life-threatening consequences; urgent intervention indicated (eg, continuous intravenous therapy or mechanical support)
LV systolic dysfunction	—	—	Symptomatic due to drop in EF responsive to intervention	Refractory or poorly controlled HF due to drop in EF; intervention such as VAD, intravenous vasopressor, or heart transplant indicated
Ejection fraction decreased	—	EF, 40%–50%; 10%–19% drop from baseline	EF, 20%–39%; >20% drop from baseline	EF<20%

Stanford Cardiology Recommended New Criteria

Adverse Event	Grade 1	Grade 2	Grade 3	Grade 4
LV systolic dysfunction/ Heart Failure	Laboratory abnormality (eg, abnormal troponin or BNP) without symptoms or imaging abnormalities	Asymptomatic; LVEF drop 10%–19% to an absolute level <55%	Asymptomatic LVEF drop ≥20% to an absolute level <55% or symptomatic heart failure with LVEF drop <20%	Symptomatic heart failure with LVEF drop ≥20%

Abbreviations: BNP, B-type natriuretic peptide; EF, ejection fraction; LV, left ventricular; LVEF, left ventricular ejection fractions; VAD, ventricular assist device.

Data from Common Terminology Criteria for Adverse Events (CTCAE) Version 4.0. U.S. Department of Health and Human Services, published May 28, 2009. (Available at: http://evs.nci.nih.gov. Accessed November 16, 2010.)

> **Box 2**
> **Stanford cardiology recommendations for asymptomatic cardiac monitoring[a]**
>
> - Anthracyclines: Baseline, 200 mg/m^2 (or at end of 240 mg/m^2 if planned total dose), 300 mg/m^2, 400 mg/m^2, and every 50 mg/m^2 thereafter (doxorubicin equivalents)
> - Trastuzumab: Baseline (post-anthracycline), every 3 months while on therapy
>
> [a] Cardiac imaging is recommended in all patients with signs/symptoms concerning for cardiotoxicity regardless of the cumulative dose.

This confusion makes these events impossible for clinicians/investigators to consistently and properly grade, and makes interpreting clinical trial results in this context exceedingly difficult.

SUMMARY

With the tremendous growth in effective antineoplastic agents, a concomitant concerning increase has occurred in off-target side effects. Cardiotoxicity, and specifically left ventricular dysfunction, remains the limiting factor for many of these agents, and is the focus of growing research and clinical emphasis.

Ultimately winning the battle to allow patients to safely receive indicated doses of increasingly effective anti-neoplastic therapies will require the following conditions:

1. Consistent definitions used across clinical trials regarding what constitutes meaningful left ventricular dysfunction, taking advantage of a 21st century understanding of cardiac injury/heart failure (and therefore not focusing exclusively or near-exclusively on symptoms) (see **Table 1**).
2. Routine cardiac screening (including imaging of asymptomatic patients) must be uniformly used in clinical trials for new anticancer agents. In addition, routine assessment of LVEF should be obtained in patients who receive anthracyclines, at minimum, after the completion of standard-dose breast cancer adjuvant therapy (240 mg/m^2 of doxorubicin), when strong evidence shows a 6% to 7% prevalence of significant reductions in left ventricular systolic function (**Box 2**).
3. Confirmatory studies are urgently needed to determine the role of biomarker (eg, troponin) screening and prophylactic treatment with standard heart failure therapies (eg, ACE-Is, β-blockers) before clinical injury is detected.

Because the therapies are aimed at the myocardium rather than the antineoplastic agent, these studies should be focused across a broad array of tumor types and antineoplastic agents so they have the broadest applicability.
4. For high-risk patients, numerous options are available to reduce cardiotoxicity, although potentially at a cost of money, time, or antineoplastic activity. These options include liposomal anthracycline preparations, continuous anthracycline infusions, dexrazoxane, and the potential for substituting less-cardiotoxic anti-HER2 agents.
5. The authors advocate that patients who have developed left ventricular dysfunction, or who have a preexisting cardiomyopathy, be treated according to current ACC/AHA heart failure guidelines, including the initiation of β-blockers and ACE-Is or ARBs unless a contraindication exists.

REFERENCES

1. Blum RH, Carter Adriamycin SK. A new anticancer drug with significant clinical activity. Ann Intern Med 1974;80:249–59.
2. Lefrak EA, Pitha J, Rosenheim S, et al. A clinicopathologic analysis of adriamycin cardiotoxicity. Cancer 1973;32:302–14.
3. Tan C, Etcubanas E, Wollner N, et al. Adriamycin—an antitumor antibiotic in the treatment of neoplastic diseases. Cancer 1973;32:9–17.
4. Von Hoff DD, Layard MW, Basa P, et al. Risk factors for doxorubicin-induced congestive heart failure. Ann Intern Med 1979;91:710–7.
5. Von Hoff DD, Rozencweig M, Layard M, et al. Daunomycin-induced cardiotoxicity in children and adults. A review of 110 cases. Am J Med 1977;62:200–8.
6. Hunt SA, Abraham WT, Chin MH, et al. ACC/AHA 2005 Guideline Update for the Diagnosis and Management of Chronic Heart Failure in the Adult: a report of the American College of Cardiology/American Heart Association Task Force on Practice Guidelines (Writing Committee to Update the 2001 Guidelines for the Evaluation and Management of Heart Failure): developed in collaboration with the American College of Chest Physicians and the International Society for Heart and Lung Transplantation: endorsed by the Heart Rhythm Society. Circulation 2005;112:e154–235.
7. Swain SM, Whaley FS, Ewer MS. Congestive heart failure in patients treated with doxorubicin: a retrospective analysis of three trials. Cancer 2003;97:2869–79.
8. Romond EH, Perez EA, Bryant J, et al. Trastuzumab plus adjuvant chemotherapy for operable

HER2-positive breast cancer. N Engl J Med 2005; 353:1673–84.

9. Torti FM, Bristow MM, Lum BL, et al. Cardiotoxicity of epirubicin and doxorubicin: assessment by endomyocardial biopsy. Cancer Res 1986;46:3722–7.

10. Jensen BV, Skovsgaard T, Nielsen SL. Functional monitoring of anthracycline cardiotoxicity: a prospective, blinded, long-term observational study of outcome in 120 patients. Ann Oncol 2002;13: 699–709.

11. Ryberg M, Nielsen D, Skovsgaard T, et al. Epirubicin cardiotoxicity: an analysis of 469 patients with metastatic breast cancer. J Clin Oncol 1998;16:3502–8.

12. van Dalen EC, Michiels EM, Caron HN, et al. Different anthracycline derivates for reducing cardiotoxicity in cancer patients. Cochrane Database Syst Rev 2006;4:CD005006.

13. Casper ES, Gaynor JJ, Hajdu SI, et al. A prospective randomized trial of adjuvant chemotherapy with bolus versus continuous infusion of doxorubicin in patients with high-grade extremity soft tissue sarcoma and an analysis of prognostic factors. Cancer 1991;68:1221–9.

14. van Dalen EC, van der Pal HJ, Caron HN, et al. Different dosage schedules for reducing cardiotoxicity in cancer patients receiving anthracycline chemotherapy. Cochrane Database Syst Rev 2006;4:CD005008.

15. Lipshultz SE, Rifai N, Dalton VM, et al. The effect of dexrazoxane on myocardial injury in doxorubicintreated children with acute lymphoblastic leukemia. N Engl J Med 2004;351:145–53.

16. van Dalen EC, Caron HN, Dickinson HO, et al. Cardioprotective interventions for cancer patients receiving anthracyclines. Cochrane Database Syst Rev 2005;1:CD003917.

17. Nakamae H, Tsumura K, Terada Y, et al. Notable effects of angiotensin II receptor blocker, valsartan, on acute cardiotoxic changes after standard chemotherapy with cyclophosphamide, doxorubicin, vincristine, and prednisolone. Cancer 2005;104:2492–8.

18. Hequet O, Le QH, Moullet I, et al. Subclinical late cardiomyopathy after doxorubicin therapy for lymphoma in adults. J Clin Oncol 2004;22:1864–71.

19. Hershman DL, McBride RB, Eisenberger A, et al. Doxorubicin, cardiac risk factors, and cardiac toxicity in elderly patients with diffuse B-cell non-Hodgkin's lymphoma. J Clin Oncol 2008;26:3159–65.

20. Shapiro CL, Hardenbergh PH, Gelman R, et al. Cardiac effects of adjuvant doxorubicin and radiation therapy in breast cancer patients. J Clin Oncol 1998;16:3493–501.

21. Steinherz LJ, Steinherz PG, Tan CT, et al. Cardiac toxicity 4 to 20 years after completing anthracycline therapy. JAMA 1991;266:1672–7.

22. Pein F, Sakiroglu O, Dahan M, et al. Cardiac abnormalities 15 years and more after adriamycin therapy in 229 childhood survivors of a solid tumour at the Institut Gustave Roussy. Br J Cancer 2004;91:37–44.

23. Pinder MC, Duan Z, Goodwin JS, et al. Congestive heart failure in older women treated with adjuvant anthracycline chemotherapy for breast cancer. J Clin Oncol 2007;25:3808–15.

24. Ewer MS, Vooletich MT, Durand JB, et al. Reversibility of trastuzumab-related cardiotoxicity: new insights based on clinical course and response to medical treatment. J Clin Oncol 2005;23:7820–6.

25. Guarneri V, Lenihan DJ, Valero V, et al. Long-term cardiac tolerability of trastuzumab in metastatic breast cancer: the M.D. Anderson Cancer Center experience. J Clin Oncol 2006;24:4107–15.

26. Telli ML, Hunt SA, Carlson RW, et al. Trastuzumabrelated cardiotoxicity: calling into question the concept of reversibility. J Clin Oncol 2007;25: 3525–33.

27. Ross JS, Slodkowska EA, Symmans WF, et al. The HER-2 receptor and breast cancer: ten years of targeted anti-HER-2 therapy and personalized medicine. Oncologist 2009;14:320–68.

28. Crone SA, Zhao YY, Fan L, et al. ErbB2 is essential in the prevention of dilated cardiomyopathy. Nat Med 2002;8:459–65.

29. Lee KF, Simon H, Chen H, et al. Requirement for neuregulin receptor erbB2 in neural and cardiac development. Nature 1995;378:394–8.

30. Slamon DJ, Leyland-Jones B, Shak S, et al. Use of chemotherapy plus a monoclonal antibody against HER2 for metastatic breast cancer that overexpresses HER2. N Engl J Med 2001;344:783–92.

31. Rastogi P, Jeong J, Geyer CE, et al. Five year update of cardiac dysfunction on NSABP B-31, a randomized trial of sequential doxorubicin/cyclophosphamide (AC)→ paclitaxel (T) vs AC→ T with trastuzumab (H) Chicago, IL, [abstract]. J Clin Oncol 2007;25(Suppl 1):Abstract LBA513.

32. Mehra MR, Rockman HA, Greenberg BH. Highlights of the 2007 Scientific Meeting of the Heart Failure Society of America. Washington, DC, September 16–19, 2007. J Am Coll Cardiol 2008;51:320–7.

33. Tan-Chiu E, Yothers G, Romond E, et al. Assessment of cardiac dysfunction in a randomized trial comparing doxorubicin and cyclophosphamide followed by paclitaxel, with or without trastuzumab as adjuvant therapy in node-positive, human epidermal growth factor receptor 2-overexpressing breast cancer: NSABP B-31. J Clin Oncol 2005;23:7811–9.

34. Smith I, Procter M, Gelber RD, et al. 2-year follow-up of trastuzumab after adjuvant chemotherapy in HER2-positive breast cancer: a randomised controlled trial. Lancet 2007;369:29–36.

35. Suter TM, Procter M, van Veldhuisen DJ, et al. Trastuzumab-associated cardiac adverse effects in the herceptin adjuvant trial. J Clin Oncol 2007; 25:3859–65.

36. Slamon D, Eiermann W, Robert N, et-al. BCIRG 006: Phase III trial comparing AC-T with AC-TH and with TCH in the adjuvant treatment of HER2 positive early breast cancer patients: second interim efficacy analysis. 2006. Available at: http://wwwbcirgorg/NR/rdonlyres/eqkdodg2dy7t557o7s6uvj7ytpe6gcfg5gmh2ely6hnhh5pjlabz3nd6jddlnao7qoikej3edohsijyiisfvp367uuc/BCIRG006+2nd+Interim+Analysispdf. Accessed January 14, 2009.

37. Slamon DJ, Eiermann W, Robert N, et al. Phase III randomized trial comparing doxorubicin and cyclophosphamide followed by docetaxel (ACT) with doxorubicin and cyclophosphamide with docetaxel and trastuzumab (ACTH) with docetaxel, carboplatin and trastuzumab (TCH) in HER2-positive early breast cancer patients: BCIRG 006 study. Breast Cancer Res Treat 2005;94:S5.

38. de Korte MA, de Vries EG, Lub-de Hooge MN, et al. 111Indium-trastuzumab visualises myocardial human epidermal growth factor receptor 2 expression shortly after anthracycline treatment but not during heart failure: a clue to uncover the mechanisms of trastuzumab-related cardiotoxicity. Eur J Cancer 2007;43:2046–51.

39. Perik PJ, Lub-De Hooge MN, Gietema JA, et al. Indium-111-labeled trastuzumab scintigraphy in patients with human epidermal growth factor receptor 2-positive metastatic breast cancer. J Clin Oncol 2006;24:2276–82.

40. Geyer CE, Forster J, Lindquist D, et al. Lapatinib plus capecitabine for HER2-positive advanced breast cancer. N Engl J Med 2006;355:2733–43.

41. Blackwell KL, Burstein HJ, Storniolo AM, et al. Randomized study of Lapatinib alone or in combination with trastuzumab in women with ErbB2-positive, trastuzumab-refractory metastatic breast cancer. J Clin Oncol 2010;28:1124–30.

42. Johnston S, Pippen J Jr, Pivot X, et al. Lapatinib combined with letrozole versus letrozole and placebo as first-line therapy for postmenopausal hormone receptor-positive metastatic breast cancer. J Clin Oncol 2009;27:5538–46.

43. Toko H, Oka T, Zou Y, et al. Angiotensin II type 1a receptor mediates doxorubicin-induced cardiomyopathy. Hypertens Res 2002;25:597–603.

44. de Lemos JA, McGuire DK, Drazner MH. B-type natriuretic peptide in cardiovascular disease. Lancet 2003;362:316–22.

45. Myocardial infarction redefined–a consensus document of The Joint European Society of Cardiology/American College of Cardiology Committee for the redefinition of myocardial infarction. Eur Heart J 2000;21:1502–13.

46. Cardinale D, Sandri MT, Colombo A, et al. Prognostic value of troponin I in cardiac risk stratification of cancer patients undergoing high-dose chemotherapy. Circulation 2004;109:2749–54.

47. Cardinale D, Colombo A, Sandri MT, et al. Prevention of high-dose chemotherapy-induced cardiotoxicity in high-risk patients by angiotensin-converting enzyme inhibition. Circulation 2006;114:2474–81.

48. Kalay N, Basar E, Ozdogru I, et al. Protective effects of carvedilol against anthracycline-induced cardiomyopathy. J Am Coll Cardiol 2006;48:2258–62.

49. Skrypniuk JV, Bailey D, Cosgriff PS, et al. UK audit of left ventricular ejection fraction estimation from equilibrium ECG gated blood pool images. Nucl Med Commun 2005;26:205–15.

50. Wassmuth R, Lentzsch S, Erdbruegger U, et al. Subclinical cardiotoxic effects of anthracyclines as assessed by magnetic resonance imaging-a pilot study. Am Heart J 2001;141:1007–13.

51. Cardinale D, Lamantia G, Cipolla CM. Troponin I and cardiovascular risk stratification in patients with testicular cancer. J Clin Oncol 2006;24:3508 [author reply: 3508–9].

52. Cardinale D, Sandri MT, Martinoni A, et al. Myocardial injury revealed by plasma troponin I in breast cancer treated with high-dose chemotherapy. Ann Oncol 2002;13:710–5.

53. Cardinale D, Sandri MT, Martinoni A, et al. Left ventricular dysfunction predicted by early troponin I release after high-dose chemotherapy. J Am Coll Cardiol 2000;36:517–22.

54. Common Terminology Criteria for Adverse Events (CTCAE) Version 4.0. U.S. Department of Health and Human Services, published May 28, 2009. Available at: http://evs.nci.nih.gov. Accessed November 16, 2010.

Stem Cell Therapy for Cardiac Disease: What Can Be Learned from Oncology

Allen J. Naftilan, MD, PhD*, Friedrich G. Schuening, MD

KEYWORDS
- Hematopoietic stem cells • Stem cell • Bone marrow
- Cardiovascular disease

Hematopoietic stem cells (HSCs) are the most well-characterized tissue-specific stem cells. They were the first tissue-specific stem cells to be isolated.[1] Decades of basic research and clinical application provide profound insight into the principles of HSC biology. To date, HSCs are the only stem cells in routine clinical use. HSC-containing grafts are used worldwide for the treatment of a variety of benign and malignant hematologic disorders such as severe aplastic anemia, leukemias, lymphomas, and multiple myeloma. More than 800,000 patients have received HSC transplants so far, and it is estimated that annually 55,000 to 60,000 HSC transplants are performed worldwide.[2] There are now about 150,000 patients surviving 5 years or more after HSC transplant. Most of these 5-year survivors are well, without evidence of their original disease, and leading normal lives.

OVERVIEW OF STEM CELL BIOLOGY

HSCs

The hematopoietic system has the impressive ability to generate billions of mature hematopoietic cells daily, which occurs over the lifetime of an individual.[3] This balanced production includes red blood cells, platelets, and white blood cells involved in oxygen transport, blood clotting, and protection from infections, respectively. These mature cells are short lived (except for some types of lymphocytes), with life spans ranging from hours for granulocytes to several weeks for erythrocytes. It is, therefore, necessary to continuously replenish these mature cells for the lifetime of an individual. The cells responsible for this tremendous task are the HSCs. HSCs are characterized by their ability to self-renew as well as to differentiate into all mature hematopoietic cell lineages. The ability of HSCs to self-renew, that is, to divide without maturation thereby producing progeny identical to the parent cell, is essential to provide a continuous lifelong supply of mature, functional hematopoietic cells. As HSCs differentiate into different types of progenitor cells, the resulting progenitor cells gradually display an increasingly limited capacity to self-renew as well as more and more restricted differentiation abilities.

HSCs are rare cells, occurring at a frequency of 1 in 10,000 to 100,000 in mouse bone marrow.[4] At steady state, most of the HSCs are quiescent[5]; only a small fraction (1.5%–8%) of HSCs enter a cycling state each day to proliferate and differentiate into progenitor cells, which further differentiate into mature blood cells.[6,7] However, when the hematopoietic system is perturbed by stressors, such as infection or acute bleeding, these cells proliferate more extensively to produce sufficient numbers of progenitor cells and mature blood cells that provide the supply of required blood cells.

HSCs are difficult to study because of their scarcity in the marrow and the relative lack of specific markers and tests for identifying them.

Plasticity of HSCs

Several reports in the past few years have described that bone marrow–derived cells can contribute to

Vanderbilt Heart and Vascular Institute, Hematology Division, Department of Medicine, Vanderbilt University, Nashville, TN 37240, USA
* Corresponding author.
E-mail address: allen.j.naftilan@Vanderbilt.edu

Heart Failure Clin 7 (2011) 345–355
doi:10.1016/j.hfc.2011.03.006
1551-7136/11/$ – see front matter

the regeneration and repair of various organs and tissues, such as the heart, brain, or liver.[8] These observations were predominantly explained by the hypothesis that HSCs can transdifferentiate into various nonhematopoietic cells such as muscle, neuronal, or liver cells. However, experiments with highly purified populations of HSCs in mice were not able to demonstrate repair of the damaged heart or brain. Experiments using single purified HSCs showed that even over long time intervals, these HSCs cannot contribute to any nonhematopoietic tissue.[8] It is, therefore, important for such experiments to purify HSCs to phenotypic and functional homogeneity and to mark these cells with retroviral or other genetic markers to be able to follow the fate of the transplanted HSCs. In addition, it is important to take into account that the bone marrow contains at least 2 or 3 different types of stem cell populations: HSCs, mesenchymal stem cells (MSCs), and endothelial progenitor cells (EPCs). Therefore, the presence of non-HSCs in the bone marrow could explain some of the positive results of nonhematopoietic tissue regeneration when using marrow-derived cells, which were not observed when single purified HSCs were used.

MSCs

MSCs are rare in the bone marrow, comprising 0.01% to 0.001% of the marrow cells.[9] MSCs are self-renewing clonal progenitor cells of nonhematopoietic stromal tissues. They adhere to plastic and are expanded in culture. Cultures of MSCs are highly heterogeneous with only rare multipotent cells and a majority of more-differentiated progenitor cells. MSCs are able to differentiate into osteoblasts, chondroblasts, adipocytes, fibroblasts, smooth muscle cells, and skeletal muscle cells. Cultured MSCs are spindlelike cells with a fibroblastlike appearance. They yield positive results for CD44, CD29, CD90, CD105, and CD73 but negative results for the hematopoietic markers CD34, CD45, and CD14.

The role of MSCs within the bone marrow is not clear. They are likely responsible for replacing osteoblasts and adipocytes. MSCs secrete a multitude of different cytokines and growth factors that play a role in supporting hematopoiesis. This ability to secrete cytokines and growth factors may be beneficial for tissue repair. Several reports have described the trophic effects of MSCs on damaged tissues such as ischemic heart, central nervous system, or renal lesions.[10,11]

EPCs

Cells with endothelial progenitor activities have been identified in the bone marrow and peripheral blood. Accumulating evidence suggests that these EPCs residing in the bone marrow can be released into the peripheral blood and may play a role in vascularization of damaged organs. At present, no specific marker can prospectively identify an EPC, which makes it difficult to clearly define the origin of EPCs. EPCs share many phenotypic and functional characteristics with HSCs. Evidence that EPCs are present in bone marrow comes from murine and human bone marrow transplant studies, which demonstrated that at least some endothelial cells are of donor origin after marrow transplant.[12] Following transplant of a single murine long-term repopulating HSC, perfusable donor-derived endothelial cells were found in the retina of a mouse after vascular injury.[13] However, recent studies have demonstrated that HSC-derived macrophages can also generate cells with features of endothelial cells.[14] The observation that the progeny of HSCs can acquire features of endothelial cells makes evaluation of the possible lineage relationship between EPCs and HSCs more difficult. At present, it is postulated that bone marrow is a source of EPCs and the more-differentiated circulating endothelial cells (CECs). EPCs and CECs are subsequently released from the bone marrow into the peripheral blood where they circulate at very low levels of 0.0001% and 0.01%, respectively. They may play a role in the repair of damaged endothelium and contribute to postnatal neoangiogenesis. The level of contribution of bone marrow–derived EPCs and CECs to organ and tissue vascularization, however, is the subject of current research.

Induced Pluripotent Stem Cells

Perhaps the most important recent contribution to stem cell biology has been the description of induced pluripotent stem (iPS) cells by Takahashi and Yamanaka.[15] These investigators reprogrammed mouse fibroblasts to iPS cells by the ectopic expression of 4 transcription factors linked to pluripotency in embryonic stem (ES) cells: octamer 3/4 (Oct4), SRY box–containing gene 2 (Sox2), Kruppellike factor 4 (Klf4), and Myc. These iPS cells closely resemble ES cells, which can differentiate into every somatic cell type and have the capacity of unlimited replication. iPS cells, like ES cells, can form teratomas, which are neoplastic tumors characterized by the presence of cells corresponding to all 3 embryonic germ layers, after injection into immunodeficient mice. iPS cells have also been shown to support the full-term development of all-iPS-cell mice, indicating that they have the full development potential of ES cells.[16] Transcription factor–based reprogramming of differentiated cells from a patient enables the generation of pluripotent stem cells for this specific patient, thereby bypassing potential issues of allogeneic immune rejection after transplantation of, for instance, cardiomyocytes derived from such patient-specific iPS cells. iPS cells also avoid the ethical concerns related to the derivation of ES cells. It is theorized that disease-specific iPS cells may allow investigators to analyze and replay the disease process and potentially serve as the basis of drug development. Initial protocols for producing iPS cells using viral vectors to exogenously express the transcription factors allows integration of the differentiated somatic cells of origin into the genome. However, it is now possible to produce iPS cells with safer, nonintegrating methods, although not yet as efficiently as with viral vectors.[17] iPS cells have so far been produced from primary mouse, pig, nonhuman primate, and human cells. Human iPS cells have been generated from skin fibroblasts, bone marrow mesenchymal cells, keratinocytes, melanocytes, peripheral blood cells, and adipose stem cells using retroviral vectors, episomal vectors, plasmid transfection, piggyback transposons, or recombinant proteins. Although retroviral vectors are currently the most effective method to generate iPS cells, they lead to genomic integration of the transcription factor genes. Because both Klf4 and c-MYC are oncogenes, these transcription factors may induce cancers in the host. In addition, insertional mutagenesis may be associated with transgene integration in the host genome, potentially leading to tumorigenicity in the patient. Several recent studies have therefore used different approaches to avoid genomic integration of the reprogramming genes. This has been done using adenoviruses, repeated plasmid transfection, or episomal vectors.[17] Ultimately, iPS cells generated by these different methods have be examined thoroughly at the genomic, epigenomic, and functional levels to determine which reprogramming methods are safe for clinical cell therapy. The final goal is to generate safe, virus-free, and transgene-free autologous iPS cells at sufficiently high efficiency for human patients in the future. Human iPS cells have so far been differentiated into a diversity of functional cell types including cardiomyocytes,[18] smooth muscle and vascular endothelial cells,[19] neuronal cells,[20] and insulin-secreting isletlike clusters.[21] Before possible clinical application, iPS cell–derived cell therapies have to be validated not only in small animals but also in large animal models that are more phylogenetically similar to humans. Both monkey[22] and pig[23] iPS cells have been generated, which provide excellent models for iPS cell–derived cell transplant studies.

iPS cell–based therapies are still in their infancy, and many hurdles need to be overcome before possible clinical application. However, the potential of patient-specific iPS cell–derived somatic cells for cell replacement therapy, disease modeling, and drug discovery is tremendous.

DEVELOPMENT OF HSC TRANSPLANT

After the atomic bomb explosion at the end of World War II, there was great interest in investigating how radiation damages living organisms. It soon became evident that the bone marrow is the organ most sensitive to radiation and that ultimately death, following low-lethal radiation exposures, was because of marrow failure. The possibility of rescue from marrow failure by HSC transplant came first from seminal studies in the mouse. First published in 1949, Jacobson and colleagues[24] demonstrated that mice could survive an otherwise-lethal exposure to total body irradiation (TBI) if the spleen (a hematopoietic organ in the mouse) was protected by a lead foil. Lorenz and colleagues[25] found shortly thereafter that similar radiation protection could be conferred by infusion of bone marrow cells. At first, it was thought that the radioprotective effect was because of a humoral factor derived from transplanted spleen or marrow cells, which stimulated marrow recovery. In 1956, Ford and colleagues[26] demonstrated that the marrow of lethally irradiated mice, given infusion of syngeneic marrow cells marked by a cytogenetic marker, was made up of cells of the cytogenetic type of the donor. These and other similar experiments demonstrated that the protection from the lethal marrow-toxic effects of TBI was because of colonization of the recipient by donor HSCs. These observations suggested that bone marrow transplant might be of benefit not only for rescue after an otherwise-lethal irradiation but also for treatment of diseases of the marrow and lymphoid system, such as leukemia, lymphoma, or marrow failure. A lethal TBI would destroy the malignant cells in the patient, and the bone marrow transplant from a normal donor would reestablish normal hematopoiesis. In 1956, Barnes and colleagues[27] described the treatment of mice with leukemia by lethal irradiation followed by marrow transplantation.[27] Thomas and colleagues[27] reported, in 1957, the treatment of 6 patients with refractory hematologic malignancies using lethal TBI and marrow transplants from normal donors.[28] Only 1 patient showed a transient marrow engraftment, and all patients died of infections, graft-versus-host disease (GVHD), or relapse of the malignancy. These failures were duplicated by many investigators. In 1970, Bortin[29] reviewed approximately 200 published attempts at alloge-neic bone marrow grafting, all of which had failed. Most of the bone marrow transplants were performed in patients with end-stage refractory leukemia who either failed to engraft or, when successful marrow engraftment occurred, often died of GVHD or infections. Many of those patients received marrow grafts from donors who were either not evaluated for HLA antigen matching or were tissue typed with methods found later to be unreliable. The discouraging results led many investigators to leave the field and others to ques-tion whether such studies should continue. However, work in animal models continued.

Studies in inbred mice had shown that histo-compatibility matching was important for success-ful HSC transplant, but the dog was the first outbred animal in which the prospective relevance of histocompatibility matching for the outcome of HSC transplant was demonstrated. Dogs that were conditioned with TBI and given bone marrow grafts from HLA-identical littermates survived significantly better than animals receiving grafts from DLA-nonidentical littermates.[30] The addition of methotrexate as an immunosuppressive drug given intermittently for 100 days after HSC trans-plantation to prevent GVHD resulted in successful engraftment and long-term survival in almost all recipients of DLA-identical littermate marrow.[31] Demonstration of successful marrow transplants in the dog model using littermate marrow donors, matched for the major histocompatibility complex, thus paved the way for successful marrow trans-plants between human siblings. It is, therefore, obvious that only a long series of experimental studies, first in inbred rodents and then predomi-nantly in outbred dogs, ultimately made human marrow transplant possible. In 1977, the Seattle team published a landmark report in which they described the outcome of 100 patients with end-stage acute leukemia, treated by high-dose chemotherapy and TBI followed by a marrow graft from an HLA antigen–identical sibling.[32] A total of 13 patients were alive at the time of the report, up to 4.5 years after transplantation, off any anti-leukemic therapy, and without recurrent leukemia. The follow-up of the transplant patients, at the time of the report, was long enough to show a plateau in the survival curve, suggesting that some of the patients were cured of their disease. The investi-gators concluded that marrow transplant should be undertaken earlier in the management of patients with acute leukemia before their disease becomes refractory to chemotherapy. Indeed, a much-improved outcome was subsequently demonstrated in patients transplanted in first or second remission, when no signs of acute leukemia were detectable.[33] A major limitation, at this time, was that only about one-fourth of the patients in need of an HSC transplant would have an HLA-identical sibling as marrow donor. To cover the needs of patients without matched related donors, marrow donor registries were es-tablished in the mid-1980s, which store HLA antigen typing data of volunteer donors who agreed to serve as HSC donors for unrelated patients. There are now more than 11 million HLA antigen–typed volunteer HSC donors world-wide. The largest donor registry is the US National Marrow Donor Program, which has about 7 million donors on its file. Caucasian patients now have an 80% or greater chance of finding an HLA antigen–identical unrelated volunteer donor through exist-ing donor panels. Non-Caucasian patients have a significantly lower probability of finding an unre-lated HLA antigen–matched HSC donor because of greater HLA antigen polymorphism and fewer ethnically similar donors. Survival after an HLA antigen–matched unrelated HSC donor transplant is now similar to that after an HLA antigen–iden-tical sibling transplant because of improved HLA antigen typing and supportive care.

Recent studies suggest that umbilical cord blood, rich in hematopoietic progenitor and stem cells, may be an alternative source of HSCs for patients without an HLA antigen–matched related or unrelated donor. Cord blood banks have, there-fore, been established worldwide, with more than 300,000 units cryopreserved. Unrelated cord blood grafts have the advantage of being rapidly available without the need for screening, HLA antigen typing, and collecting cells from live related or unrelated HSC donors. Cord blood units can also be collected and stored to preferentially represent ethnic groups underrepresented in the unrelated volunteer HSC donor registries. This feature of cord blood units would improve the chances of finding sufficiently matched HSC grafts for ethnic minorities.

Transplant-related morbidity and mortality increase with increasing age of the patient. There-fore, transplant centers have upper age limits for myeloablative HSC transplants, which are usually between 55 and 60 years for related HSC trans-plants and between 50 and 55 years for unrelated HSC transplants. In contrast, the median age at which most malignant hematologic diseases occur, for which HSC transplants are performed, is about 65 years. The recent development of reduced-intensity HSC transplants addresses this discrepancy. The intensity of the conditioning chemotherapy and TBI regimens is greatly reduced to just allow engraftment of the HSC graft by suppressing the patient's immune system and prevent graft rejection. The antitumor effect after the HSC transplant results, therefore, not from the intensity of the conditioning regimen, but from the immunotherapeutic effect of the immunocompetent cells of the donor in the graft. These donor lymphocytes exert a graft-versus-tumor effect on any malignant hematopoietic cell remaining in the patient at the time of HSC transplant. This approach has permitted potentially curative HSC transplants to patients up to the age of 70 to 75 years, thereby greatly expanding the number of patients who can benefit from this potentially curative treatment.

PRECLINICAL AND ANIMAL TRIALS IN CARDIOVASCULAR DISEASE

Ischemic cardiovascular disease, despite recent advances, remains a leading cause of morbidity and mortality worldwide. One major roadblock to overall improvement is the apparent inability of cardiac cells to regenerate after an ischemic injury and the resultant left ventricular (LV) dysfunction and heart failure (HF). In light of the success of HSC transplant, there is a great interest in cardiac regeneration. Early studies in animals have fueled these efforts because it seemed that transfer of cells from bone marrow could significantly improve cardiac function after infarction.[34,35] Further studies in animals have suggested that this benefit may because of paracrine effects[36–38] and that iPS cells may be induced to repair myocardial cells.[39] With early human studies demonstrating feasibility and safety of this approach,[40,41] there has been an explosion of studies trying to demonstrate the effectiveness of this method along with efforts to determine the proper cell type and the best timing for this therapy.

STEM CELL TRIALS IN ACUTE MYOCARDIAL INFARCTION

There have been many trials in patients using different cell types, delivery methods, or timing after myocardial infarction (MI). For the purpose of this article, the authors limit their discussion to randomized controlled trials and trials that demonstrate important points of emphasis. In an early trial in humans, Strauer and colleagues[42] investigated 10 patients who received autologous mononuclear bone marrow cells infused into the infarct-related artery 5 to 9 days after MI, with the mononuclear bone marrow cells isolated by Ficoll density gradient separation. When compared with 10 patients treated with the standard therapy, the perfusion defect was reduced by 26% and the stroke index volume index was increased, as was

LV contractility. There were no serious adverse events, suggesting that this may be a safe and feasible intervention.

The Transplantation of Progenitor Cells and Regeneration Enhancement in Acute Myocardial Infarction (TOPCARE-AMI) trial[40] was a similar feasibility and safety trial in 20 patients who were reperfused post-MI. They were treated by injection into the infarct-related artery 4 days after MI with either bone marrow–derived cells (n = 9) or circulating blood–derived progenitor cells (n = 11). There was an increase in LV ejection fraction (LVEF), wall motion score in the infarcted zone, and a reduction in end-systolic volume in the treated group when compared with a nonrandomized control group. This trial reemphasized the feasibility and safety of this intervention and suggested a benefit, which led to a larger randomized trial. This same group then conducted a randomized trial in a larger group of patients, the TOPCARE-Coronary Heart Disease (TOPCARE-CHD) trial.[43] In this trial, patients were infused with no cells (n = 23), bone marrow–derived progenitor cells (HSCs) (n = 28), or circulating blood–derived progenitor cells (EPCs) (n = 24) 3 months after an acute MI into the artery supplying the most dyskinetic area. They reported an increase in the overall global cardiac function due in large part to an enhanced contractility in the targeted area. This effect was only seen in the patients treated with the HSCs?, with no improvement seen in the control group or those infused with EPCs? derived from circulating blood (**Table 1**).

In the Bone Marrow Transfer to Enhance ST-Elevation Regeneration (BOOST) trial,[44] 60 patients were randomized after stent deployment to receive either routine post-MI care (control) or infusion of autologous unfractionated HSCs into the infarct-related artery 4 days after intervention. Cardiac magnetic resonance imaging (MRI) was performed at 3 days, 6 months, and 18 months post-MI. The difference in the global LVEF was significant after 6 months in patients receiving the infusion when compared with the controls (0.6% vs 3.1%), but the difference was not significant at 18 months (3.1% vs 5.9%). This was the first trial to look as far out as 18 months and suggested that a single dose of cells is not enough to offer sustained benefit.

In a somewhat different strategy, the Stem Cells in Myocardial Infarction (STEMMI) trial explored the effects of stimulation of MSC by injection of granulocyte colony-stimulating factor (G-CSF).[45] A set of 78 patients who had an intervention less than 12 hours after onset of symptoms were randomized to either subcutaneous injections of

Table 1
Stem cell populations with potential for cardiac cell therapy

Cell Type	Origin	Advantages	Disadvantages
HSCs	Bone marrow, peripheral blood, cord blood	Proved to be safe to transplant; easy to obtain	Only modest benefit in clinical trials
MSCs	Bone marrow, adipose tissue	Easy to obtain and expand in culture; less immunogenic	Possible differentiation into osteoblasts producing bone
EPCs	Bone marrow, peripheral blood	Relatively easy to obtain from bone marrow or peripheral blood; important for neovascularization	Rare, heterogeneous population
iPS cells	Epigenetically reprogrammed skin fibroblasts, keratinocytes, peripheral blood cells, adipose stem cells, neural stem cells, marrow mesenchymal cells	Give rise to all somatic cell types including cardiomyocytes; patient-specific thereby avoiding allogeneic immune rejection	Still in infancy; safety and long-term efficacy need to be demonstrated first in large animal models.

G-CSF (10 μg/kg) for 6 days or placebo. This resulted in a significant increase in concentration of circulating leukocytes and CD34$^+$ cells. The primary end point was systolic function measured at baseline and 6 months by cardiac MRI. No association was found between the number of CD34$^+$ cells and the change in LVEF, and there was an inverse relationship between the LVEF and the number of CD45$^-$/CD34$^-$ cells. This result was in contrast in that reported in the TOPCARE study[40] and the percutaneous coronary intervention with stent implantation (PCI) post-MI study[46] and suggested that the stimulated MSC might not be a successful cellular strategy.

In the PCI post-MI study,[46] 67 patients were randomized in a double-blind placebo-controlled study to either placebo or HSC infusion. HSCs were harvested in all patients, isolated by Ficoll density gradient centrifugation, and then infused into the infarct-related artery within 24 hours of reperfusion. Cardiac MRI was performed at baseline and 4 months after infusion, as were whole body positron emission tomographic scans to assess cardiac metabolism. The investigators found a slightly greater increase in the LVEF with bone marrow cell infusion (2.2% vs 3.3%) and a decrease in infarct size. However, it was concluded that there was no incremental effect of autologous HSCs on LV function recovery and that HSCs could not be recommended at this time.

The Autologous Stem Cell Transplantation in Acute Myocardial Infarction (ASTAMI) trial[47] was another attempt at using autologous HSCs in patients approximately 6 days after MI. Patients were randomized after an acute anterior MI to either autologous HSCs or placebo. Cells were separated by Ficoll density gradient centrifugation and infused into the infarct-related artery with distal occlusion. There were 47 patients in the treatment group, and 50 received placebo. Baseline single-photon emission computed tomographic (SPECT) scan, echocardiography, and cardiac MRI were preformed 2 to 3 weeks after infarction and at 6 months. End points included LVEF and end-diastolic volume by all 3 methods and infarct size by SPECT and MRI. No effect was found on any of these 3 measurements between the 2 groups. This study was powered to detect a 5% difference in the LVEF. Although it was not clear why this study was different from the TOPCARE-AMI[40] or BOOST studies,[44] it was postulated by the investigators that differences in cell number or in cell subpopulations may explain the differences. In the same issue of the *New England Journal of Medicine*, the Reinfusion of Enriched Progenitor Cells and Infarct Remodeling in Acute Myocardial Infarction (REPAIR-MI) trial was reported.[48] In this trial, 204 patients were randomized to receive either HSCs or placebo infused 3 to 6 days after reperfusion from their MI. All patients had bone marrow aspiration, and progenitor cells were isolated by Ficoll-Hypaque centrifugation. Cells were infused into the infarct-related artery using the stop-flow technique. Quantitative LV angiography was performed at the time of the infusion and at 4 months. At the 4 month time point, the increase in LVEF was significantly greater in the cell group, 5.5% ± 7.3% versus 3.0% ± 6.5%, P = .01. This improvement was inversely proportional to the baseline LVEF, indicating that patients with the most-severe deficit benefited the most. At 1 year, bone marrow infusion was associated with a reduction in death, recurrent MI, and need for revascularization. The REPAIR-AMI group has recently published its 2-year follow-up result,[49] and it was reported that the clinical end point of death, MI, or need for revascularization was significantly reduced in the cell group compared with the placebo group. In a subgroup of 59 patients, MRI imaging was available, but only 27 had a baseline MRI. Although not statistically significant, the HSC-treated group had a higher LVEF than the placebo group (50.1 vs 43.6, mean difference of 6.5% ± 2.4% between the 2 groups).

There have been several more recent studies. The Clinical Benefit and Long-Term Outcome after Intracoronary Autologous Bone Marrow Cell Transplantation Study in Patients with Acute Myocardial Infarction (BALANCE) trail[50] studied the effect of bone marrow cell infusion into the infarct artery in 62 patients and 62 patients with comparable LVEF at baseline. This study was not randomized. The LVEF improved by 7.9% (by quantitative ventriculography) and the infarct size decreased by 8% a total of 3 months after infusion in their patients. The investigators followed up their patients at 12 and 60 months postinfusion and continued to see an improvement in LVEF compared with the control group and also reported a decrease in mortality in the treated group. In the Myocardial Regeneration by Intracoronary Infusion of Selected Population of Stem Cells in Acute Myocardial Infarction (REGENT) trial,[51] patients were randomized in an open-label design to unselected bone marrow mononuclear cells (n = 80), cells selected for CD34+/CXCR4+ to enhance the population of HSCs (n = 80), or control (n = 40). Patients with an anterior MI, successful stent placement, and an LVEF of 40% or less were included. The primary end point was LVEF and LV volume determined by cardiac MRI at 6 months' follow-up. There was no difference in these parameters or in major cardiovascular events in any of the groups. There was a trend, however, for improvement in the groups of patients given either cellular product who had a baseline LVEF less than 37%. This trial was plagued by a high dropout rate, so the final analysis was possible in less than 60% of the total population.

Two recent studies have used different methods and cell types to treat patients after MI. Co and colleagues[52] treated 120 patients with acute ST elevation infarctions with EPC capture stents. These stents are coated with monoclonal human CD34 antibodies designed to attract circulating EPCs. There was 1 patient with an acute stent thrombosis and 1 with a subacute thrombosis, but no late stent thrombosis was reported. All that can be concluded from this study is that these stents are safe and need to be studied in a randomized trial. Hare and colleagues[53] used precultured bone marrow–derived human MSCs. These cells have the advantage over autologous HSCs in that they can be infused intravenously and should hone to an area of injury and lack various major histocompatibility complex antigens. However, they also have disadvantages in that it is not clear how many cells actually cross over the pulmonary vasculature to the arterial circulation. They performed a dose-escalating phase 1 safety trial (0.5, 1.6, and 5 million cells/kg) in 53 patients who had been reperfused after an acute MI. There were no adverse events, and there was a suggestion of an increase in the LVEF in treated patients compared with untreated patients by both echocardiogram and cardiac MRI. Again, a larger, randomized trial is needed to fully assess the value of this approach.

It is apparent from all of these trials that the efficacy of stem cells after an MI is not established. Not only are there questions of the overall effectiveness but also as to the optimal cell type, the timing of the therapy, the correct method of delivery, as well as the mechanism by which the cell therapy may be helping. There are currently several larger trials being conducted that may help answer these questions before this type of therapy can become an accepted treatment strategy.

STEM CELLS TRIALS FOR HF

Overall, the current clinical trial evidence for the use of HSCs for HF has limited numbers of patients and conflicting results.[53–59] These studies did demonstrate the safety and feasibility of HSCs in these patients but certainly did not establish efficacy. In the first randomized trial, Hendrikx and colleagues[60] studied 20 patients who were undergoing coronary artery bypass grafting and had autologous HSCs directly injected into the border zone of the infarcted area at the time of surgery. This trial revealed a trend toward a greater increase in LVEF determined by cardiac MRI in the treated group. In a larger study, Assmus and colleagues[43,61] randomized 75 patients at least 3 months post-MI to infusion with circulating EPCs, HSCs? or no cell infusion. Cells were infused into the infarct-related artery using balloon occlusion. The primary end point was the LVEF determined by angiography. There was no increase in the LVEF in either the control group or with EPCs, but there was an increase of 3.7% ± 4.0% in the HSC-treated group. In a subset of patients who had cardiac MRI, the increase in LVEF was 4.8% ± 6.0% in the bone marrow–treated group compared with 2.8% ± 5.2% in the peripheral cell group (?significant). At 3 months, the patients were crossed over, and in both the peripheral treated group and the control, infusion of HSCs resulted in a significant increase in the LVEF at 3 months follow-up.

Another moderately sized study reported by van Ramshorst and colleagues[62] randomized 50 patients (25 treated and 25 placebo injected) with chronic angina not eligible for revascularization to HSCs injected into the ischemic zone identified by SPECT scanning using the NOGA (Biologics Delievery Systems Group, Cordis; Bridgewater, NJ, USA) catheter-guiding system. The primary end point was a summed stress score determined by SPECT scanning with secondary end points of LVEF assessed by MRI, cardiovascular society class score, and Seattle angina quality of life score. At the 3-month follow-up, there was an improvement in all end points in the treated group compared with the controls (are they true controls?). Although these improvements in cardiac testing were modest, these parameters provide impetus for further investigation.

There is only 1 small study in patients with dilated nonischemic cardiomyopathy. Seth and colleagues[63] reported on a study of 44 patients with LVEF less than 35% and normal coronary arteries. Using a balloon occlusion of the coronary sinus to slow coronary blood flow, 2of 3 of the HSCs were infused into the left coronary artery and the remaining 1of 3 into the right coronary artery. There were 24 patients in the treated group and 20 in the control group (sham or no procedure?). These investigators demonstrated a small but significant increase in the LVEF by echocardiography in the treated group of 5.4% and a decrease in the end-diastolic volume only in the treated group compared with the control population.

Again, although these trials are provocative, they do not provide a definitive answer. Currently several larger trials are being conducted or planned in an attempt to answer the question of efficacy of HSC therapy in patients with HF and recent MI.

WHAT CAN BE LEARNED FROM ONCOLOGY REGARDING STEM CELL THERAPY FOR CARDIOVASCULAR DISEASE?

HSCs are the most well-characterized tissue-specific stem cells with decades of basic research and clinical application. HSCs were the first tissue-specific stem cells to be prospectively isolated.[1] They are the only stem cells, to date, in routine clinical use for the treatment of a variety of malignant and benign blood cell diseases. So far, HSC therapy represents the most successful cell-based therapy. Emerging new stem cell fields can, therefore, benefit greatly from the lessons learned from the study of the biology and transplant of HSCs.

First, well-planned preclinical studies in animal models have been key to the development of HSC transplantation. Dr Thomas[64] described this well in his speech when accepting the Nobel Prize for Medicine in 1990 in Stockholm: "It should be noted that marrow grafting could not have reached clinical application without animal research, first in inbred rodents and then in outbred species, particularly the dog." The moderate effects of current cellular therapy for cardiovascular diseases, such as post-MI or in HF, have been obtained with little understanding of the biologic mechanisms involved. Using marrow cells, it is unclear which of the different cell types in the bone marrow results in best outcomes: hematopoietic cells, MSCs, or EPCs. It is also unclear which is the best route of transplanting these cells, and when specifically to improve myocardial function, either early or later after injury. Systematic preclinical animal studies are likely the key to enhance the current understanding of these experimental treatment approaches and thereby to improve the so-far modest treatment results.

Second, breakthroughs do not occur in biomedical research, but scientific progress results, small step by small step, from well designed and executed preclinical and clinical studies. As described previously, about 2 decades went by from the time of the first description by Barnes and colleagues[27] in 1956 that mice with leukemia could be treated with otherwise-lethal TBI followed by transplantation of bone marrow from healthy syngeneic mice until the landmark article by Thomas and colleagues[32] in 1977 (the description of the likely cure of 13 of 100 patients with end-stage acute leukemia). During this period of 2 decades, the efforts to transplant allogeneic bone marrow grafts had to overcome significant hurdles such as graft failure, GVHD, or infections. Bortin[29] reviewed in 1970, 14 years after Barnes and colleagues' initial report on bone marrow transplants for mice with leukemia, 200 published attempts at allogeneic bone marrow transplant in patients, all of which had failed. These discouraging results caused many investigators to leave the field and others to question whether such studies should continue. Fortunately, from today's perspective, work in animal models, especially in the dog, has showed that histocompatibility matching was important for successful HSC transplantation.

These preclinical observations then paved the way for successful HSC transplants in humans. Given the current enormous attention and hype surrounding stem cell therapy and regenerative medicine, it is wise to remember that it took about 2 decades for HSC transplant to become the standard treatment for a significant number of otherwise-incurable hematologic diseases. Thus, if history is our guide, it will likely take at least 2 decades for stem cell therapy for cardiovascular disease to develop into a widely successful therapeutic approach. To achieve this goal, step by step, carefully designed, and well executed preclinical and clinical studies, supported by sufficient long-term funding, will be crucial.

REFERENCES

1. Spangrude GJ, Heimfeld S, Weissman IL. Purification and characterization of mouse hematopoietic stem cells. Science 1988;241:58–62.

2. Horowitz MM. Uses and growth of hematopoietic cell transplantation. In: Applebaum FR, Forman SJ, Negrin RS, et al, editors. Thomas' hematopoietic cell transplantation. 4th edition. Chichester (UK): Wiley-Blackwell; 2009. p. 9–15.

3. Ogawa M. Differentiation and proliferation of hematopoietic stem cells. Blood 1993;81:2844–53.

4. Harrison DE, Stone M, Astle CM. Effects of transplantation on the primitive immunohematopoietic stem cell. J Exp Med 1990;172:431–7.

5. Wilson A, Laurenti E, Oser G, et al. Hematopoietic stem cells reversibly switch from dormancy to self-renewal during homeostasis and repair. Cell 2008; 135:1118–29.

6. Passegue E, Wagers AJ, Giuriato S, et al. Global analysis of proliferation and cell cycle gene expression in the regulation of hematopoietic stem and progenitor cell fates. J Exp Med 2005;202:1599–611.

7. Bhatia M, Wang JC, Kapp U, et al. Purification of primitive human hematopoietic cells capable of repopulating immune-deficient mice. Proc Natl Acad Sci U S A 1997;94:5320–5.

8. Wagers AJ, Sherwood RI, Christensen JL, et al. Little evidence for developmental plasticity of adult hematopoietic stem cells. Science 2002;297:2256–9.

9. Pittenger MF, Mackay AM, Beck SC, et al. Multilineage potential of adult human mesenchymal stem cells. Science 1999;284:143–7.

10. Caplan JED, Dennis JE. Mesenchymal stem cells as trophic mediators. J Cell Biochem 2006;98:1076–84.

11. Mangi AA, Noiseux N, Kong D, et al. Mesenchymal stem cells modified with Akt prevent remodeling and restore performance of infarcted hearts. Nat Med 2003;9:1195–201.

12. Lin Y, Weisdorf DJ, Solovey A, et al. Origins of circulating endothelial cells and endothelial outgrowth from blood. J Clin Invest 2000;105:71–7.

13. Grant MG, May WS, Caballero S, et al. Adult hematopoietic stem cells provide functional hemangioblast activity during retinal neovascularization. Nat Med 2002;8:607–12.

14. Yoder MC, Mead LE, Prater D, et al. Redefining endothelial progenitor cells via clonal analysis and hematopoietic stem/progenitor cell principals. Blood 2007;109:1801–9.

15. Takahashi K, Yamanaka S. Induction of pluripotent stem cells from mouse embryonic and adult fibroblast cultures by defined factors. Cell 2006;126(4):663–76.

16. Stadtfeld M, Apostolou E, Akutsu H, et al. Abberant silencing of imprinted genes on chromosome 12qFl in mouse induced pluripotent stem cells. Nature 2010;465:175–81.

17. Yu J, Hu K, Smuga-Otto K, et al. Human induced pluripotent stem cells free of vector and transgene sequences. Science 2009;324:797–801.

18. Zhang GF, Wilson GF, Soerens AG, et al. Functional cardiomyocytes derived from human induced pluripotent stem cells. Circ Res 2009;104:e30–41.

19. Taura D, Sone M, Homma K, et al. Induction and isolation of vascular cells from human induced pluripotent stem cells: brief report. Arterioscler Thromb Vasc Biol 2009;29:1100–3.

20. Karumbayaram S, Novitch BG, Patterson M, et al. Directed differentiation of human-induced pluripotent stem cells generates active motor neurons. Stem Cells 2009;27:806–11.

21. Tateishi K, He J, Taranova O, et al. Generation of insulin-secreting islet-like clusters from human skin fibroblasts. J Biol Chem 2008;283:31601–7.

22. Liu H, Zhu F, Zhang P, et al. Generation of induced pluripotent stem cells from adult rhesus monkey fibroblasts. Cell Stem Cell 2008;3:587–90.

23. Ezashi T, Telugu BP, Alexenko AP, et al. Derivation of induced pluripotent stem cells from pig somatic cells. Proc Natl Acad Sci U S A 2009;106:10993–8.

24. Jacobson LO, Simmons EL, Marks EK, et al. Recovery from radiation injury. Science 1951;113: 510–1.

25. Lorenz E, Uphoff D, Reid TR, et al. Modification of irradiation injury in mice and guinea pigs by bone marrow injections. J Natl Cancer Inst 1951;12:197–201.

26. Ford CE, Hamerton JL, Barnes DWH, et al. Cytological identification of radiation-chimeras. Nature 1956;177: 452–4.

27. Barnes DW, Corp MJ, Loutit JF, et al. Treatment of murine leukemia with X-rays and homologous bone marrow. Preliminary communication. Br Med J 1956;2:626–7.

28. Thomas ED, Lochte HL, Lu WC, et al. Intravenous infusion of bone marrow in patients receiving radiation and chemotherapy. N Engl J Med 1957;25:491–6.

29. Bortin MM. A compendium of reported human bone marrow transplants. Transplantation 1970;9:571–87.

30. Storb R, Rudolph RH, Thomas ED. Marrow grafts between canine siblings matched by serotyping and mixed leukocyte culture. J Clin Invest 1971;50:1272–5.

31. Storb R, Epstein RB, Graham TC, et al. Methotrexate regimens for control of graft-versus-host disease in dogs with allogeneic marrow grafts. Transplantation 1970;9:240–6.

32. Thomas ED, Buckner CD, Banaji M, et al. One hundred patients with acute leukemia treated by chemotherapy, total body irradiation, and allogeneic marrow transplantation. Blood 1977;49:511–33.

33. Thomas ED, Buckner CD, Clift RA, et al. Marrow transplantation for acute nonlymphoblastic leukemia in first remission. N Engl J Med 1979;301:597–9.

34. Orlic D, Kajstura J, Chimenti S, et al. Bone marrow cells regenerate infracted myocardium. Nature 2001;410:701–5.

35. Kocher AA, Schuster MD, Szabolcs MJ, et al. Neovascularization of ischemic myocardium by human bone-marrow derived angioblasts prevents cardiomyocyte apoptosis, reduces remodeling and improves cardiac function. Nat Med 2001;7:430–6.

36. Gnecchi M, He H, Liang OD, et al. Paracrine action accounts for marked protection of ischemic heart by modified Akt-modified mesenchymal stem cells. Nat Med 2005;11:367–8.

37. Wang X, Jameel N, Li Q, et al. Stem cells for myocardial repair with use of a transarterial catheter. Circulation 2009;120(Suppl 1):S238–46.

38. Zeng L, Hu Q, Wang X, et al. Bioenergetic and functional consequences of bone marrow-derived multipotent progenitor cell transplantation in hearts with post-infarction left ventricular remodeling. Circulation 2007;115:1866–75.

39. Nelson TJ, Martinex-Fernandez A, Yamada S, et al. Repair of acute myocardial infarction human stemness factors induced pluripotent stem cells. Circulation 2009;120:408–16.

40. Assmus B, Schachinger V, Teupe C, et al. Transplantation of progenitor cells and regeneration enhancement in acute myocardial infarction (TOPCARE-MI). Circulation 2002;106:3009–17.

41. Wollert KC, Meyer GP, Lotz J, et al. Intracoronary autologous bone-marrow cell transfer after myocardial infarction: the BOOST randomized controlled clinical trial. Lancet 2004;364:141–8.

42. Strauer BE, Brehm M, Zeus T, et al. Repair of myocardium bu autologous intracoronary mononuclear bone marrow cell transplantation in humans. Circulation 2002;106:1913–8.

43. Assmus B, Honold J, Schachinger V, et al. Transcoronary transplantation of progenitor cells after myocardial infarction. N Engl J Med 2006;355:1222–32.

44. Meyer GP, Wollert KC, Lotz J, et al. Intracoronary bone marrow cell transfer after myocardial infarction: eighteen months' follow-up data from the randomized, controlled BOOST (Bone Marrow Transfer to Enhance ST-Elevation Infarct Regeneration) trial. Circulation 2006;113:1287–94.

45. Ripa RS, Haack-Sorensen M, Wang Y, et al. Bone marrow derived mesenchymal cell mobalization by granulocyte-colony stimulating factor after acute myocardial infarction: results form the Stem Cell in Myocardial Infarction (STEMMI) trial. Circulation 2007;116:I24–34.

46. Janssens S, Dubois C, Theunissen K, et al. Autologous bone marrow-derived stem-cell transfer in patients with ST-segment elevation myocardial infarction: double-blind, randomized controlled trial. Lancet 2006;367:113–21.

47. Lunde K, Solheim S, Aakhus S, et al. Intracoronary injection of mononuclear bone marrow cells in acute myocardial infarction. N Engl J Med 2006;355:1199–209.

48. Schachinger V, Erbs S, Elsasser A, et al. Inracoronary bone marrow-derived progenitor cells in acute myocardial infarction. N Engl J Med 2006;355:1210–21.

49. Assmus B, Rolf A, Erbs S, et al. Clinical outcome 2 years after intracoronary administration of bone marrow-derived progenitor cells in acute myocardial infarction. Circ Heart Fail 2010;3:89–96.

50. Yousef M, Schannwell M, Kostering M, et al. The BALANCE study: clinical benefit and long-term outcome after intracoronary autologous bone marrow cell transplantation in patients with acute myocardial infarction. J Am Coll Cardiol 2009;53:2262–9.

51. Tendera M, Wojakowski W, Euzyllo W, et al. Intracoronary infusion of bone marrow-derived selected CD34+CXCR4+ cells and non-selected mononuclear cells in patients with acute STEMI and reduced left ventricular ejection fraction: results of randomized, multicentre Myocardial Regeneration by Inracoronary Infusion of Selected Population of Stem Cells in Acute Myocardial Infarction (REGENT) trial. Eur Heart J 2009;30:1313–21.

52. Co M, Tay E, Lee CH, et al. Use of endothelial cell capture stent (Genous bio-engineered R stent) during primary percutaneous coronary intervention in acute myocardial infarction: intermediate-to long-term clinical follow up. Am Heart J 2008;155:128–32.

53. Hare JM, Traverse JH, Henry TD, et al. A randomized, double-blind, placebo-controlled, dose-escalation study of intravenous adult mesenchymal stem cells (prochymal) after acute myocardial infarction. J Am Coll Cardiol 2009;54:2277–86.

54. Tse HF, Kwong YL, Chan JK, et al. Angiogenesis in ischemic myocardium by intramyocardial autologous cell implantation. Lancet 2003;361:47–9.

55. Fuchs S, Satler LF, Kornowski R, et al. Catheter-based autologous bone marrow myocardial injection in no-option patients with advanced coronary artery disease. J Am Coll Cardiol 2003;41:1721–4.

56. Perin EC, Dohmann HF, Borojevic R, et al. Transendocardial, autologous bone marrow cell transplantation for severe, chronic ischemic heart failure. Circulation 2003;107:2294–302.

57. Silva GV, Perin EC, Dohmann HF, et al. Catheter-based trans-endocardial delivery of autologous bone-marrow derived mononuclear cells in patients listed for heart transplantation. Tex Heart Inst J 2004;31:214–9.

58. Kuethe F, Richartz BM, Kasper C, et al. Autologous intracoronary mononuclear bone marrow cell transplantation in chronic ischemic cardiomyopathy in humans. Int J Cardiol 2005;100:485–91.

59. Strauer BE, Brehm M, Zeus T, et al. Regeneration of human infarcted heart muscle by intracoronary autologous bone marrow cell transplantation in chronic coronary artery disease. The ICAT study. J Am Coll Cardiol 2005;46:1651–8.

60. Hendrikx M, Hensen K, Clijsters C, et al. Recovery of regional but not global contractile function by the direct intramyocardial autologous bone marrow transplantation: results from a randomized controlled clinical trial. Circulation 2006;114:I101–7.

61. Assmus B, Fischer-Rasokat U, Honold J, et al. Transcoronary transplantation of functionally competent BMCs in associated with a decrease in natriuretic peptide serum levels and improved survival of patients with chronic postinfarction heart failure: results of the TOPCARE-CHD registry. Circ Res 2007;100:1234–41.

62. van Ramshort JA, Bax JJ, Beeres SL, et al. Intramyocardial bone marrow cell injection for chronic myocardial ischemia: a randomized controlled trial. JAMA 2009;301:1997–2004.

63. Seth S, Narang R, Bhargava B, et al. Percutaneous intracoronary cellular cardiomyoplasty for nonischemic-cardiomyopathy: clinical and histopathological results: the first-in-man ABCD (Autologous Bone Marrow Cells in Dilated Cardiomyopathy) trial. J Am Coll Cardiol 2006;48:2350–1.

64. Thomas ED. The Nobel prizes, 1990. In: Tryckeri AB, editor. Les prix Nobel. Stockholm (Sweden): Norstedts; 1991. p. 227.

Cardiac Disease and Heart Failure in Cancer Patients: Is Our Training Adequate to Provide Optimal Care?

Carol L. Chen, MD[a],*, Richard Steingart, MD[b]

KEYWORDS

- Cardiotoxicity • Prevention • Training programs

Cardiac disease within the realm of cancer care is an aspect of cardiology that has been seen in the past as a rare anomaly. With the advent of new biologic cancer therapies and increasing cancer survival, growing interest has been shown in the unique cardiac manifestations of cancer care. However, this expertise is concentrated mainly in survivorship clinics and academic cancer centers. As cancer care is increasingly delivered in the community, treatment of cardiac disease in the setting of active cancer treatment and surveillance for cardiac toxicity will fall into the hands of a variety of health care providers. Clinicians who treat these patients have very limited resources available to help them become familiar with the issues of cardiac toxicity in patients with cancer and cancer survivors. It has now become apparent that health care providers who care for these patients must be knowledgeable about at least six main topics: left ventricular dysfunction, rhythm management (particularly atrial fibrillation and arrhythmias associated with QT prolongation), myocardial ischemia, hypertension, cardiac risk assessment and management around the time of chemotherapy and cancer surgery, and survivorship. Therefore, these topics must be incorporated into medical training at the earliest exposure to clinical medicine, because postgraduate education in pediatrics, internal medicine, family medicine, and specialized fellowship training in oncology and cardiology are some of the disciplines in which these clinical expectations arise. Additionally, because nurse practitioners, advanced nurse specialists, and physician assistants are playing a more important role in the management of cardiovascular disease in patients with cancer, their curriculum also requires retooling.

INCREASING POPULATION AT RISK

In January 2007, 11.7 million people diagnosed with cancer were living in the United States. Because of advances in the early detection and treatment of cancer, approximately 66% of people diagnosed with cancer are expected to live at least 5 years after diagnosis.[1] Although in the general population deaths from both heart disease and cancer have been declining over the past decade, cardiac deaths remain more prevalent than cancer deaths in people older than 65 years (**Fig. 1**). In an investigation of the National Cancer Institute's Surveillance, Epidemiology, and End Results database for patients diagnosed between 1973 and 1987, cardiovascular disease accounted for almost half of non–cancer-related mortality after diagnosis. The highest risk populations are men

The authors have nothing to disclose.

[a] Cardiology Division, Memorial Sloan-Kettering Cancer Center, 1275 York Avenue, Howard-809, New York, NY 10065, USA

[b] Cardiology Division, Memorial Sloan-Kettering Cancer Center, 1275 York Avenue, Howard-818, New York, NY 10065, USA

* Corresponding author.

E-mail address: chenc@mskcc.org

Heart Failure Clin 7 (2011) 357–362

doi:10.1016/j.hfc.2011.03.007

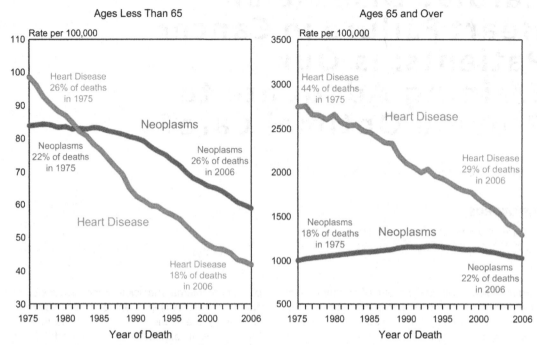

Fig. 1. US Death Rates 1975–2006. (*Data from* Horner MJ, Ries LAG, Krapcho M, et al, editors. SEER Cancer statistics review, 1975–2006, National Cancer Institute. Bethesda (MD). Based on November 2008 SEER data submission 2008. Available at: http://seer.cancer.gov/csr/1975_2006/. Accessed September 1, 2009.)

who undergo hormone therapy for prostate cancer and patients receiving anthracyclines and chest radiation.[2] Similarly, a Dutch study of more than 2000 testicular cancer survivors showed a twofold increased risk of myocardial infarction in survivors younger than 45 years compared with the age-matched general population.[3] The 10-year risk of a serious cardiovascular event was as high as breast cancer recurrence in almost 80% of patients in a postmenopausal cohort of patients with breast cancer studied by Bardia.[4]

Another special population that continues to grow because of the success of cancer treatment is the group of pediatric cancer survivors. More than 80% of children and adolescents who are treated for cancer become long-term survivors.[1] In 2003, there were approximately 270,000 survivors of pediatric cancer in the United States, or approximately 1 in 640 adults between the ages of 20 and 39.[5] Many younger survivors will live long enough to develop typical cardiovascular diseases, particularly heart failure, at an earlier age than their siblings or other age-matched controls. These patients may also survive long enough to manifest other late toxicities of cancer treatment. In the Childhood Cancer Survivor Study (CCSS) cohort, cardiac mortality is estimated to be sevenfold higher than that of an age-matched population.[6] The Children's Oncology Group recently formulated long-term follow-up guidelines

to standardize care and surveillance for toxicities of therapy.[7,8] Surveillance for the development of cardiac disease by pediatricians, family physicians, and survivorship clinics is an important component of these guidelines.

THE CHALLENGES OF DELIVERING CARDIAC CARE

During active cancer treatment, patients and their families are primarily focused on cancer care even if they have serious comorbid conditions such as cardiac disease. Because of the frequent oncology visits for follow-up, other health care visits are often postponed or neglected. Symptoms of heart failure, such as fatigue, dyspnea on exertion, and lower extremity edema, are very similar to the expected adverse effects of cancer therapy, and likely delay or mask the diagnosis of heart failure in these patients. Patients undergoing cancer therapy often limit their physical activity for a variety of reasons, and this can promote cardiovascular disease or limit detection. Challenges in communication among specialists, especially those in different institutions, easily results in fragmented care. Multispecialty groups incorporating cardiovascular and cancer care under one health care umbrella are rare.

Albini and colleagues[9] suggest that patients who have both undiagnosed cardiovascular disease and cancer could have a different course and outcome depending on whether they present first to a cardiologist or an oncologist. Diagnosis of occult cancer and initiation of treatment by an oncologist may result in delay in diagnosis and treatment of coronary artery disease (CAD), which may be exacerbated by treatment-related hypertension, ischemia, or heart failure. Often the patients themselves, especially pediatric cancer survivors, have no specific knowledge of their cancer treatment and late toxic effects. Long-term follow-up by oncologists primarily focus on disease recurrence. Sedentary lifestyles may mask symptoms of heart failure or CAD.

Non-oncologists cannot be expected to know the standard treatments for various cancers and the specific risk of cardiac toxicity. To this end, survivorship clinics are becoming more prevalent in many academic cancer centers to provide annual surveillance for late effects of cancer treatment in response to the Institute of Social Medicine's 2009 International Meeting on Integrated Care.[10] However, fewer than one in eight patients with cancer are estimated to be admitted to academic medical centers in the United States, and most new cancer cases continue to be treated in hospitals and physician offices located close to the patient's home.[11] The CCSS reported that survivors receive most of their care from primary care providers.[12] Because of these dynamics, an improved awareness is required and has resulted in the development of the International CardiOncology Society, a group committed to improving care in patients with cancer and cardiac disease.[13]

Several examples of patients for whom the intersection of cardiac disease and cancer therapy illustrate the need for enhanced understanding are presented below.

Case 1

A 46-year-old woman with stage II Her2+ breast cancer received adjuvant doxorubicin (240 mg/m²) and cyclophosphamide, followed by trastuzumab and paclitaxel. According to published treatment guidelines, she underwent a multigated acquisition scan before starting trastuzumab. Her left ventricular ejection fraction (LVEF) was 60%. During routine surveillance at her 3-month follow-up visit while on trastuzumab therapy, her echocardiography showed a 45% LVEF. She reported being less active than previously and is more fatigued on exertion. Her oncologist believed that given her multiple positive lymph nodes and Her2+ status, she was at high risk for recurrence and would derive great benefit from continued treatment with trastuzumab. The cooperative agreement was that trastuzumab would be held, and the patient began a heart failure treatment regimen of carvedilol and lisinopril. After 4 weeks, a repeat echocardiogram showed that her LVEF was 55%. She resumed trastuzumab and was followed closely for symptoms, and underwent frequent echocardiographic assessment of LVEF. Over the next year she completed trastuzumab as prescribed by her oncologist, and her LVEF remained normal. She has no other CAD risk factors; however, she is now menopausal. Some important clinical questions remain, such as how her left ventricular function should be followed up and whether should she continue carvedilol and lisinopril.

Case 2

43 year old man was treated at 15 years of age for non-Hodgkin's lymphoma with 18 Gy to lung and mediastinal areas, daunorubicin (197 mg/m²), and a myriad of other therapies. He enrolled in the survivorship clinic and at 30 years of age he had an echocardiogram that showed an LVEF of 55% with mild septal hypokinesis. Repeat echocardiogram 2 years later was not significantly changed. At 39 years of age, he was admitted to a community hospital with pneumonia, and subsequently experienced recurrent upper respiratory infections manifested as cough and wheezing over the next 3 months. Because of the history of lymphoma involving in his lung and his past radiation treatment, his primary care physician contacted the adult survivorship clinic. Ultimately, when the patient was evaluated, he described the classic symptoms of heart failure, including orthopnea, paroxysmal nocturnal dyspnea, and dyspnea on minimal exertion. His echocardiography showed an LVEF of 22%. Over the next several months he was treated for heart failure, he received a biventricular pacemaker/defibrillator, and his symptoms have resolved; however, his systolic function only mildly improved. The question remains whether earlier recognition of heart failure might have resulted in greater improvement of LVEF.

Case 3

A 65-year-old woman with history of hypertension, diabetes, and nonobstructive CAD was diagnosed with colorectal cancer. She began treatment with 5-fluorouracil (5-FU)via intrahepatic pump over 72 hours. She developed chest pain and presented to a community emergency room. Electrocardiograms and cardiac enzymes were unremarkable and she was discharged home, continuing on the 5-FU infusion because it was

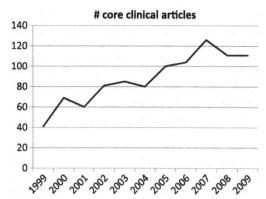

 # core clinical articles

Fig. 2. PubMed search of MeSH terms (anthracyclines or antineoplastic protocols or antineoplastic agents) and (cardiovascular disease or heart disease) from 1999–2009.

apparently not recognized as a potential contributor to the clinical presentation. Over the next 12 hours she develops worsening chest pain and presents to the cancer center emergency room. Her electrocardiogram shows ST depressions, and the 5-FU infusional pump is immediately discontinued. Her chest pain continues and she is sent for coronary angiography, ultimately showing no significant CAD. Again, some important clinical questions remain, such as whether she can resume 5-FU–based therapy in any form, and whether calcium channel blockers or nitrates would be helpful.

HOW CAN CLINICIANS BE EQUIPPED TO CARE FOR THIS SPECIAL AND GROWING POPULATION?

The authors investigated the typical methods of education: peer-reviewed journals, annual scientific sessions, and specialized conferences. Searching the overlap of Medical Subject Heading terms *antineoplastic protocols* and *heart diseases* in PubMed over the past 10 years showed that the numbers of articles have increased minimally despite the significant rise in cardiotoxic therapy (**Fig. 2**). The authors also searched the abstracts and session topics of the annual meetings of the American Society of Oncology (ASCO), the American College of Cardiology, and the Heart Failure Society of America over the past 2 years (**Box 1**). The intersection of cardiology and oncology also remains minimal in these national meetings. A small number of specialized international meetings are now dedicated to the care of cardiac disease in patients with cancer; however, these meetings are relatively small and physicians who attend often are already well aware of the issues.

How can clinicians be exposed to these critical clinical decisions so that patients with cancer receive optimal cardiovascular care? Because all oncology and cardiology trainees must go through internal medicine residency and fellowship training, the authors propose that purposeful and thoughtful exposure be initiated in these curricula.

Currently, the American College of Graduate Medical Education (ACGME) mandates the minimal educational program requirements for housestaff training. The requirements for hematology-oncology specialists refer to the intersection of cancer and cardiology in the following statement:

Fellows must have formal instruction, clinical experience, and demonstrate competence in the prevention, evaluation and management of chemotherapeutic drugs, biologic products, and growth factors; their mechanisms

---

Box 1
Presentations at recent national meetings

Meeting/Year	Title Words Searched	# of Presentations (Abstracts + Sessions)
Heart Failure Society of America, (HFSA) Annual Scientific Meeting 2009	"chemotherapy" or "cancer"	14
HFSA, 2010	"chemotherapy" or "cancer"	13
American College of Cardiology (ACC), Annual Scientific Session 2009	"chemotherapy" or "cancer"	6
ACC, 2010	"chemotherapy" or "cancer"	6
American Society of Clinical Oncology (ASCO) Annual Meeting, 2009	"cardiotoxicity" or "cardiac"	23
ASCO, 2010	"cardiovascular" or "cardiac"	21

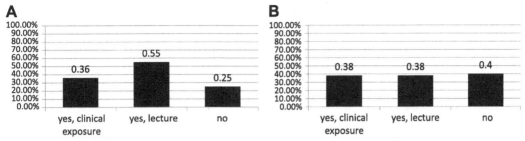

Fig. 3. (*A*) Does your oncology training program systematically expose fellows to cardiac disease in cancer patients? (n = 60). (*B*) Does your cardiology training program systematically expose fellows to cardiac care of cancer patients? (n = 60).

of action, pharmacokinetics, clinical indications, and limitations, including their effects, toxicity, and interactions.[14]

Within the ACGME requirements for cardiovascular disease specialty training, the cardiotoxic effects of cancer therapy also has a limited presence in the curriculum and is summarized by the following statement: "The training program must provide formal instruction for the fellows to acquire knowledge of the following areas…cardiovascular pharmacology, including …the effects of non-cardiovascular drugs upon the cardiovascular function."[15]

ASCO released a core curriculum in 2005. In response to a growing knowledge base and the need to ensure uniform quality training, a comprehensive education template was written to serve as the gold standard for training oncology physicians. In an almost 10,000-word document, cardiovascular disease is referenced only four times; two were regarding Hodgkin lymphoma and the potential for treatment-related cardiovascular toxicity and long-term cardiac complications, one was regarding palliation of symptoms of carcinoid cardiac disease, and one was listed among 20 other complications of treatment ranging from rash to neurotoxicity.[16]

The authors conducted a brief online survey of both cardiology (n = 180) and hematology/oncology (n = 132) fellowship directors to gauge current practices of training and interest in the incorporation of a single didactic lecture into their curriculum (**Fig. 3**). Of the oncology programs that responded (n = 60), 35% reported exposure to cardiovascular disease education in lecture form, 56% in clinical practice, and 25% reported no formal exposure. Most responders indicated they would be interested in incorporating one didactic lecture given by an acknowledged expert in the field. Cardiology program directors who responded (n = 60) were evenly divided among lecture exposure, clinical exposure, and no

exposure to cardiac toxicity of cancer care. Again, most stated they would be interested in adding a core didactic lecture on oncologic diseases and their treatment into the curriculum (**Fig. 4**).

PROPOSAL FOR HOUSESTAFF AND OTHER PROVIDER EDUCATION CURRICULUM

The authors propose six main topics be included in a core curriculum for housestaff in internal medicine, cardiology, and oncology, and other providers entering the field (nurse practitioners, advanced practice nurses, and physician assistants):

1. Left ventricular dysfunction
2. Myocardial ischemia
3. Arrhythmia
4. Treatment-related hypertension
5. Pretreatment cardiac risk assessment (both medical and surgical therapy)
6. Cancer survivorship care.

Goals for oncologists and primary care providers would focus more on awareness and surveillance, whereas goals for cardiovascular specialists would focus more on appropriate identification and early treatment. Vital to this

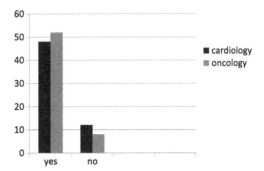

Fig. 4. If offered by expert in the field, would you be interested in incorporating one didactic lecture covering this topic into your core curriculum?

education is the concept that the team of clinicians must communicate and work collaboratively in the care of these patients.

SUMMARY

The care of patients with cancer who have cardiac disease is dispersed both sequentially and concurrently across multiple providers, and an important goal of education is communication among the providers regarding change of therapy, toxicity of therapy, and symptom assessments. Changes must be made to improve the delivery of cardiac care in patients with cancer and cancer survivors. Therefore, the authors propose a multilevel approach that includes short, targeted curriculum for housestaff training programs in internal medicine, family medicine, pediatrics, cardiology and oncology, increasing presence at national meetings of internists, oncologists and cardiologists, and an Internet-based repository of core information.

REFERENCES

1. Horner MJ, Ries LAG, Krapcho M, et al, editors. SEER Cancer statistics review, 1975–2006, National Cancer Institute. Bethesda (MD). Based on November 2008 SEER data submission 2008. Available at: http://seer.cancer.gov/csr/1975_2006/. Accessed September 1, 2009.
2. Brown BW, Brauner C, Minnotte MC. Noncancer deaths in white adult cancer patients. J Natl Cancer Inst 1993;85(12):979–87.
3. van den Belt-Dusebout AW, Nuver J, de Wit R, et al. Long-term risk of cardiovascular disease in 5-year survivors of testicular cancer. J Clin Oncol 2006; 24(3):467–75.
4. Bardia A. Comparison of breast cancer recurrence risk and cardiovascular disease risk among postmenopausal breast cancer survivors. Presented at: ASCO Breast Cancer Symposium, San Francisco, October, 2009 [abstract 1332009].
5. Hewitt MWS, Simone JV, editors. Childhood cancer survivorship: improving care and quality of life. Washington, DC: National Academics Press; 2003.
6. Mertens AC, Yasui Y, Neglia JP, et al. Late mortality experience in five-year survivors of childhood and adolescent cancer: the Childhood Cancer Survivor Study. J Clin Oncol 2001;19(13):3163–72.
7. Long-term follow-up care for pediatric cancer survivors. Pediatrics 2009;123(3):906–15.
8. Tukenova M, Guibout C, Oberlin O, et al. Role of cancer treatment in long-term overall and cardiovascular mortality after childhood cancer. J Clin Oncol 2010;28(8):1308–15.
9. Albini A, Pennesi G, Donatelli F, et al. Cardiotoxicity of anticancer drugs: the need for cardio-oncology and cardio-oncological prevention. J Natl Cancer Inst 2010;102(1):14–25.
10. Stein KV, Rieder A. Lost in transition-meeting the challenge through integrated care. Highlights from the 9th International Conference on Integrated Care in Vienna. Int J Integr Care 2009;9:e109.
11. Green LA, Fryer GE Jr, Yawn BP, et al. The ecology of medical care revisited. N Engl J Med 2001; 344(26):2021–5.
12. Oeffinger KC, Mertens AC, Hudson MM, et al. Health care of young adult survivors of childhood cancer: a report from the Childhood Cancer Survivor Study. Ann Fam Med 2004;2(1):61–70.
13. Lenihan DJ, Cardinale D, Cipolla CM. The compelling need for a cardiology and oncology partnership and the birth of the International CardiOncology Society. Prog Cardiovasc Dis 2010;53(2):88–93.
14. Hoff VP, Vick U. The value of eosinophilia in the diagnosis of allergic otitis media. Z Arztl Fortbild (Jena) 1975;69(5):235–7 [in German].
15. Haugh PJ, Levy CS, Hoff-Sullivan E, et al. Pyomyositis as the sole manifestation of disseminated gonococcal infection: case report and review. Clin Infect Dis 1996;22(5):861–3.
16. Muss HB, Von Roenn J, Damon LE, et al. ACCO: ASCO core curriculum outline. J Clin Oncol 2005; 23(9):2049–77.

A Historical Perspective of Anthracycline Cardiotoxicity

Michael S. Ewer, MD, JD[a],*, Daniel D. Von Hoff, MD[b],
Robert S. Benjamin, MD[c]

KEYWORDS

- Anthracyclines • Cardiotoxicity • History of anthracyclines
- Oncologic benefit of anthracyclines

The history of the anthracycline antibiotics goes back more than half a century, when the Italian company, Pharmitalia Research Laboratories, sought to investigate potential antineoplastic agents that might be derived from microorganisms found in the soil near the Adriatic Sea. A spore-producing *Streptomycete* was subsequently categorized as a bacterium and eventually identified. Interestingly, it produced a red pigment that expressed antibacterial properties. This pigment was purified and studied, thus becoming the first recognized anthracycline antibiotic. The agent, as have all agents in this class, proved far too toxic when used as an antibacterial, but was later synthesized and became an important anticancer therapy. Notwithstanding the fact that none of the anthracyclines have ever been used as antibacterial agents, members of this group are still referred to as the anthracycline antibiotics. As anticancer drugs, they have found an exceedingly important niche and are widely used and highly effective in the treatment of both hematologic malignancies and solid tumors.

Clinical trials using anthracyclines were conducted in the 1960s. The first anticancer anthracycline to be introduced clinically was daunomycin in the late 1960s. The compound now carries the compromise name, daunorubicin, because an identical drug discovered in France was called rubidomycin. Unfortunately, the new name loses the term "mycin," which identified it as an antibiotic. The agent is still widely used in the treatment of some forms of leukemia. A second anthracycline, derived from *Streptomyces peucetius var. caesius*, and now known as doxorubicin (the name that is used in this article), remains a therapeutic mainstay for the treatment of breast cancer, lymphoma, and most forms of sarcoma. Doxorubicin was originally called adriamycin; however, the scientific name was changed to conform with the structure. The name *adriamycin* was retained and replaced the initial trade name, Adriablastina, in part in recognition of the locality of its discovery along the shores of the Adriatic Sea. The name adriamycin is still encountered in the medical literature and when not capitalized, refers to the initial generic name of the compound. Through a sequence of acquisitions and mergers, doxorubicin migrated through a number of corporate entities before being acquired by Bedford Laboratories in Ohio, the present source in the United States. Although both daunorubicin and doxorubicin were noted to have significant oncologic effects soon after their discovery and synthesis, both

[a] Department of Cardiology, The University of Texas MD Anderson Cancer Center, 1515 Holcombe Boulevard, Houston, TX 77030, USA
[b] Translational Genomics Research Institute's (TGen), Translational Drug Development Division, US Oncology and the Scottsdale Clinical Research Institute, 445 N. Fifth Street, Phoenix, AZ 85004, USA
[c] Department of Sarcoma Medical Oncology, The University of Texas MD Anderson Cancer Center, 1515 Holcombe Boulevard, Houston, TX 77030, USA
* Corresponding author.
E-mail address: mewer@mdanderson.org

Heart Failure Clin 7 (2011) 363–372
doi:10.1016/j.hfc.2011.03.001

agents also were recognized to elicit serious cardiotoxicity that was a limiting factor for their use.[1] The cardiomyopathy that accompanied them was a consistent finding in that it affected all patients who received sufficiently large amounts of these agents.[2] Although some patients could clearly tolerate larger cumulative doses than others, with sufficient exposure cardiotoxicity was always present. Even for patients treated with cumulative doses that were usually tolerated, heart failure could be severe. Although afflicted patients sometimes responded to interventions to stabilize cardiac function, anthracycline-associated heart failure proved to be a chronic disorder and sometimes resulted in death. It is the evolution of our thoughts regarding this unusual form of cardiotoxicity related to the anthracyclines that is the subject of this article.

ANTHRACYCLINES OVER THE YEARS

A number of facts regarding doxorubicin cardiotoxicity were recognized quite early, even though the full impact of these findings surfaced much more gradually.[3,4] Among the early thoughts was that doxorubicin exposure resulted in both early and late cardiotoxicity, and that these 2 expressions of toxicity were different. For many years, the early toxicity was considered unimportant; patients had transient nonspecific repolarization changes on their electrocardiogram and occasionally experienced symptoms of mild myopericarditis. These manifestations almost always resolved promptly and until quite recently were deemed to be inconsequential; their full impact was not appreciated until decades after the early recognition and description of this phenomenon. It was the later manifestations of toxicity, termed subacute, late, chronic, and even "late-late" cardiac dysfunction that was associated with clinically relevant heart failure and was a major focus of the then new and poorly understood entity of doxorubicin-associated cardiotoxicity.[5]

Early observations noted that this subacute or late cardiotoxicity was related to the cumulative dose administered rather than to the dose given at any individual treatment cycle, and that this relationship was, at least to some extent, predictable. The depiction of this relationship in a curve plotting the likelihood of developing heart failure as a function of the cumulative dose of doxorubicin represented the work of Von Hoff and colleagues.[6] When looking at cardiac sequelae of more than 4000 patients who had been treated with doxorubicin, the likelihood of developing this devastating complication formed the basis of estimating the likelihood of developing cardiotoxicity for patients exposed to the agent.[6] Several other facts

emerged from this and other early clinical experience: first, the relationship, when integrated with efficacy data, allowed a cumulative dose to be defined with the intent to maximize disease-free and overall survival. It was intuitive that excessive cumulative doses would shorten survival in that increasingly large numbers of patients would succumb to heart failure; low cumulative doses would not optimize survival in that malignancy was not inhibited to the extent possible by the anthracycline. Based on what was known at the time, it was thought that if 5% of patients developed heart failure from doxorubicin, and only a small percentage of those with heart failure went on to die a cardiac death, disease and overall survival would be maximized. According to the Von Hoff curve, the cumulative dose that correlated with 5% of the patients developing heart failure was approximately 550 mg/m^2, somewhat lower than what was originally thought, and this became the nominal upper limit for doxorubicin administration for nearly 2 decades. This utilitarian approach to maximize the effect of therapeutic intervention did not take into account that an arbitrary ratio of 1:20 for developing heart failure might not apply equally for all tumors; that concept evolved more gradually.

Additionally, it was noted that the cumulative-dose versus congestive heart failure relationship was not linear; at low cumulative doses in the range of 100 to 300 mg/m^2, heart failure was unusual, and the curve was essentially flat (**Fig. 1**). It was at cumulative doses of greater than 300 mg/m^2 where the incidence of heart failure rose much more rapidly. Another factor that emerged was that not all patients who developed cardiotoxicity did so at the same cumulative dose. Although the curve defined what was thought to be the likelihood of developing cardiotoxicity for an average patient, it was very clear that some who were treated developed cardiotoxicity at much lower cumulative doses than the norm, whereas others seemed to tolerate cumulative doses far in excess of those estimated by the Von Hoff curve.

It was this variation in susceptibility of patients to the cardiotoxic effects of these agents that led to strategies for assessing early damage that had been caused by the anthracyclines, and for ways to predict who might be especially likely to develop toxicity at lower cumulative doses. The most successful strategy for assessing actual myocardial damage evolved as a consequence of the morphologic studies performed by Margaret Billingham and colleagues[7–9] of Stanford University in California. They recognized that doxorubicin caused ultrastructural changes in the myocardial

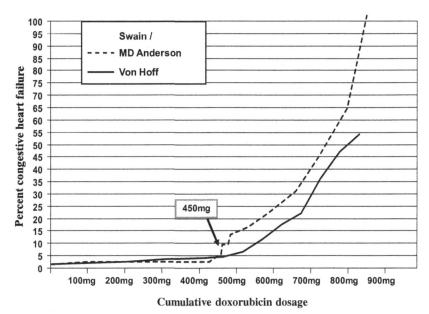

Fig. 1. The original Von Hoff curve (*solid*) showing low expression of cardiotoxicity at low cumulative doses with rapid rise as cumulative doses exceeded 500 mg/m². Subsequent analysis demonstrated that doxorubicin was more cardiotoxic than initially appreciated, as depicted by the dashed curve based on data from Swain and colleagues[21] and from the MD Anderson Cancer Center. (*Data from* Von Hoff D, Layard M, Basa P, et al. Risk factors for doxorubicin-induced congestive heart failure. Ann Intern Med 1979;91:710–7; Swain S, Whaley F, Ewer M. Congestive heart failure in patients treated with doxorubicin: a retrospective analysis of three trials. Cancer 2003;97:2869–79.)

muscle cell that were characteristic, that progressed as the cumulative dose increased, and that could serve as a toxicity scale. Their technique required myocardial specimens to be evaluated by electron microscopy after preservation in glutaraldehyde. As cells in the biopsy specimens were not all equally affected to the same extent, a toxicity grade was based on the number of cells in an electron microscopic grid that demonstrated certain characteristics. The Billingham grading scale encompassed 4 points designated as 0, 1, 2, and 3, whereby a grade of 0 was applied when no cellular changes were detected, and the scores increased according to the appearance of vacuoles, myofibrillar dropout, and myocyte necrosis.[7–9]

As more patient data accumulated it became clear that 4 points on the grading scale were insufficient to fully characterize the extent of damage sustained by patients who had been exposed to doxorubicin. Bruce Mackay and colleagues[10] at the M.D. Anderson Cancer Center in Houston modified the scale to include 2 additional points, defining them as 0.5 and 1.5. This addition allowed comparison of scores regardless of which system was used, as Billingham grades remained fundamentally unchanged through this modification. The criteria for both grading scales are provided in **Table 1**, and typical structural alterations are

depicted in **Fig. 2**. During the 1980s, many patients underwent myocardial biopsies after having received cumulative doses of doxorubicin that approached 300 mg/m²; if the grade was below 1.5, administration of the anthracycline could continue with low likelihood of developing cardiotoxicity with the next 1 or 2 cycles of drug. It was not unusual for patients, especially those who had low biopsy grades and who therefore could be expected to tolerate additional exposure to doxorubicin beyond what an average patient could tolerate, to undergo repeated cardiac biopsies during the course of their anthracycline-based treatment.

Although the cardiac biopsy was exceedingly helpful in making clinical decisions as to whether an anthracycline could or could not be safely continued, it proved to have additional value on 2 fronts: first, it allowed direct comparison of the relative cardiotoxicity of various anthracyclines, and, second, it provided very strong evidence as to whether or not newly introduced agents exhibited similar biopsy changes. The first of these facilitated a comparison of the cardiotoxicity of the 4-prime epimer of doxorubicin (epirubicin) and later of the liposomal preparations with that of the parent compound, demonstrating that on a milligram-to-milligram basis, and more importantly on the basis of dosages that resulted in equivalent

Table 1
Morphologic grading systems for anthracycline cardiotoxicity

	Billingham Scoring System[8]	Mackay Scoring System[10a]		
Grade	Morphologic Characteristics	Vacuoles	Myofibrillar Dropout	Necrosis
0	Normal myocardial ultrastructural morphology	0	0	0
0.5	Not completely normal but no evidence of anthracycline-specific damage	<4	0	0
1	Isolated myocytes affected and/or early myofibrillar loss; damage to <5% of all cells	4–10	<3	0
1.5	Changes similar to grade 1 except damage involves 6%–15% of all cells	<10	3–5	<2
2.0	Clusters of myocytes affected by myofibrillar loss and/or vacuolization, with damage to 16%–25% of all cells	~[b]	6–8	2–5
2.5	Many myocytes (26%–35% of all cells) affected by vacuolization and/or myofibrillar loss	Not included in Mackay Scoring System		
3.0	Severe, diffuse myocytes damage (>35% of all cells)	~	>8	>5

[a] Average number of abnormal muscle fibers per grid based on an examination of a minimum of 6 grids obtained from 6 blocks.
[b] Any number.

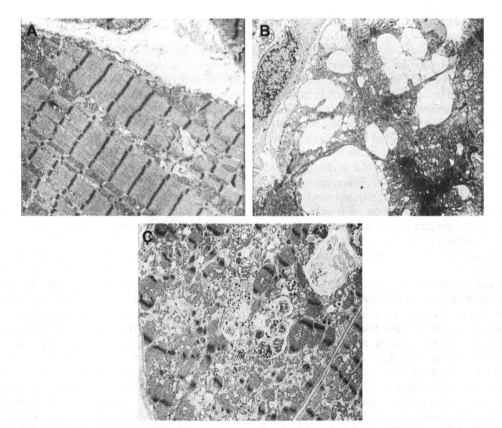

Fig. 2. (A) Normal-appearing myocyte. (B) Endomyocardial specimen showing a cell with vacuole formation following doxorubicin administration. (C) Endomyocardial specimen showing myocardial necrosis following doxorubicin administration.

myelosuppression, both epirubicin and the pegy-lated liposomal formulation were associated with lower biopsy grades than was the case with the parent compound.[11] Second, demonstrating that an agent did not exhibit the electron microscopic changes characteristic of the anthracyclines helped to formulate the concept that some of the newer agents known to affect the heart were inherently different, as the anthracyclinelike changes on the myocardial biopsy did not exist. Such comparisons demonstrate that the cardiotoxicity associated with trastuzumab, and perhaps other newer anticancer agents, was not the same as that of the anthracyclines, leading to the proposed categorization of agents in type I (anthracyclinelike cardiotoxicity) or type II (not cumulative dose–related and without anthracyclinelike morphologic changes) cardiotoxic agents (see later in this article).[12]

Interestingly, cardiac biopsies were almost always undertaken just before the anticipated next administration of the anthracycline-based chemotherapy, and the vital piece of information, ie, that the abnormalities seen on cardiac biopsy were transient and resolved over time, was not appreciated until considerably later. This came about after patients who had been treated with anthracyclines in the past, and who later developed metastatic disease, underwent cardiac biopsy before reintroduction of an anthracycline-containing regimen; such biopsies frequently were normal, suggesting that abnormal cells had either undergone repair and appeared normal, or had experienced cell death and were replaced by fibrous tissue. Unfortunately, the 2 situations showing similar biopsies are quite different. When doxorubicin is given with cardioprotective strategies and stopped early, the myocardium can repair the damage, and retreatment, albeit with caution, is possible. When sufficient cardiac damage occurs so that the damaged cells die, cardiac reserve is severely compromised. In that situation, if patients are rechallenged under the misconception that the heart has become normal, they will develop cardiotoxicity with left ventricular dysfunction early following reintroduction of the anthracycline. The concept that the maximal cumulative dose constituted a lifetime limitation was thereby clearly reinforced.

The third characteristic of anthracycline toxicity that gained considerable attention was the identification of subgroups of patients who were noted to develop cardiotoxicity at cumulative doses below those predicted by the Von Hoff curve. Initially these risk factors were enumerated and later grouped together; prior anthracycline administration was the most consistent, but exposure to radiation, extremes of age, and a variety of other underlying cardiac abnormalities joined what seemed to be an ever-expanding list of cardiac risk factors and identified groups of patients where more careful scrutiny of possibly early cardiotoxicity was deemed prudent.[6,13,14]

Based on these facts, by the early 1980s, anthracyclines were widely used and considered to have an acceptable safety profile up to cumulative doses of 550 mg/m^2 for patients without the recognized risk factors. Cardiac biopsy could help define a subset of patients who exhibited less myocyte damage and who could therefore tolerate higher cumulative doses.

Noninvasive Surveillance and Monitoring

Although noninvasive testing for early toxicity had been used extensively and had the decided advantages of not subjecting patients to the risk and expense of the invasive biopsy, the limitations of noninvasive parameters became increasingly clear. It is unknown how many patients were prematurely removed from their effective anticancer treatment on the basis of falsely positive decreases in their left ventricular ejection fraction (LVEF); however, in centers that made wide use of biopsies, the correlation between morphologic change and functional abnormalities was determined to be clearly suboptimal. Although systolic time intervals enjoyed only limited application, changes in LVEF ultimately became the mainstay both for monitoring individual patients receiving anthracyclines as well as for evaluating cardiac safety in large multicenter clinical trials. Gradually, the weaknesses in these monitoring techniques were appreciated with regard to the monitoring of individual patients, but when used in large clinical trials where false positive and false negative results were likely to be statistically compensated for in the mean LVEF, differences in mean ejection fractions for various arms, or mean changes from baseline were considered highly relevant.[15–17]

For individual patients, the misconceptions that reductions in LVEF from baseline during chemotherapy with anthracyclines always were caused by the chemotherapy, or that noting that no change in this parameter had taken place implied that cardiotoxicity did not occur were widespread. It mattered little if the method used to estimate LVEF was based on cardiac ultrasound or one of several nuclear techniques, LVEF studies lacked sensitivity and specificity. Nevertheless, in the absence of more reliable noninvasive tests, countless patients were followed with serial LVEF determinations with assessments undertaken before, during, and after anthracycline-based regimens.

Many attempts were made to improve the predictive value of noninvasive testing. These included adding exercise testing or relying more heavily on abnormalities of diastolic dysfunction. Although each of these variants had their proponents, the weaknesses of noninvasive testing could not be overcome to a sufficiently satisfactory level where they could be fully relied on in making clinical decisions regarding the use of an anthracycline. Today, even with higher resolution imaging and greater sensitivity of the methodology, and appreciating that progress has been made in this regard, noninvasive imaging remains suboptimal as a parameter to follow patients who have received, or to assess those who are about to receive, an anthracycline.

Because of the suboptimal nature of noninvasive testing, Bayes' law analysis was applied, and suggested that because toxicity was much less common at low cumulative doses, that a different threshold for defining anthracycline toxicity be used at different cumulative doses. For example, at cumulative doses below 200 mg/m^2, a drop of more than 20 percentage points might be deemed relevant, whereas at doses between 200 and 400 mg/m^2, a drop of more than 15 percentage points might be a more appropriate decrease to raise concern; at cumulative arms of more than 400 mg/m^2, a drop of more than 10 percentage points might be significant where at lower doses this might not be the case. This concept, although advocated, never caught on, perhaps, in part, because regimens using lower cumulative doses were being used increasingly.

Other Clinical Considerations

Clinically, the pieces of the puzzle fell into place, albeit gradually. The explanation as to why the biopsy changes occurred at cumulative doses that were so much lower than those that were associated with overt heart failure emerged through 2 additional findings. First was that the Von Hoff curve could be approximated by a simple mathematical formula, suggesting when extrapolated to those portions of the curve where little clinical evidence of heart failure existed, that damage had to be taking place much earlier in the process than had heretofore been appreciated, and that myocardial reserves compensated for the loss of myocyte; the extent of cardiac reserve used could not be quantitated by the available noninvasive testing.[18] The hypothesis that damage took place early was later underscored and substantiated by the finding that troponin I was released shortly after exposure to the anthracycline, and that the extent of cardiotoxicity was seen later correlated with the extent of troponin I release.[19,20] It is now appreciated that anthracycline-associated cardiac damage occurs at the time of exposure. What had been thought of as early anthracycline-associated cardiotoxicity, and that was initially considered to be of little importance, represented the actual insult that starts the relentless process, that if sufficiently severe, cascades toward myocardial dysfunction, heart failure, and in some instances, cardiac death.

In part through improved assessment of cardiac function by noninvasive testing, and in part as a consequence of information obtained through long-term follow-up and surveillance of patients, the cumulative dose that resulted in a likelihood of heart failure of approximately 5% decreased. Although in the early 1970s it had been thought that this threshold was reached with a cumulative dose of 600 mg/m^2, this number decreased following the publication of the Von Hoff analysis to the range of 500 to 550 mg/m^2, and was adjusted downward further by the analysis by Swain and colleagues[21] in 2003 to about 400 to 450 mg/m^2. Now, with the recognition that cell damage takes place at the time of exposure, one can assert that any amount of an anthracycline has the capacity to cause cell injury, but that damage is unlikely, albeit not invariably so, to be clinically problematic at cumulative doses below 240 to 300 mg/m^2 in patients who do not have cardiac risk factors; in the modern era, most patients are treated to this level.

As has been noted, until quite recently, even when cardiac damage was quite extensive, especially when high cumulative doses had been administered, the damage usually remained clinically silent in that patients were asymptomatic and the LVEF neither changed significantly nor declined into the abnormal range. It was only when endomyocardial biopsy studies were undertaken was there any hint as to the extent of the actual damage to the myocyte. As we move forward, troponin I measurements, although not yet incorporated into our everyday management strategies, are likely to provide a much more useful metric relative to myocardial damage; they are only now becoming part of our clinical armamentarium.[22] Noninvasive assessments of cardiac function are continuing to evolve, albeit gradually. M-mode echocardiography, of course, was supplanted by 2-dimensional studies, and Doppler imaging and flow measurements became able to provide a semiquantitative estimate of diastolic dysfunction. We now have parameters for evaluating localized myocardial abnormalities, and can get an excellent depiction of wall motion by incorporating computer-generated 3-dimensional images. Nevertheless, the true extent of cardiac damage remained elusive; the impact that any given abnormality has for the future of an individual patient can be estimated only imperfectly. Many centers incorporate their own algorithms of testing, but none of these methods, short of the biopsy, have been able to define who could or could not tolerate the next 1 or 2 cycles of their anthracycline-containing regimen without early or late cardiac sequelae. Even with modern methods of ultrasound, the true extent of myocardial damage and remaining compensatory reserves cannot be measured or estimated accurately. Furthermore, when early changes or abnormalities are noted, they have not proven to be especially helpful in that clinicians have little impetus to modify treatment schedules on that basis without strong data to support a change in regimen; this is especially so in the present era where the cumulative doses of anthracycline used in many regimens is declining.

Mechanistic Considerations and the Concept of Remodeling

The enigma of what anthracyclines were actually doing to the heart, both mechanistically and clinically, was extensively studied and partially elucidated. Although mechanistic questions still exist, myocyte toxicity is, at least in part, related to iron-dependent oxidative stress. Reduction of the quinone groups on the anthracycline B ring results in a semiquinone radical before reduction to the alcohol, which in the case of doxorubicin, is doxorubicinol. Free radicals induce peroxidation of the membranes of the myocyte, and subsequent influx of intracellular calcium ensues.[23–25]

As in the case of cardiomyopathy of other etiologies, the heart undergoes remodeling as a compensatory mechanism following the insult, yet the LVEF may remain in the normal range even though significant damage at the cellular level has taken place.[26] It is only when the myocardial reserves are depleted and compensation is not possible that LVEF becomes significantly reduced. These instances may, in cases of severe toxicity, appear soon after exposure, but when the damage is extreme, it may come to the forefront much later, sometimes becoming apparent only after other stressors, either natural or iatrogenic, overwhelm the already burdened myocardium.[27]

Risk Factors

As noted previously, not all patients experience cardiac damage to an equal degree at similar cumulative doses of an anthracycline. It was the appreciation of that fact that led to the exploration of cardiac risk factors. Initially, specific factors were identified, and among them were the classic concerns of exposure to ionizing radiation, children, the elderly, and prior exposure to anthracyclines. Later additional risk factors were identified that included hypertension, valvular disorders, diabetes, and left-ventricular hypertrophy.[28] These factors were then grouped into conditions that were associated with increased left-ventricular end-diastolic pressure, and more recently the concept evolved to appreciate that any factor that has previously damaged the heart, or any factor that is likely to make the heart more vulnerable to on-going damage should be considered a risk factor for increased anthracycline-associated cardiac injury. Such a concept takes into account that increases in risk are gradual, albeit not linear, and clearly additive, in that patients with more than one condition are more vulnerable than those with only a single abnormality. The one risk factor that proved to be sufficiently unique in this regard was the pediatric age group, where, along with the toxic damage noted previously, the developing heart may experience inhibition of myocyte development. The specific problems related to the pediatric patient during and following treatment with anthracyclines has been studied and reported extensively by Lipshultz and colleagues.[29–32]

Cardioprotection

In addition to identifying groups that demonstrated increased cardiac vulnerability, strategies for cardioprotection were also explored with the intent that sparing the heart at the time of administration might allow larger cumulative doses of an anthracycline to be administered. Only much later was it also appreciated that if the heart could be protected, it would be much less vulnerable to sequential stresses that might amplify the expression of cardiac damage. Very strong evidence for the prevention of early damage was suggested by the observation that weekly administration of doxorubicin resulted in lower biopsy grades at equivalent cumulative doses than was the case when the drug was administered according to the usual 3-weekly dosage schedule as demonstrated by the Von Hoff curve; oncologic efficacy was not substantially affected.[33,34] Benjamin and colleagues[35,36] studied this phenomenon and recognized that cardiotoxicity was related more to the peak plasma level of the anthracycline, whereas oncologic efficacy was related more to the area under the curve of plasma concentration. This led to the exploration of continuous infusion regimens that proved to be highly successful in reducing cardiotoxicity. Benjamin and colleagues[35,36] also studied both efficacy and cardiotoxicity of infusional doxorubicin and established protocols for 72-hour and 96-hour infusions using ambulatory infusional pumps. Biopsy grades indicated that about twice the number of chemotherapy cycles could be given by using this strategy; additional benefits were a reduction in nausea and vomiting associated with more rapid infusions. Stomatitis became problematic with infusions of longer than 96 hours, but infusions of 72 hours were widely used in some centers and were highly effective in reducing the devastating effects of cardiotoxicity associated with the standard 20-minute infusion.

A number of substances were studied with the intent of reducing cardiotoxicity, and dexrazoxane, an EDTA analog free-radical scavenger, was found to be highly effective, reaching, by some estimations, the degree of cardioprotection achieved by 72-hour infusion. Although animal studies and most studies in humans found that dexrazoxane did not alter efficacy, one study reported by Swain and colleagues[37] suggested that efficacy was reduced. The agent was ultimately approved for use in the United States, but had a limited indication in that it was approved for patients who had received 300 mg/m^2 of doxorubicin without dexrazoxane, but for whom additional anthracyclines were to be administered. Early damage had not yet been appreciated when the administration-limitations were introduced; it now seems intuitive that reducing toxicity at the time of initial exposure, rather than after damage has already taken place, might have been a superior strategy. In part because of the labeling limitation, dexrazoxane was not widely used in the adult population; largely through the efforts of Lipshultz and colleagues,[29–32] who studied the agent in children, dexrazoxane found an important niche in that population. The concern regarding reduced efficacy was not confirmed in children.

Other strategies for reducing cardiotoxicity of anthracyclines emerged, among them those that altered the structure of the molecule and the implementation of liposomal delivery systems. Epirubicin, the 4-prime isomer of the parent compound, mentioned previously, is the most successful of these alternatives that have been deemed to be less cardiotoxic; in equivalent myelosuppressive dosages, epirubicin allows about one-third more cycles to be given than is the case with doxorubicin. Recent meta-analysis, however, did not confirm a statistically significant reduction in cardiotoxicity, although there was a tendency toward less cardiotoxicity. The oncologic spectrum is not generally thought to have been substantially altered. Liposomal delivery systems were designed to take both pharmacodynamics and molecule size

into account in an effort to reduce cardiotoxicity. Although clearly less cardiotoxic than the parent compound, these agents, however, have a sufficiently different spectrum of oncologic efficacy so that they should not be considered universally interchangeable with conventional forms of anthracyclines.

Among the more interesting aspects of anthracycline cardiotoxicity is the interaction with trastuzumab, a monoclonal antibody; considerable discussion has taken place as to the nature of cardiac dysfunction that has been associated with this agent. Trastuzumab blocks the HER2 neu pathway, a pathway that is probably essential for cell repair. Initially trastuzumab was not expected to demonstrate cardiotoxicity, but the pivotal trial demonstrated decreases in ejection fraction in 28% of the exposed population.[15] Later studies where the drug was administered in the adjuvant setting revealed far fewer instances of cardiotoxicity, but were nevertheless in the 2% to 4% range.[16,17,38] Furthermore, a substantial number of patients had trastuzumab withdrawn and therefore could not benefit from the full intended course of that agent. Initial biopsy studies did not demonstrate the cell destruction that was characteristic of anthracycline toxicity, and that, along with the fact that extended duration of therapy was often tolerated, presented strong evidence against a cumulative dose-related toxicity. Toxicity was distinguished from that of the anthracyclines in that it appeared that trastuzumab did not destroy myocytes, but resulted in myofibrillar disarray that was reversible, and resulted in a state analogous to the stunning or hibernation seen in some cases of ischemic heart disease. These distinguishing features led to the previously noted designations of type I and type II treatment-related cardiac dysfunction, where type I was characteristic of the anthracyclines and resulted in cell death, whereas type II was predominantly transient and depicted cell dysfunction. These generalities were proposed originally for trastuzumab-related toxicity and caution should be applied when considering newer medications that may have a completely different mechanism of toxicity.

Later experience demonstrated that those who had not received anthracyclines before receiving trastuzumab had an extremely low probability of experiencing cardiotoxicity.[39] De Kort and colleagues,[40] in an elegant study, showed that hearts that had been exposed to doxorubicin had upregulated the HER2 receptor with increased binding of trastuzumab to the myocardium and may have partially saturated the receptor, thereby interfering with cell repair. It is now believed that trastuzumab modulates the cardiotoxicity of doxorubicin, and has an additional but modest direct and probably reversible effect on the myocardium in the absence of an anthracycline. Furthermore, the temporal relationship between the administration of doxorubicin and trastuzumab as a factor of synergistic interaction between the agents strongly suggests a mechanism of the type described.[41]

As other agents have entered into the therapeutic armamentarium, the need for high-dose anthracyclines has diminished. The cardiac biopsy is now rarely necessary as an evaluative tool for accepting or rejecting very high cumulative doses. Interestingly, the very strategies that have been demonstrated to clearly mitigate the cardiotoxicity of the anthracyclines, ie, continuous infusion and dexrazoxane, are implemented infrequently, yet newer and inadequately studied strategies are often proposed. Theoretically, any intervention that reduces wall stress is likely to provide some degree of protection, and both beta-blockers and afterload reducing agents such as angiotensin-converting enzyme inhibitors and angiotensin-receptor blocking agents have been advocated.[42]

SUMMARY

Many aspects of medical care go through a cycle, whereby use initially increases, levels off, and gradually declines. Countless highly touted therapies have come and gone, going through these phases, only to be recalled in the context of historical interest. The use of anthracyclines has clearly leveled off, but it is unlikely that this group of agents will cease to be an important class of anticancer drugs over the next years or even, perhaps, decades. Nevertheless, they are used less than in the past, as new agents and new combinations are gaining broader usage. The age of high-dose anthracyclines, with few exceptions, is waning. Nevertheless, anthracyclines at lower cumulative doses are widely used. Although we no longer perform heart biopsies on a regular basis, we are starting to look at cardiac biomarkers with greater interest. Although we protect less because of the decreasing use of continuous infusion administration schedules to prevent cardiotoxicity, we monitor more closely in an effort to detect myocyte damage earlier. Additionally, we follow patients for longer periods to quantitate the extent and affect of late damage. Anthracyclines remain a highly toxic group of very effective oncologic agents. Although we have learned quite a bit about how they can be used with increasing safety, there is still definitely room for further evolution with regard to our knowledge of protective strategies.

Anthracyclines will remain part of our oncologic armamentarium, at least for some time to come.

REFERENCES

1. Tan C, Tasaka H, Yu K, et al. Daunomycin, an antitumor antibiotic, in the treatment of neoplastic disease. Clinical evaluation with special reference to childhood leukemia. Cancer 1967;20:333–53.
2. Ritchie J, Singer J, Thorning D. Anthracycline cardiotoxicity: clinical and pathological outcome assessed by radionuclide ejection fraction. Cancer 1970;46:1109–16.
3. Lefrak E, Pitha J, Rosenheim S, et al. A clinicopathologic analysis of adriamycin cardiotoxicity. Cancer 1973;32:302–14.
4. Benjamin R, Wiernik P, Bachur N. Adriamycin chemotherapy—efficacy, safety, and pharmacologic basis of an intermittent single high-dosage schedule. Cancer 1974;33:19–27.
5. Gottlieb SL, Edmiston WA Jr, Haywood LJ. Late, late doxorubicin cardiotoxicity. Chest 1980;78:880–2.
6. Von Hoff D, Layard M, Basa P, et al. Risk factors for doxorubicin-induced congestive heart failure. Ann Intern Med 1979;91:710–7.
7. Billingham M, Bristow M, Glastein E, et al. Adriamycin cardiotoxicity: endomyocardial biopsy evidence of enhancement by irradiation. Am J Surg Pathol 1977; 1:17–23.
8. Billingham M, Mason J, Bristow M, et al. Anthracycline cardiomyopathy monitored by morphologic changes. Cancer Treat Rep 1978;62:865–72.
9. Billingham M, Bristow M. Evaluation of anthracycline cardiotoxicity: predictive ability and functional correlation of endomyocardial biopsy. Cancer Treat Symp 1984;3:71–6.
10. Mackay B, Ewer M, Carrasco C, et al. Assessment of anthracycline cardiomyopathy by endomyocardial biopsy. Ultrastruct Pathol 1994;18:203–11.
11. Valero V, Buzdar A, Theriault R. Phase II trial of liposome-encapsulated doxorubicin, cyclophosphamide, and fluorouracil as first-line therapy in patients with metastatic breast cancer. J Clin Oncol 1999;17:1425–34.
12. Ewer M, Lippman S. Type II chemotherapy-related cardiac dysfunction: time to recognize a new entity. J Clin Oncol 2005;23:2900–2.
13. Minow R, Benjamin R, Gottlieb J. Adriamycin (NSC 123127) cardiomyopathy—an overview with determination of risk factors. Cancer Chemother Rep 1975;6:195–201.
14. Minow R, Benjamin R, Lee E, et al. Adriamycin cardiomyopathy—risk factors. Cancer 1977;39:1397–402.
15. Slamon D, Leyland-Jones B, Shak S, et al. Use of chemotherapy plus a monoclonal antibody against HER2 for metastatic breast cancer that overexpresses HER2. N Engl J Med 2001;344:783–92.

16. Tan-Chiu E, Yothers G, Romond E, et al. Assessment of cardiac dysfunction in a randomized trial comparing doxorubicin and cyclophosphamide followed by paclitaxel, with or without trastuzumab as adjuvant therapy in node-positive, human epidermal growth factor receptor 2-overexpressing breast cancer: NSABP B31. J Clin Oncol 2005;23:7811–9.

17. Suter T, Procter M, Van Veldhuisen D, et al. Trastuzumab-associated cardiac adverse effects in the herceptin adjuvant trial. J Clin Oncol 2007;25:3859–65.

18. Ewer M, Vooletich M, Benjamin R. A mathematical model for doxorubicin cardiotoxicity: added evidence for the concept of sequential stress. Proceedings of the 40th Annual Meetings of the American Society of Clinical Oncology (post-meeting edition). Journal of Clinical Oncology 2004; vol 22, No 14S (July 15 Supplement) [abstract: 2086].

19. Cardinale A, Sandri M, Martinoni A, et al. Myocardial injury revealed by plasma troponin I in breast cancer treated with high-dose chemotherapy. Ann Oncol 2002;13:710–5.

20. Cardinale D, Colombo A, Torrisi R, et al. Trastuzumab-induced cardiotoxicity: clinical and prognostic implication of troponin I elevation. J Clin Oncol 2010;28:3910–6.

21. Swain S, Whaley F, Ewer M. Congestive heart failure in patients treated with doxorubicin: a retrospective analysis of three trials. Cancer 2003;97:2869–79.

22. Ewer M, Lenihan D. Left ventricular ejection fraction and cardiotoxicity: is our ear really to the ground? J Clin Oncol 2008;26:1201–3.

23. Gianni L, Meyers C. The role of free radical formation in the cardiotoxicity of anthracycline. In: Muggia F, Green M, Speyer J, editors. Cancer treatment and the heart. Baltimore (MD): The John Hopkins University Press; 1992. p. 9–46.

24. Simunek T, Sterba M, Popelova O, et al. Anthracycline-induced cardiotoxicity: overview of studies examining the roles of oxidative stress and free cellular iron. Pharmacol Rep 2009;61:154–71.

25. Zhang Y, Shi J, Li Y, et al. Cardiomyocyte death in doxorubicin-induced cardiotoxicity. Arch Immunol Ther Exp 2009;57:435–45.

26. Moore D. Mechanisms and models in heart failure: a combinatorial approach. Circulation 1999;100:999–1008.

27. Ewer M, Gibbs H, Swafford J, et al. Cardiotoxicity in patients receiving trastuzumab (Herceptin): primary toxicity, synergistic or sequential stress, or surveillance artifact? Semin Oncol 1999;26:96–101.

28. Buzdar A, Marcus C, Smith T, et al. Early and delayed clinical cardiotoxicity of doxorubicin. Cancer 1985;55:2761–5.

29. Lipshultz S, Colan S, Gelber R. Late cardiac effects of doxorubicin therapy for acute lymphoblastic leukemia in childhood. N Engl J Med 1991;324:808–15.

30. Lipshultz S, Lipsitz S, Mone S, et al. Female sex and higher drug dose as risk factors for late cardiotoxic effects of doxorubicin therapy for childhood cancer. N Engl J Med 1995;332:1738–43.

31. Lipshultz S, Colan S, Silverman L, et al. Dexrazoxane reduces incidence of doxorubicin-associated acute myocardiocyte injury in children with acute lymphoblastic leukemia (ALL.). Proc Am Soc Clin Oncol 2002;21 [abstract: 1557].

32. Lipshultz S. Exposure to anthracyclines during childhood causes cardiac injury. Semin Oncol 2006;33:S8–14.

33. Weiss A, Metter G, Fletcher W, et al. Studies on adriamycin using a weekly regimen demonstrating its clinical effectiveness and lack of cardiac toxicity. Cancer Treat Rep 1976;60:813–22.

34. Torti F, Bristow M, Howes A, et al. Reduced cardiotoxicity of doxorubicin delivered on a weekly schedule. Assessment by endomyocardial biopsy. Ann Intern Med 1983;99:745–9.

35. Benjamin R, Chawla S, Hortobagyi G, et al. Continuous-infusion adriamycin. In: Rosenthal C, Rotman M, editors. Clinical applications of continuous infusion chemotherapy and concomitant radiation therapy. New York: Plenum Press; 1986. p. 19–25.

36. Chawla S, Benjamin R, Hortobagyi G, et al. Decreased cardiotoxicity of 96 hour continuous infusion adriamycin compared with epirubicin. Proc Am Soc Clin Oncol 1986;5:44.

37. Swain S, Whaley F, Gerber M, et al. Cardioprotection with dexrazoxane for doxorubicin-containing chemotherapy in advanced breast cancer. J Clin Oncol 1997;15:1318–32.

38. Perez E, Suman V, Davidson N, et al. Cardiac safety analysis of doxorubicin and cyclophosphamide followed by paclitaxel with or without trastuzumab in the North Central Cancer Treatment Group N9831 adjuvant breast cancer trial. J Clin Oncol 2008;26:1231–8.

39. Slamon D, Eiermann W, Robert N, et al. BCIRG 006 phase III trial comparing AC-T with AC-TH and with TCH. In: The adjuvant treatment of HER2-amplified early breast cancer patients: third planned efficacy analysis, San Antonio Breast Cancer Symposium. San Antonio (TX): 2009.

40. de Korte M, de Vries E, Lub-de Hooge M, et al. 111Indium-trastuzumab visualises myocardial human epidermal growth factor receptor 2 expression shortly after anthracycline treatment but not during heart failure: a clue to uncover the mechanisms of trastuzumab-related cardiotoxicity. Eur J Cancer 2007;43:2046–51.

41. Ewer SM, Ewer MS. Cardiotoxicity profile of trastuzumab. Drug Saf 2008;31:459–67.

42. Cardinale D, Colombo A, Lamantia G, et al. Anthracycline-induced cardiomyopathy: clinical relevance and response to pharmacologic therapy. J Am Coll Cardiol 2010;55:213–20.

The Importance of Clinical Grading of Heart Failure and Other Cardiac Toxicities During Chemotherapy: Updating the Common Terminology Criteria for Clinical Trial Reporting

Akm Hossain, MD, MPH[a], Alice Chen, MD[b],*, Percy Ivy, MD[b],
Daniel J. Lenihan, MD[c], Jonathan Kaltman, MD[d],
Wendy Taddei-Peters, PhD[e], Scot C. Remick, MD[f]

KEYWORDS

- Common terminology criteria for adverse events
- Cardiac side effects of chemotherapy • Cardiooncology
- Adverse events

The natural history for most types of human malignancy is changing. This trend is substantiated by the emergence of more durable complete response rates, improved survival especially with the observance of more prolonged periods of freedom from progressive disease, and even cure. With the development and emergence of novel biologically targeted agents in the treatment of cancer, new treatment paradigms are emerging, which include revisiting the use of maintenance regimens with biologically active agents. Coincident with these observations, the time-honored traditional cytotoxicity profile of myelosuppression, alopecia, and mucositis is giving way to new systemic side effects and, in particular, cardiovascular toxicities.

The views expressed in this article do not necessarily represent the views of the National Cancer Institute, the National Heart, Lung, and Blood Institute, the National Institutes of Health, the Department of Health and Human Services, or the US government.
Financial disclosures: None.
[a] Departments of Medicine, Hematology and Oncology, Ellis Fischel Cancer Center, University of Missouri, 15 Business Loop 70 West, DC 116.71 Columbia, MO 65203, USA
[b] Investigational Drug Branch, Cancer Therapy Evaluation Program, Division of Cancer Treatment and Diagnosis, National Cancer Institute, Suite 7131, 6130 Executive Boulevard, Rockville, MD 20852, USA
[c] Vanderbilt Heart and Vascular Institute, 1215 21st Avenue South, Suite 5209, Nashville, TN 37232-8802, USA
[d] Division of Cardiovascular Sciences, National Heart, Lung, and Blood Institute, 6701 Rockledge Drive, MSC 7940, Bethesda, MD 20892-7940, USA
[e] Division of Cardiovascular Sciences, National heart, Lung, and Blood Institute, RKL2, 6701 Rockledge Drive, Bethesda, MD 20817, USA
[f] Department of Medicine, West Virginia University School of Medicine, Mary Babb Randolph Cancer Center, 1801 Health Sciences South, PO Box 9300, Morgantown, WV 26506, USA
* Corresponding author.
E-mail address: chenali@mail.nih.gov

Heart Failure Clin 7 (2011) 373–384
doi:10.1016/j.hfc.2011.03.008
1551-7136/11/$ – see front matter. Published by Elsevier Inc.

According to Surveillance Epidemiology and End Results (SEER) database information, cancer survivorship has increased by 100% in the last decade and is expected to triple in the next decade.[1] As patients are living longer, significant late-term treatment-related sequelae are becoming more evident in cancer patients.[2] Anticancer chemotherapeutic agents and other modalities are often associated with and complicated by the development of acute and chronic cardiac toxicities.[3] The common cardiac complications associated with anticancer therapies are arrhythmia, left ventricular dysfunction (systolic and diastolic) (LVD) and/or heart failure (HF), myocardial ischemia or acute coronary syndrome (ACS), hypertension (HTN), and QT (corrected) (QTc) prolongation.[4] These complications have both short-term and long-term consequences affecting selection and administration of subsequent anticancer therapy, and may exacerbate other comorbid medical conditions and impair quality of life. The socioeconomic burden of emerging cardiovascular toxicities on the health care system is significant.[3,4]

Given this backdrop it is very important for oncologists, cardiologists, and other specialists to prevent, recognize, and treat these cardiac complications during or after anticancer treatment, as it is understood that early recognition and treatment may prevent long-term consequences.[5] Thus, a consistent description and grading of cardiac toxicity allows for a more uniform assessment of consequences of treatment. The Common Terminology Criteria for Adverse Events (CTCAE), used by virtually all oncology therapeutic trials, permits uniform detection and grading of these toxicities.

SCOPE OF THE PROBLEM: CARDIOVASCULAR TOXICITIES WITH ANTICANCER THERAPY

With increasing numbers of cancer survivors and patients with multiple medical comorbidities, treatment-related cardiac toxicities can be extremely challenging not only for the oncology community but also for cardiologists and other medical professionals to appropriately manage. Cardiac disease and cancer are by far the two leading causes of mortality in the United States, accounting for more than 50% of all deaths. It is anticipated that these two diseases will remain the leading causes of death over the next several decades. Moreover, recognition of long-term cancer-related morbidities has been conceptualized in most European countries, where significant efforts have been made to use common terminology and grading not only of cardiac toxicity associated with anticancer therapy but also side effects in other body systems.[6,7] Developing

countries in Asia and South America are also embracing these ideas for regulatory and clinical purposes.[8] Clinical trials with cytotoxic therapy have identified a wide spectrum of cardiovascular side effects. It is anticipated that with the development of targeted therapies that have antiangiogenic effects, such as small-molecule tyrosine kinase vascular endothelial growth factor (VEGF) inhibitors and vascular disrupting agents, cardiac toxicities are likely to be a significant issue. For example, both fatal and nonfatal cardiac events have been seen in vascular disrupting agents such as fosbretabulin (CA4P), DMXAA, and ZD6126; and significant hypertension has been observed with agents targeting the VEGF signaling cascade, such as bevacizumab.[9]

It has been estimated that the incidence and prevalence of fatal and nonfatal cardiac complications ranges between 12% and 18%, but it is very difficult to accurately assess true cardiovascular toxicity related to chemotherapy as opposed to exacerbation of previously existing but clinically silent cardiac disease.[7] Nonuniform reporting, disparities in reporting, and/or omission of cardiovascular side effects entirely, and their respective assessment and toxicity grading, present challenges in the medical literature.[8,10] The CTCAE, a grading system of common adverse events encountered in oncology therapeutic trials, allows for better understanding of toxicities and severity of cardiac toxicity due to oncologic investigational agents.

COMMON CARDIOVASCULAR TOXICITIES WITH ANTICANCER AGENTS
Left Ventricular Dysfunction and/or Heart Failure

The most common class of agents associated with LVD and HF are the anthracyclines. LVD and/or HF has been reported during anthracycline exposure as either acute (reported incidence is <1%), early-onset chronic progressive (reported incidence is 1.6%–2.1%), or late-onset chronic progressive (reported incidence is 1.6%–5%).[11] The overall incidence of LVD, estimated based on cumulative dose of doxorubicin, is 3% to 5% with 400 mg/m^2, 7% to 26% with 550 mg/m^2, and 18% to 48% with 700 mg/m^2.[10] Epirubicin and idarubicin appear to have lower incidence of LVD and/or HF.[12] Cyclophosphamide-related LVD and/or HF is related to total dose administered (>150 mg/kg and 1.5 g/m^2/d) and usually occurs within 1 to 10 days after the first dose.[2] In a study comparing docetaxel plus doxorubicin and cyclophosphamide (TAC) with fluorouracil plus doxorubicin and cyclophosphamide (FAC) in breast cancer patients, the incidence of LVD and/or HF at 55 months was 1.6% in the TAC arm versus 0.7% in the FAC arm.[13] At 70 months' follow-up, LVD and/or HF were reported in 2.3% of the TAC group compared with 0.9% of the FAC group.[14] With trastuzumab, the incidence of LVD and or HF ranges from 2% to 7% when used as monotherapy, 2% to 13% when used in combination with paclitaxel, and may be up to 27% when used concurrently with anthracyclines plus cyclophosphamide. Small-molecule tyrosine kinase inhibitors (sunitinib, desatinib, lapatinib) have been associated with the development of HF and LVD.[14–17] **Table 1** summarizes the approximate incidence of LVD, principally defined by changes in left ventricular ejection fraction (LVEF) with common anticancer agents.

Cardiac Ischemia or Acute Coronary Syndrome

The chemotherapy agent that is most commonly associated with cardiac ischemia is 5-fluorouracil (5-FU). 5-FU causes angina-like chest pain, classically Prinzmetal or vasospastic angina. The incidence of cardiac ischemia associated with 5-FU may be anywhere from 1% to 68%. High doses (>800 mg/m²) and continuous infusion of 5-FU have been associated with higher rates of ischemia (7.6%) when compared with bolus injection (2%).[18] Capecitabine, an oral medication with similarities mechanistically to 5-FU, is also associated with cardiac ischemia, at times reported as high as 3% to 9%.[19] Other medications potentially related to cardiac ischemia include paclitaxel (has been reported to be up to 5%) and docetaxel (only 1.7%). In addition, bevacizumab, a monoclonal antibody that inhibits VEGF, has a slight increase in cardiac ischemia compared with placebo (1.5% vs 1%) in a pooled analysis of 5 randomized controlled trials. Another anti-VEGF based therapy, sorafenib, has been associated with an increased risk of cardiac ischemia.[20–23] In a pancreatic cancer treatment trial, cardiac ischemia was reported in 2.3% of cases who received erlotinib 100 mg/d with gemcitabine versus 1.2% of cases who received gemcitabine alone.[24] **Table 2** summarizes the estimated incidence of chemotherapy associated cardiac ischemia.

QT/QTc Interval Prolongation

It is difficult to accurately relay the degree of QT prolongation during chemotherapy for a host of reasons. First, 16% to 36% of cancer patients will have baseline electrocardiogram (ECG) abnormalities at diagnosis. The incidence and prevalence of other comorbid conditions including structural and functional heart diseases are also higher than the general population.[25] Often patients will be on other medications that can cause or worsen QT interval prolongation.[26] Accompanying electrolyte abnormalities (especially hypocalcemia and hypomagnesemia) may also increase the QT interval. Nonetheless, in

Table 1
Chemotherapeutic agents associated with left ventricular dysfunction

Chemotherapeutic Drug Class	Agent(s)	Incidence (%)
Anthracyclines	Doxorubicin (At a cumulative dose of 550 mg/m²) Idarubicin Epirubicin	3–26 5–18 0.9–3.3
Alkylating agents	Cyclophosphamide Ifosfamide	7–28 17
Antimicrotubule agent	Docetaxel	2.3–8
Antimetabolite	Clofarabine	27
Monoclonal antibody-based tyrosine kinase signal inhibitors	Bevacizumab Trastuzumab	1.7–3 2–28
Proteasome inhibitor	Bortezomib	2–5
Small-molecule tyrosine kinase inhibitors	Dasatinib Lapatinib Sunitinib Imatinib mesylate	2–4 1.5–2.2 2.7–11 0.5–1.7

Table 2
Chemotherapy agents associated with cardiac ischemia or acute coronary syndrome

Chemotherapeutic Drug Class	Agent(s)	Incidence (%)
Antimetabolites	Fluorouracil Capecitabine	1–68 3–9
Antimicrotubule agents	Paclitaxel Docetaxel	<1–5 1.7
Small-molecule tyrosine kinase inhibitors	Erlotinib Sorafenib	2.3 2.7–3
Monoclonal antibody–based tyrosine kinase signal inhibitor	Bevacizumab	0.6–1.5

a trial using lapatinib the incidence of either QTc >480 ms or an increase in QTc >60 ms from baseline on ECG was 16%. The incidence of QTc prolongation is 1% to 10% with nilotinib and 3.5% to 6% with vorinostat. Thalidomide has also been associated with QTc prolongation. With arsenic treatment, the incidence of QTc prolongation varies in the literature anywhere from 26% to 93%.[24,27–34] **Table 3** summarizes the incidence of chemotherapy-associated QT interval prolongation.

Other Arrhythmias

There are reports of arrhythmias such as sinus bradycardia, sinus tachycardia, and atrial fibrillation that occur in association with chemotherapy. However, the incidence is not well documented in direct relation to the chemotherapy and although all of these categories were created in the CTCAE tool, these are not commonly reported.

Hypertension

The popularity of anti-VEGF therapy has brought HTN, and its sequelae and management, into the forefront for cancer patients. The rapid onset and significant HTN has led to cardiovascular events including heart failure and myocardial infarction. Urgent management of HTN is frequently needed. The incidence of HTN can range from 4% to 35% with bevacizumab. About 11% to 18% of cases treated with bevacizumab had grade 3 HTN in different clinical trials.[19] As a major adverse effect of sorafenib therapy, HTN was reported in 17% to 43% cases in different clinical trials. With sunitinib, the incidence of HTN was 5% to 24% and reported grade 3 HTN was 2% to 8%.[26,30] **Table 4** summarizes the incidence of chemotherapy-associated hypertension.

Table 3
Chemotherapy agents associated with QT interval prolongation

Chemotherapeutic Drug Class	Agent(s)	Incidence (%)
Small-molecule tyrosine kinase inhibitors	Lapatinib Dasatinib Nilotinib	16 <1–3 1–10
Histone deacetylase inhibitor	Vorinostat	3.5–6
Others	Arsenic trioxide	26–93
	Vascular disrupting agents (eg, fosbretabulin)	6–7

Table 4
Chemotherapy agents associated with hypertension

Chemotherapeutic Drug Class	Agent(s)	Incidence (%)
Small-molecule tyrosine kinase inhibitors	Sunitinib Sorafenib	5–47 17–43
Monoclonal antibody–based tyrosine kinase signal inhibitor	Bevacizumab	4–35

Sinus bradycardia

Sinus bradycardia is not common with anticancer treatment and frequently does not require management. The incidence of sinus bradycardia secondary to paclitaxel varies considerably in reports, ranging from less than 0.1% to 31%. The rate of sinus bradycardia associated with thalidomide therapy has been reported to range from 5% to 55%.[35] Any degree of heart block is very uncommon with anticancer therapy.[35–37] **Table 5** summarizes the incidence of chemotherapy-associated bradycardia.

APPROACH TO COMMON TERMINOLOGY CRITERIA FOR ADVERSE EVENTS IN VERSION 4.0

The CTCAE is a National Cancer Institute (NCI) "dictionary" of adverse events and grading criteria that is widely used for reporting adverse events in oncology therapeutic clinical trials. The original purpose for the Common Toxicity Criteria (CTC) was to assist uniform cataloging and grading of toxicity in NCI-sponsored oncology therapeutic trials. There have been 4 versions, with the latest being released in May 2009. The CTCAE encompasses toxicities seen in all modalities of cancer therapy, namely, surgery, radiation, and chemotherapy. The first 2 versions, known as the CTC, focused on toxicity grading criteria from

Table 5
Chemotherapy agents associated with bradycardia

Chemotherapeutic Drug Class	Agent(s)	Incidence (%)
Antimicrotubule agent	Paclitaxel	<0.1–31
Angiogenesis inhibitor	Thalidomide	0.12–55

Table 6
Comparison of left ventricular systolic dysfunction in CTCAE version 3.0 versus version 4.0

Grading	CTCAE v.3.0	CTCAE v.4.0	Remarks
1	Asymptomatic, resting ejection fraction (EF) <60%–50%; shortening fraction (SF) <30%–24%	—	Omitted in version 4.0
2	Asymptomatic, resting EF <50%–40%; SF <24%–15%	—	
3	Symptomatic congestive heart failure (CHF) responsive to intervention, EF <40%–20%; SF <15%	Symptomatic due to drop in EF responsive to intervention	Version 4.0 is symptoms and intervention oriented
4	Refractory CHF or poorly controlled; EF <20%; intervention such as ventricular assist device, ventricular reduction surgery, or heart transplant indicated	Refractory or poorly controlled heart failure due to drop in EF; intervention such as ventricular assist device, intravenous vasopressor support, or heart transplant indicated	
5	Death	Death	No change

many vantage points including clinical, research, and regulatory settings. The CTCAE has been widely accepted by the oncology community and is used by many regional and national institutions, research organizations, industry, and individual investigators conducting cancer clinical trials outside of NCI sponsorship. Medical Dictionary for Regulatory Activities (MedDRA) terminologies, a catalog of more than 80,000 terms (not all related to adverse events), is more expansive and has been accepted by the International Conference on Harmonisation (ICH, Geneva, Switzerland). The use of MedDRA is mandatory for adverse event reporting to regulatory authorities in and outside of the United States; however, MedDRA does not provide grading of any of its terms.

Approximately 70% of CTCAE version 3.0 terminologies are MedDRA terms. The remaining 25% requires mapping to a MedDRA term, which had been done by NCI with each prior CTC and CTCAE versions released. Thus, there was a need for harmonization of CTCAE terminology and grading with MedDRA terminologies. Under leadership of the NCI's Cancer Therapy Evaluation Program (CTEP) and the Center for Bioinformatics Technology and Training (CBIIT), revision and generation of new CTCAE version 4.0 was undertaken between July 2008 and June 2009. With this revision, CTCAE terms were completely harmonized with MedDRA. Experts were drawn from CTEP, other National Institutes of Health institutes, the CBITT, the Food and Drug Administration (FDA),

Table 7
Comparison of heart failure in CTCAE version 3.0 versus version 4.0

Grading	CTCAE v.3.0	CTCAE v.4.0	Remarks
1	—	Asymptomatic with laboratory (eg, brain natriuretic peptide) or cardiac imaging abnormalities	New category in version 4.0
2	—	Symptoms with mild to moderate activity or exertion	
3	—	Severe with symptoms at rest or with minimal activity or exertion; intervention indicated	
4	—	Life-threatening consequences; urgent intervention indicated (eg, continuous intravenous therapy or mechanical hemodynamic support)	
5	—	Death	

Table 8
Comparative correlation of heart failure grading between CTCAE version 4.0 and other major societies

Grade/Class	CTCAE v.4.0	NYHA Functional Classification	CCS Functional Classification	ACC/AHA Stages of Heart Failure	Specific Activity Scale
I/A	Asymptomatic with laboratory (eg, BNP) or cardiac imaging abnormalities	Patients with cardiac disease but without resulting limitations of physical activity. Ordinary physical activity does not cause undue fatigue, palpitation, dyspnea, or anginal pain	Ordinary physical activity, such as walking and climbing stairs, does not cause angina. Angina with strenuous or rapid prolonged exertion at work or recreation	At high risk for developing heart failure. No identified structural or functional abnormality; no signs or symptoms	Patients can perform to completion any activity requiring ≥7 metabolic equivalents; eg, can carry 24 lb up 8 steps; do outdoor works (shovel snow, spade soil); do recreational activities (skiing, basketball, squash, handball, jog/walk 5 mph)
II/B	Symptoms with mild to moderate activity or exertion	Patients with cardiac disease resulting in slight limitation of physical activity. They are comfortable at rest. Ordinary physical activity results in fatigue, palpitation, dyspnea, or anginal pain	Slight limitation of ordinary activity. Walking or climbing stairs rapidly, walking uphill, walking or stair climbing after meals, in cold, in wind, or when under emotional stress, or only during the few hours after awakening. Walking more than 2 blocks on the level and climbing more than 1 flight of ordinary stairs at a normal pace and in normal conditions	Developed structural heart disease that is strongly associated with the development of heart failure, but without signs or symptoms	Patients can perform to completion any activity requiring ≤5 metabolic equivalents, eg, have sexual intercourse without stopping, garden, rake, weed, roller skate, dance fox trot, walk at 4 mph on level ground, but cannot and do not perform to completion activities requiring ≥7 metabolic equivalents

III/C	Severe with symptoms at rest or with minimal activity or exertion; intervention indicated	Patients with cardiac disease resulting in marked limitation of physical activity. They are comfortable at rest. Less than ordinary physical activity causes fatigue, palpitation, dyspnea, or anginal pain	Marked limitation of ordinary physical activity. Walking 1–2 blocks on the level and climbing more than 1 flight in normal conditions	Symptomatic heart failure associated with underlying structural heart disease	Patients can perform to completion any activity requiring ≤2 metabolic equivalents, eg, shower without stopping, strip and make bed, clean windows, walk 2.5 mph, bowl, play golf, dress without stopping, but cannot and do not perform to completion any activities requiring >5 metabolic equivalents
IV/D	Life-threatening consequences; urgent intervention indicated (eg, continuous intravenous therapy or mechanical hemodynamic support)	Patient with cardiac disease resulting in inability to carry on any physical activity without discomfort. Symptoms of cardiac insufficiency or of the anginal syndrome may be present even at rest. If any physical activity is undertaken, discomfort is increased	Inability to carry on any physical activity without discomfort; anginal syndrome may be present at rest	Advanced structural heart disease and marked symptoms of heart failure at rest despite maximal medical therapy	Patients cannot or do not perform to completion activities requiring >2 metabolic equivalents. Cannot carry out activities listed above (Specific activity scale III)
V	Death	—	—	—	—

Abbreviations: ACC/AHA, American College of Cardiology/American Heart Association; BNP, brain natriuretic peptide; CCS, Canadian Cardiovascular Society; CTCAE v.4.0, Common Terminology Criteria for Adverse Events version 4.0; NYHA, New York Heart Association.

clinical investigators, and pharmaceutical companies, among others. Twelve working groups were assembled to harmonize toxicity grading across 23 system organ classes (SOCs) (ie, the Cardiac Working Group revised the cardiac and vascular SOCs). This article contains a brief review and orientation to the new terminology for reporting major cardiovascular toxicities.[38,39]

In general, CTCAE content revision for version 4.0 has emphasized improved comprehensibility and usability by the entire research team, and improves clinical applicability for the clinical investigator. Earlier versions of the CTC grading criteria were more devoted to grading objective signs and symptoms by history and physical examination; or objective findings by laboratory or imaging studies. The current version attempts to correlate the grade of CTCAE to the clinical situation, that is, dose modification. Management and intervention (urgency and type) are used to indicate the severity of the event. Also, activities determined by basic self care or advanced daily care are also used to indicate severity of any event. Symptoms are also used to determine the grade. There was an attempt to link grading whenever feasible to either progressive symptomatic/functional status deterioration (eg, no symptoms, mild, moderate, and severe) or temporal medical/other therapeutic intervention (eg, none, indicated, urgent, and emergent). In general, Grade 1 was defined as an observable side effect with no significant clinical consequences. Grades 2 and 3 were defined as immediately observed adverse events with mild and moderate, respectively, clinical consequences. Grade 4 generally has life-threatening consequence, and Grade 5 was defined as death or not compatible with life.[39,40]

COMPARISON OF COMMON CARDIAC TOXICITIES BETWEEN CTCAE VERSIONS 3.0 AND 4.0

The CTCAE version 4.0 was released in May 2009. In this section the common cardiac toxicities in CTCAE versions 3.0 and 4.0 are presented and compared.[38–41] Moreover, a mapping document linking each CTCAE version 3.0 AE term and grade to CTCAE version 4.0 AE term and grade can be found at http://ctep.cancer.gov/protocolDevelopment/ electronic_applications/ctc.htm#ctc_mapping_ docs.

Left Ventricular Systolic Dysfunction

Left ventricular systolic dysfunction (LVSD) is a disorder characterized by reduced left ventricular function, as assessed by imaging techniques, and commonly results in heart failure. Clinical

manifestations may include dyspnea, orthopnea, and other signs and symptoms of pulmonary congestion and edema. In version 3.0, LVSD was correlated to changes in ejection fraction evident by objective testing. There are significant changes in version 4.0. Grades 1 and 2 were omitted in version 4.0. Grades 3 and 4 were defined solely on symptoms and interventions. Ejection fraction is placed into a separate terminology and is under the SOC of Investigations. These changes will help investigators with quick and appropriate grading of LVSD and trial management. **Table 6** summarizes the comparison between versions 3.0 and 4.0 regarding LVSD.

Heart Failure

As per CTCAE, HF is characterized by the inability of the heart to pump blood at an adequate volume to meet tissue metabolic requirements, or the ability to do so only at an elevation in the filling pressure. HF was not defined or graded in version 3.0, so this is a completely new entity for version 4.0. The necessity to include this terminology was acknowledged by all reviewers. With an increased number of cancer survivors who are likely to experience HF, it was also practical to add HF in version 4.0. Like all other CTCAE criteria, the grading system was focused on scaled interventions. **Table 7** summarizes the comparison between versions 3.0 and 4.0 regarding HF.

Several major societies in the United States and Europe have published extensive guidelines for the functional grading and treatment of HF. These recommendations include the 2005 American College of Cardiology/American Heart Association (ACC/AHA) guidelines with a 2009 focused update; the 2006 Canadian Cardiovascular Society consensus conference; the 2006 Heart Failure Society of America guidelines; and the 2008 European Society of Cardiology (ESC) guidelines. There is harmonization of categorizations of HF and its treatment among these societies. There was an attempt in CTCAE version 4.0 to synthesize this information and incorporate more functional or physiologic descriptors of the grading scales, and also to integrate tiers of therapeutic intervention to indicate severity. Some differences in the grading of functional classifications across these different guidelines persist (**Table 8**).

Acute Coronary Syndrome

ACS may be defined by signs and symptoms related to acute ischemia of the myocardium, most commonly secondary to coronary artery disease. The clinical presentation covers a spectrum of heart diseases from unstable angina to

Table 9
Comparison of acute coronary syndrome in CTCAE version 3.0 versus version 4.0

Grading	CTCAE v.3.0	CTCAE v.4.0	Remarks
1	—	Asymptomatic arterial narrowing without ischemia	New in version 4.0
2	Symptomatic, progressive angina; cardiac enzymes normal; hemodynamically stable	Asymptomatic and testing suggesting ischemia; stable angina	Version 4.0 is symptoms and intervention oriented
3	Symptomatic, unstable angina and/or acute myocardial infarction, cardiac enzymes abnormal, hemodynamically stable	Symptomatic and testing consistent with ischemia; unstable angina; intervention indicated	
4	Symptomatic, unstable angina and/or acute myocardial infarction, cardiac enzymes abnormal, hemodynamically unstable	Levels consistent with myocardial infarction as defined by the manufacturer	
5	Death	Death	No change

myocardial infarction. Regarding ACS, version 3.0 was already oriented to symptoms and clinical status. In version 4.0, objective laboratory findings were included to define and distinguish ACS from other acute coronary entities. **Table 9** shows the comparisons between versions 3.0 and 4.0 regarding ACS.

Atrial Fibrillation

Atrial fibrillation is defined as an arrhythmia without discernible P waves and an irregular ventricular response due to multiple atrial reentry circuits. There was no change in Grades 1, 2, and 5 between versions 3.0 and 4.0. Ablation was added to Grade 3 to indicate the evolution in the treatment management of this disorder. For Grade 4, an indication for intervention was included.

Table 10 summarizes the comparison between versions 3.0 and 4.0 regarding atrial fibrillation and these changes.

Hypertension

HTN is characterized by a pathologic increase in blood pressure with repeated elevation in the blood pressure exceeding 140 over 90 mm Hg. The grading of hypertension has been associated with international and national (Joint National Committee) guidelines. The Joint National Committee on Prevention, Detection, Evaluation and Treatment of High Blood Pressure released its seventh report and version 4.0 adopted that guideline.[42] There was an attempt to harmonize this grading of hypertension among the different authorities and assist medical scientists in both clinical and experimental

Table 10
Comparison of atrial fibrillation in CTCAE version 3.0 versus version 4.0

Grading	CTCAE v.3.0	CTCAE v.4.0	Remarks
1	Asymptomatic, intervention not indicated	Asymptomatic, intervention not indicated	No significant changes
2	Nonurgent medical intervention indicated	Nonurgent medical intervention indicated	
3	Symptomatic and incompletely controlled medically, or controlled with device (eg, pacemaker)	Symptomatic and incompletely controlled medically, or controlled with device (eg, pacemaker), or ablation	
4	Life-threatening (eg, arrhythmia associated with CHF, hypotension, syncope, shock)	Life-threatening consequences; urgent intervention indicated	Intervention oriented
5	Death	Death	No change

settings. **Table 11** summarizes the comparisons between versions 3.0 and 4.0 regarding hypertension and these changes. One issue not addressed in CTCAE version 4.0 is how to manage and grade abnormal baseline blood pressure.

QT Prolongation (Corrected)

QTc is an ECG finding characterized by an abnormally long corrected QT interval. Significant prolongation of the QT interval may predispose patients to ventricular arrhythmia. Grade 5 was omitted in version 4.0 because this is in the Investigation SOC, which is a laboratory finding that

could not lead to death by itself. In the past few years, there have been minor changes (regarding duration of QT interval) made in the definition of prolonged QTc.[25] Version 4.0 adopted these changes and is aligned with more conventional definitions. **Table 12** summarizes the comparisons between versions 3.0 and 4.0 regarding QTc and these changes.

Cardiac Disorders, Not Otherwise Specified

This terminology has the potential to include a significant number of conditions that are not

Table 11
Comparison of hypertension in CTCAE version 3.0 versus version 4.0

Grading	CTCAE v.3.0	CTCAE v.4.0	Remarks
1	Asymptomatic, transient (<24 h) increase by >20 mm Hg (diastolic) or to >150/100 if previously within normal limit (WNL); intervention not indicated Pediatric: Asymptomatic, transient (<24 h) blood pressure (BP) increase >upper limit of normal (ULN); intervention not indicated	Prehypertension (systolic BP 120–139 mm Hg or diastolic BP 80–89 mm Hg)	Version 4.0 adopted seventh report of The Joint National Committee on Prevention, Detection, Evaluation and Treatment of High Blood Pressure
2	Recurrent or persistent (≥24 h) or symptomatic increase by >20 mm Hg (diastolic) or to >150/100 if previously WNL; monotherapy may be indicated Pediatric: Recurrent or persistent (≥24 h) BP >ULN; monotherapy may be indicated	Stage 1 hypertension (systolic BP 140–159 mm Hg or diastolic BP 90–99 mm Hg); medical intervention indicated; recurrent or persistent (≥24 h); symptomatic increase by >20 mm Hg (diastolic) or to >140/90 mm Hg if previously WNL; monotherapy indicated Pediatric: recurrent or persistent (≥24 h) BP >ULN; monotherapy indicated	
3	Requiring more than one drug or more intensive therapy than previously Pediatric: Same as adult	Stage 2 hypertension (systolic BP ≥160 mm Hg or diastolic BP ≥100 mm Hg); medical intervention indicated; more than one drug or more intensive therapy than previously used indicated Pediatric: Same as adult	
4	Life-threatening consequences (eg, hypertensive crisis) Pediatric: Same as adult	Stage 2 hypertension (systolic BP ≥160 mm Hg or diastolic BP ≥100 mm Hg); medical intervention indicated; more than one drug or more intensive therapy than previously used indicated Pediatric: Same as adult	
5	Death	Death	No change

Table 12
Comparison of QT prolongation (corrected) in CTCAE version 3.0 versus version 4.0

Grading	CTCAE v.3.0	CTCAE v.4.0	Remarks
1	QTc >0.45–0.47 s	QTc 0.45–0.48 s	Version 4.0 adopted new criteria
2	QTc >0.47–0.50 s; ≥0.06 s above baseline	QTc 0.481–0.5 s	
3	QTc >0.50 s	QTc ≥0.501 s on at least 2 separate ECGs	
4	QTc >0.50 s; life-threatening signs or symptoms (eg, arrhythmia, CHF, hypotension, shock syncope); Torsade de pointes	QTc ≥0.501 or >0.60 s; change from baseline and Torsade de pointes or polymorphic ventricular tachycardia or signs/symptoms of serious arrhythmia	
5	Death	—	Omitted in version 4.0

defined elsewhere in the cardiac or Investigation SOCs.

SUMMARY

It is well documented that cardiac toxicities are becoming some of the most important complications of contemporary systemic cancer therapy and often of cancer chemoprevention. Thus, the uniform and collaborative toxicity descriptions and grading will allow a consistent reporting of cardiac side effects. Consequently, cardiac safety outcomes of newer cancer agents can be more readily compared.

The approach of cardiologists to the definition of cardiac disease secondary to systemic cancer therapy may be quite different from that of oncologists. Therefore, it is important to foster interdisciplinary interactions but, at the same time, there is a risk that many concepts and observations may well be "lost in translation." The Cardiac Disorder and Vascular Disorder SOCs in CTCAE version 4.0 were developed by a collaboration of oncologists and cardiologists. In this regard, CTCAE version 4.0 will, it is hoped, play an important and decisive role in defining and grading cardiac toxicity in cancer clinical trials. In addition, it is anticipated that the cardiology clinical trial community will consider using a standard grading system for clinical trials in a manner similar to oncology that allows comparisons between studies and populations. In version 4.0, an effort was made to be more informative with both subjective and objective data. Timing or urgency of therapeutic intervention was also included in version 4.0. With the introduction of CTCAE version 4.0, it is the authors' hope that oncologists, cardiologists, clinical investigators, and regulatory authorities will freely adapt and use the same language regarding systemic cancer therapy–related cardiac toxicities and realize the advantages of collaboration and consistency. Using more comprehensive definitions and enhancing the understanding of emerging cardiovascular toxicities already observed with newer anticancer agents will result in undoubtedly tangible improvement in overall patient care.

REFERENCES

1. Available at: www.SEER.Cancer.Gov. Accessed April 16, 2011.
2. Oeffinger KC, Mertens AC, Sklar CA, et al. Chronic health conditions in adult survivors of childhood cancer. N Engl J Med 2006;355:1572–82.
3. Pai VB, Nahata MC. Cardiotoxicity of chemotherapeutic agents: incidence, treatment and prevention. Drug Saf 2000;22:263–302.
4. Gharib MI, Burnett AK. Chemotherapy-induced cardiotoxicity: current practice and prospects of prophylaxis. Eur J Heart Fail 2002;4:235–42.
5. Van Heeckeren WJ, Bhakta S, Remick SC, et al. Promise of new vascular-disrupting agents balanced with cardiac toxicity: is it time for oncologists to get to know their cardiologists? J Clin Oncol 2006;24(10):1485–8.
6. Sereno M, Brunello A, Chiappori A, et al. Cardiac toxicity: old and new issues in anti-cancer drugs. Clin Transl Oncol 2008;10(1):35–46.
7. Yeh ET, Bickford CL. Cardiovascular complications of cancer therapy: incidence, pathogenesis, diagnosis, and management. J Am Coll Cardiol 2009; 53(24):2231–47.
8. Cardinale D. A new frontier: cardio-oncology. Cardiologia 1996;41(9):887–91.
9. Saad A, Beta R, Abraham J, et al. Cardiovascular safety and toxicity profile of new molecular targeted

anticancer agents. Alexandria (VA): American Society of Clinical Oncology; 2008. p. 428–34.

10. Lipshultz SE, Alvarez JA, Scully RE. Anthracycline associated cardiotoxicity in survivors of childhood cancer. Heart 2008;94:525–33.

11. Grenier MA, Lipshultz SE. Epidemiology of anthracycline cardiotoxicity in children and adults. Semin Oncol 1998;25:72–85.

12. Wouters KA, Kremer LC, Lipshultz SE, et al. Protecting against anthracycline-induced myocardial damage: a review of the most promising strategies. Br J Haematol 2005;131:561–78.

13. Swain SM, Whaley FC, Gerber MC, et al. Cardioprotection with dexrazoxane for doxorubicin-containing therapy in advanced breast cancer. J Clin Oncol 1997;15:1318–32.

14. Von Hoff DD, Layard MW, Basa P, et al. Risk factors for doxorubicin-induced congestive heart failure. Ann Intern Med 1979;91:710–7.

15. Swain SM, Whaley FS, Ewer MS. Congestive heart failure in patients treated with doxorubicin: a retrospective analysis of three trials. Cancer 2003;97:2869–79.

16. Quezado ZM, Wilson WH, Cunnion RE, et al. High-dose ifosfamide is associated with severe, reversible cardiac dysfunction. Ann Intern Med 1993;118:31–6.

17. Martin M, Pienkowski T, Mackey J, et al. Adjuvant docetaxel for node-positive breast cancer. N Engl J Med 2005;352:2302–13.

18. Tan-Chiu E, Yothers G, Romond E, et al. Assessment of cardiac dysfunction in a randomized trial comparing doxorubicin and cyclophosphamide followed by paclitaxel, with or without trastuzumab as adjuvant therapy in node-positive, human epidermal growth factor receptor 2-overexpressing breast cancer: NSABP B-31. J Clin Oncol 2005;23:7811–9.

19. Miller KD, Chap LI, Holmes FA, et al. Randomized phase III trial of capecitabine compared with bevacizumab plus capecitabine in patients with previously treated metastatic breast cancer. J Clin Oncol 2005;23:792–9.

20. Marty M, Cognetti F, Maraninchi D, et al. Randomized phase II trial of the efficacy and safety of trastuzumab combined with docetaxel in patients with human epidermal growth factor receptor 2-positive metastatic breast cancer administered as first-line treatment: the M77001 study group. J Clin Oncol 2005;23:4265–74.

21. Richardson PG, Sonneveld P, Schuster MW, et al. Bortezomib or high-dose dexamethasone for relapsed multiple myeloma. N Engl J Med 2005; 352:2487–98.

22. Miller K, Wang M, Gralow J, et al. Paclitaxel plus bevacizumab versus paclitaxel alone for metastatic breast cancer. N Engl J Med 2007;357:2666–76.

23. Seidman A, Hudis C, Pierri MK, et al. Cardiac dysfunction in the trastuzumab clinical trials experience. J Clin Oncol 2002;20:1215–21.

24. Chen MH, Kerkela R, Force T. Mechanisms of cardiac dysfunction associated with tyrosine kinase inhibitor cancer therapeutics. Circulation 2008;118:84–95.

25. Schall R, Ring A. Statistical characterization of QT prolongation. J Biopharm Stat 2010;20(3):543–62.

26. Chu TF, Rupnick MA, Kerkela R, et al. Cardiotoxicity associated with tyrosine kinase inhibitor sunitinib. Lancet 2007;370:2011–9.

27. Slamon DJ, Leyland-Jones B, Shak S, et al. Use of chemotherapy plus a monoclonal antibody against HER2 for metastatic breast cancer that overexpresses HER2. N Engl J Med 2001;344:783–92.

28. Perez EA, Koehler M, Ewer MS, et al. Cardiac safety of lapatinib: pooled analysis of 3689 patients enrolled in clinical trials. Mayo Clin Proc 2008;83: 679–86.

29. Kerkela P, Grazette L, Yacobi R, et al. Cardiotoxicity of the cancer therapeutic agent imatinib mesylate. Nat Med 2006;12:908–16.

30. Khakoo AY, Kassiotis CM, Tannir N, et al. Heart failure associated with sunitinib malate: a multitargeted receptor tyrosine kinase inhibitor. Cancer 2008;112:2500–8.

31. Soignet SL, Frankel SR, Douer D, et al. United States multicenter study of arsenic trioxide in relapsed acute promyelocytic leukemia. J Clin Oncol 2001; 19:3852–60.

32. Huang SY, Chang CS, Tang JL, et al. Acute and chronic arsenic poisoning associated with treatment of acute promyelocytic leukaemia. Br J Haematol 1998;103:1092–5.

33. Ohnishi K, Yoshida H, Shigeno K, et al. Arsenic trioxide therapy for relapsed or refractory Japanese patients with acute promyelocytic leukemia: need for careful electrocardiogram monitoring. Leukemia 2002;16:617–22.

34. Kaur A, Yu SS, Chiao TB. Thalidomide-induced sinus bradycardia. Ann Pharmacother 2003;37:1040–3.

35. Morandi P, Ruffini PA, Benvenuto GM, et al. Cardiac toxicity of high-dose chemotherapy. Bone Marrow Transplant 2005;35:323–34.

36. Rajkumar SV. Thalidomide therapy and deep venous thrombosis in multiple myeloma. Mayo Clin Proc 2005;80:1549–51.

37. Rodeghiero F, Elice F. Thalidomide and thrombosis. Pathophysiol Haemost Thromb 2003;33(Suppl 1): 15–8.

38. Available at: http://ctep.cancer.gov/branches/pio/reporting_guidelines.htm. Accessed April 16, 2011.

39. Available at: https://ctep.cancer.gov/protocoldevelopment. Accessed April 16, 2011.

40. Available at: https://cabig.nci.nih.gov. Accessed April 16, 2011.

41. Available at: https://cabig-kc.nci.nih.gov/Vocab/KC/index.php/CTCAE. Accessed April 16, 2011.

42. Available at: www.nhlbi.nih.gov/guidelines/hypertension/jnc7full.pdf. Accessed April 16, 2011.

Amyloidotic Cardiomyopathy: Multidisciplinary Approach to Diagnosis and Treatment

David C. Seldin, MD, PhD[a,b,]*, John L. Berk, MD[a,c], Flora Sam, MD[a,d], Vaishali Sanchorawala, MD[a,b]

KEYWORDS

- Amyloidosis • Cardiomyopathy • Transthyretin
- Immunoglobulin light chain • Matrix metalloproteinase
- Autologous stem cell transplantation • Biomarkers

AMYLOIDOTIC CARDIOMYOPATHY: NOT A RARE DISEASE

Amyloidosis is the generic term for a family of fibrillar protein deposition diseases. In the mid-19th century, pathologist Rudolf Virchow found amorphous-appearing deposits in sections of kidney, spleen, heart, and other tissues in autopsies performed on patients succumbing to untreatable infections. The investigator called them starchlike or amyloid. It is now known that amyloid deposits are composed of regular 10-nm polymeric protein fibrils; the authors surmise that Virchow was observing amyloid composed of fibrils of serum amyloid A protein, an acute phase reactant and the cause of amyloid A amyloidosis (AA) or secondary amyloidosis. AA is still found in patients with chronic mycobacterial or bacterial infections; those with rare hereditary periodic fever syndromes, such as familial Mediterranean fever; and those with refractory autoimmune diseases. Although AA most often involves the kidney, about 10% of patients develop cardiac involvement.[1]

Other forms of amyloidosis more frequently affect the heart and are more likely to be diagnosed by cardiologists. Familial amyloidosis (AF) is caused by inheritance of mutations in DNA encoding abundant serum proteins that become prone to misfolding and aggregation. Inherited mutations of transthyretin (TTR) are the most common cause of AF, producing syndromes of familial amyloidotic cardiomyopathy (FAC) and familial amyloidotic polyneuropathy (FAP), depending on the tissue tropism of the particular mutant. TTR mutations are common in regions of Portugal, Japan, and Sweden but can be found worldwide. More than 100 polymorphisms of TTR have been reported, of which more than 80 are amyloidogenic.[2] Other serum proteins that can cause inherited amyloidoses include fibrinogen, lysozyme, gelsolin, and apolipoproteins.

Funding support: NIH R01 NS051306 (J.L.B.); HL079099, HL095891, and HL102631 (F.S.)

The authors have no conflicts of interest.

[a] Amyloidosis Treatment and Research Program, Department of Medicine, Boston University School of Medicine, Boston Medical Center, K5, 72 East Concord Street, Boston, MA 02118, USA

[b] Hematology-Oncology Section, Department of Medicine, Boston Medical Center, 72 East Concord Street, Boston, MA 02118, USA

[c] Pulmonary Section, Department of Medicine, FGH1, 72 East Concord Street, Boston, MA 02118, USA

[d] Division of Cardiology, Whitaker Cardiovascular Institute, 715 Albany Street, W507, Boston, MA 02118, USA

* Corresponding author. Amyloidosis Treatment and Research Program, Department of Medicine, Boston University School of Medicine, Boston Medical Center, K5, 72 East Concord Street, Boston, MA 02118.

E-mail address: dseldin@bu.edu

heartfailure.theclinics.com

Immunoglobulin light chain amyloidosis (AL), formerly termed primary amyloidosis, is caused by fibrils composed of immunoglobulin light chains (LCs). Immunoglobulin AL can occur not only in clonal B lymphoproliferative diseases, usually in low-grade plasma cell dyscrasias, but also in multiple myeloma, B cell lymphoma, chronic lymphocytic leukemia, or Waldenström macroglobulinemia. As many as 50% of patients with AL have cardiac involvement, which is often rapidly progressive and fatal if untreated.

The hereditary and acquired forms of amyloidosis are relatively rare. However, just as normal aging is accompanied by the development of Aβ plaques in the brain, it is also accompanied by the formation of amyloid deposits in other tissues, of which the heart is the organ in which this deposition is most clinically apparent. This syndrome is termed senile systemic amyloidosis (SSA), sometimes termed senile cardiac amyloidosis. In SSA, the fibrils are formed of wild-type TTR protein. Histopathologic evidence of SSA can be found in 10% to 25% of people older than 80 years and in almost all centenarians,[3] but how frequently SSA causes amyloidotic cardiomyopathy (ACMP) is uncertain. Nonetheless, in an aging population, SSA and the associated ACMP are increasingly recognized by cardiologists investigating diastolic or systolic hypertrophic cardiomyopathy (CMP) and heart failure (HF).

Thus, ACMP can occur as a consequence of a blood disorder, an inherited genetic disease, or a part of normal aging. As more and more effective therapies are developed for these disorders, accurate and timely diagnosis has become increasingly important for patients.

DIAGNOSIS OF ACMP: CLINICAL SUSPICION PLUS APPROPRIATE LABORATORY INVESTIGATION

First and foremost, the key to the diagnosis of amyloidosis is to consider the diagnosis. Amyloidosis, not syphilis, is the great mimic of the twenty-first century because it can masquerade as more common disorders capable of causing nephrotic syndrome and renal insufficiency, cholestatic liver failure, malabsorption and gastrointestinal bleeding, or peripheral or autonomic neuropathy. For ACMP, the typical presentation is with symptoms of HF with preserved left ventricular function, manifesting first as nonspecific symptoms of fatigue, exertional dyspnea, and hypotension (**Box 1**). These symptoms progress over time, eventually to systolic HF. As discussed later, HF due to amyloidosis is refractory to many of the usual interventions. The amyloidotic heart is also highly

---

Box 1
Symptoms and signs of cardiac amyloidosis

Common symptoms
- Fatigue
- Exertional dyspnea
- Edema

Uncommon symptoms
- Jaw or buttock claudication
- Atypical chest pain

Physical findings
- Rales
- Pitting edema
- Elevated jugular venous pressure
- Hepatojugular reflux
- Adventitious third heart sound

Electrocardiographic findings
- Low-voltage electrocardiograph
- Atrial fibrillation
- Ventricular arrhythmias

Echocardiographic findings
- Concentric hypertrophy
- Thickened interventricular septum
- Diastolic dysfunction
- Systolic dysfunction (late)

---

susceptible to heart block and arrhythmia, likely as a result of deposition of fibrils in the conducting system. Progressive HF and sudden death are the most common causes of death in patients with ACMP because of ventricular arrhythmias or pulseless electrical activity (PEA). Atrial arrhythmias are also common.

Amyloidosis should be suspected in patients who present with unexplained nephrotic syndrome, cholestatic liver disease, autonomic neuropathy, peripheral neuropathy, CMP with concentric hypertrophy, or combinations of these syndromes. Pathognomonic symptoms and signs of amyloidosis include macroglossia and periorbital purpura, and these findings should be promptly pursued.

With respect to the heart, patients usually come to the attention of cardiologists for evaluation of exertional dyspnea, fatigue, or hypotension. Chest pain due to amyloid in epicardial coronary vessels is rare, although patients with amyloidosis in small arterioles and capillaries may develop atypical chest pain, jaw claudication with chewing, or buttock claudication with ambulation. Hypotension can occur because of a combination of cardiac dysfunction and autonomic insufficiency.

Such symptoms are evaluated by echocardiography to assess cardiac structure and function.

Textbooks describe a classic "sparkly" pattern on echocardiography that was actually an artifact produced by low-resolution imaging and is not seen as commonly with modern equipment. The common echocardiographic features of ACMP are concentric hypertrophy of the ventricular walls, biatrial enlargement, and abnormal diastolic filling parameters and, commonly, mild to moderate valvular regurgitation. HF symptoms can occur with minimal ventricular wall thickening. The standard electrocardiogram can provide a tip-off to the presence of an infiltrative CMP because the limb lead voltages are often reduced rather than increased as in other hypertrophic CMPs. Cardiac magnetic resonance imaging can identify structural and functional abnormalities consistent with amyloidosis, and a phenomenon of delayed subendocardial enhancement with gadolinium has been reported.[4] The only specific scan for amyloid deposits is done using labeled serum amyloid P (SAP) component,[5] an accessory protein that binds to amyloid fibrils and has been postulated to protect amyloid fibrils from degradation. However, this scan is not useful for diagnosing cardiac amyloidosis because the tracer pools in the heart; furthermore, SAP scanning is not available in the United States.

The gold standard for diagnosing amyloidosis is a tissue biopsy demonstrating the presence of fibrils that bind the dye Congo red, producing apple-green birefringence under polarized microscopy (**Table 1**). Fibrils can also be identified by electron microscopy as rodlike bundles that are 10 nm in diameter. The most accessible site for demonstration of fibrils is in fat readily obtained by aspiration from the abdominal wall using an 18-gauge syringe needle after administering a local anesthetic. The result of the fat test is positive in 65% to 95% of cases, depending on the type of systemic amyloidosis.[6] If the result is negative in a patient suspected of having amyloidosis, the next step is usually to proceed with biopsy of an affected organ, although biopsies of salivary glands and the rectum are other sources of tissue that frequently show positive results. In patients with cardiac symptoms and signs indicating amyloidosis without clinically detectable involvement of other organs, an endomyocardial biopsy would be performed next. Biopsy material should be fixed in formalin and also in paraformaldehyde for immunoelectron microscopy, in case immunohistochemical studies fail to identify the subunit protein by light microscopy.

Once amyloid fibrils are identified, the next step is to establish the type of amyloid protein, a critical step in determining treatment. Multiple modalities are used to do this step. Patients with AL almost always have evidence of a clonal plasma cell process by one or more of the following tests: bone marrow immunohistochemistry or flow cytometry for κ and λ LCs, serum or urine immunofixation electrophoresis (the standard serum and urine immunofixation electrophoreses are usually normal because there is rarely enough monoclonal immunoglobulin to be detected with these techniques), or serum free LC testing using the Freelite Assay, a relatively new test marketed internationally by the Binding Site Co. Normally, almost all LCs are associated with immunoglobulin heavy chains to form tetramers. In plasma cell diseases, the levels of free LC are elevated and can be detected by nephelometry using specific antibodies. Unlike whole immunoglobulins, LCs are rapidly excreted by the kidney and have a half-life of only 6 hours; so, measurement of serum-free LCs provides an early measure of disease response in patients undergoing treatment, aiding diagnosis.

Table 1
Workup of cardiac amyloidosis

Assay	AL	ATTR	AA	SSA	Source
Congo Red Fibrils	+	+	+	+	Pathology laboratory
Serum and Urine Immunofixation Electrophoresis for Monoclonal Immunoglobulin	+	−	−	−	Clinical laboratory
Serum Free LCs	+	−	−	−	Binding Site, Quest
Abnormal TTR Isoelectric Focusing	−	+	−	−	Specialty laboratory
Abnormal TTR Gene Sequence	−	+	−	−	Specialty laboratory, Athena
Kappa or Lambda Immunohistochemistry	+	−	−	−	Pathology laboratory
TTR Immunohistochemistry	−	+	−	+	Pathology laboratory
Amyloid A Immunohistochemistry	−	−	+	−	Pathology laboratory
Mass Spectrometry Protein Identification	+	+	+	+	Specialty laboratory

Patients with TTR amyloidosis (ATTR) or other hereditary forms of amyloidosis have DNA mutations that can be detected by gene sequencing. However, the presence of a mutation or a plasma cell disorder is not conclusive for identifying the amyloid type, and in most cases, immunochemical or biochemical identification is essential. However, amyloid fibrils are notoriously sticky and bind many antibodies nonspecifically, so careful controls, immunoelectron microscopy with gold-labeled antibodies, and extraction or microdissection of the fibrils and identification by mass spectrometry are important confirmatory tests, which are available in specialized centers. Misdiagnosis and inappropriate application of chemotherapy should be avoided.

MECHANISMS OF CARDIAC DYSFUNCTION IN ACMP

Cardiac dysfunction in amyloidosis has been attributed to the deposition of amyloid fibrils and physical disruption of the integrity of the myocardial syncytium. However, clinical observation has shown that the degree of cardiac dysfunction is not necessarily proportional to the thickness of the walls; thus, it has been hypothesized that amyloid may have other effects on the heart. For example, CMP in AL has the worst prognosis and most rapid progression, although wall thickness in patients with this condition may be much less than in those with ATTR or SSA[7,8] in whom wall thickness can exceed 2 cm. A likely explanation is that prefibrillar LC oligomers have direct toxic effects on cardiomyocyte function, impairing excitation-contraction coupling via increased oxidant stress[9,10] mediated by p38 MAPK signaling.[11]

Extracellular amyloid fibrils also seem to disrupt cardiac matrix homeostasis and alter extracellular matrix (ECM) turnover.[12] Regulated ECM turnover is critical for the maintenance of myocyte-myocyte force coupling and proper myocardial function. Disruption of the ECM alters matrix metalloproteinases (MMPs) and their tissue inhibitors in AL CMP. As a result, matrix degradation is impaired. Reactive oxygen species alter myocardial MMP activity by translational and posttranslational mechanisms, activating MMPs and decreasing fibrillar collagen synthesis in cardiomyocytes, contributing to the accelerated clinical manifestations of the disease.

CARDIAC BIOMARKERS AND RISK STRATIFICATION IN AL

The extent of ACMP is the single most important determinant of outcome in AL.[13] The concentration of cardiac biomarkers, B-type natriuretic peptide (BNP) and troponins, has been shown to be elevated with cardiac stress and cardiomyocyte damage caused by amyloidogenic LC. These biomarkers have been useful for both diagnosis and prognosis.

Criteria for the assessment of cardiac involvement at baseline and of cardiac response after treatment have been established by an international consensus panel.[14] Short of endomyocardial biopsy, electrocardiography and echocardiography were accepted as the gold standards for the diagnosis of heart involvement by amyloidosis. Recently, it has been shown that serum cardiac troponin T (CTnT) and serum cardiac troponin I (CTnI) as well as BNPs (either BNP or N-terminal-proBNP [NT-proBNP]) are highly sensitive markers of cardiac involvement, and normal values exclude clinically significant cardiac amyloidosis.[15] Furthermore, an analysis of outcomes for 242 patients with AL demonstrated that patients could be divided into 3 prognostic groups based on elevation of NT-proBNP and troponin levels (NT-proBNP>332 ng/L, CTnT>0.035 µg/L, and CTnI>0.1 µg/L).[16] Patients with normal proBNP and troponin levels in this study had a median survival of about 2 years and were designated as stage I. Patients with either biomarker elevated were categorized into stage II and had a median survival of slightly less than a year. Patients with both cardiac biomarkers elevated were categorized into stage III, corresponding to a median survival of only 3 to 4 months (**Table 2**).

In addition, among patients with cardiac involvement, cardiac troponins provide quantitative information about myocardial damage. Median survivals of patients with elevated CTnT and CTnI levels were 6 and 8 months, respectively, and worse than that for those with undetectable values (22 and 21 months, respectively). After multivariate analysis, CTnT provided a better predictor of survival than CTnI.[17] Nonetheless,

Table 2 Cardiac biomarker staging system		
Staging	NT-proBNP, 332 ng/L; CTnT, 0.035 µg/L	Median Survival (mo)
I	Neither elevated	26
II	One elevated	11
III	Both elevated	4

Data from Dispenzieri A, Gertz MA, Kyle RA, et al. Serum cardiac troponins and N-terminal pro-brain natriuretic peptide: a staging system for primary systemic amyloidosis. J Clin Oncol 2004;22:3751.

the baseline CTnI has also been shown to be an excellent predictor of relative survival.[18]

Based on these studies, biomarker criteria for cardiac involvement and improvement and progression after therapy are now being incorporated into the consensus for organ involvement and response.[19] Furthermore, reductions in levels of cardiac biomarkers from baseline also correlate with improvement in survival after treatment in patients with cardiac involvement; a 30% or 300 ng/L decrease in the NT-proBNP level from baseline correlates with improved survival, whereas an increase of that magnitude correlates with progression and worse survival posttreatment.

AL TREATMENT

Treatment of AL is aimed at eradicating the plasma cell clone that produces the deleterious fibril-forming LC. The first attempt to do this was by using oral dosing of the alkylating chemotherapy melphalan, accompanied by prednisone. In AL, 2 outcomes are assessed: hematologic responses (reduction in the plasma cell clone and LC production) and clinical responses (improvement in organ function). Studies have demonstrated that these outcomes are linked, and treatments that significantly reduce production of the LC fibril precursor, for example, by 90% or more, are those that can be associated with clinical improvement. Melphalan and prednisone are relatively ineffective because partial (50%) responses occur in only 20% to 25% of patients and deeper responses and improvements in organ function were rare. Thus, there was little impetus to make the diagnosis and initiate therapy, and most patients died of their disease within the first 1 to 2 years of diagnosis.

About 15 years ago, the authors and other centers took advantage of accumulating data from the myeloma field indicating that high-dose intravenous melphalan (HDM) supported by transplant of autologous bone marrow stem cells (SCT) could produce complete or near-complete hematologic responses and transferred this approach, with some trepidation, to patients with AL. Over the next few years, it was learned that a high rate of complete hematologic responses can be achieved, and organ function can then improve. However, inexperienced centers have had treatment-related mortality (TRM) rates as high as 30% to 40%. In a multicenter randomized trial from France that compared outcomes of HDM/SCT to oral melphalan chemotherapy, 25% of enrolled patients in the HDM/SCT group did not receive their transplant and another 25% died because of TRM.[20] At Boston Medical Center, the authors have observed that the TRM in the early years was 14%[21] and more recently has been reduced to less than 5%. Thus, with careful selection of patients and expert multidisciplinary care, morbidity and mortality during HDM/SCT can be minimized.

The first step in this treatment involves harvesting hematopoietic stem cells. At present, this harvesting is almost always accomplished by leukapheresis of peripheral blood after administration of high-dose myeloid growth factors, usually granulocyte colony-stimulating factor (G-CSF), that promote hematopoietic stem cell division and egress from the bone marrow. It is rare to subject patients to bone marrow harvest. For those patients who fail to mobilize enough cells with G-CSF, plerixafor, an antagonist of the CXCR4 chemokine receptor, can be administered, which promotes release of stem cells from the bone marrow stroma. Hematopoietic stem cells are then cryopreserved while patients undergo treatment with high doses of antiplasma cell chemotherapy that is myeloablative. Melphalan is the most useful alkylating chemotherapy agent for this purpose. With the reinfusion of stem cells 1 to 2 days after chemotherapy, the hematopoietic system is soon reconstituted, with neutrophil engraftment typically occurring 10 days later and platelet and erythrocyte engraftments a few days after. It is this period of pancytopenia during which patients are at highest risk of infection and also mucositis and enteritis because of the melphalan. During this period, shifts in fluid and electrolyte levels, stress, fever, fatigue, cytokines, and infection provide a significant stress on the heart, and it is not infrequent for patients to have their first atrial or ventricular arrhythmia during this period. Exacerbation of HF symptoms frequently occurs. Even the administration of high doses of G-CSF during the prechemotherapy period can precipitate such events. Guidelines for the management of congestive HF (CHF) and arrhythmias in patients with amyloidosis are provided below.[22]

However, if this treatment can be administered safely, the outcomes are excellent. Patients who have cessation of LC production after HDM/SCT are able to recover organ function. The authors have demonstrated significant improvement in nephrotic syndrome and recently in wall thickness by echocardiography.[23] Hepatomegaly also regresses in many patients. More subjective symptoms of fatigue, lightheadedness, anorexia, and gut dysmotility also improve, as does quality of life. However, this improvement is a slow process, and patients often require extensive supportive care for 6 to 12 months as their performance status and immunologic function slowly improves.

Patients with advanced ACMP are at high risk of complications, and such patients should be identified using clinical criteria or biomarkers and generally excluded from undergoing HDM/SCT. The standard alternative chemotherapy regimen is considered to be pulse oral melphalan combined with dexamethasone, which is fairly well tolerated and can produce hematologic responses and organ improvement.[24] Nonetheless, patients with ACMP are poorly tolerant of multiday pulses of high-dose corticosteroids, and the authors generally use a less-intensive regimen of dexamethasone 1 day a week, instead of 4 consecutive days once or twice a month. It is also common for patients with significant ACMP or edema due to nephrotic syndrome to require dose reduction from the typical starting dose of 40 mg each day to 20 mg or even 10 mg.

Multiple myeloma treatment has undergone a transformation in the last 5 or so years with the advent of novel antiplasma cell agents. These agents fall into 2 major classes of proven efficacy: the immunomodulator drugs (so-called IMiDs), of which thalidomide was the first in class, and the proteasome inhibitors, of which bortezomib (Velcade) was the first and only one so far achieving Food and Drug Administration approval. The IMiDs are thought to act on the bone marrow microenvironment, affecting stromal-plasma cell interactions, cytokines, and angiogenesis. The proteasome inhibitors seem to be more directly plasma cytotoxic, perhaps, because plasma cells are antibody factories particularly susceptible to disruption of intracellular proteolytic pathways. Thalidomide, its newer analogs lenalidomide and pomalidomide, and bortezomib have all been studied in patients with AL and have shown to provide effective antiplasma cell activity. These drugs clearly have a role in the treatment of AL, alone or in combination. It is too soon to argue that these agents can replace HDM/SCT in good-risk patients, but further clinical trials will undoubtedly demonstrate that these agents have a role in patients who are ineligible for HDM/SCT or in those in whom the treatment fails or the condition relapses or perhaps in induction or as maintenance therapy.

However, these agents are not benign, particularly in patients with AL. Thalidomide was marketed in Europe as a sedative, until a high rate of birth defects was observed; thus, IMiDs are highly regulated, and pregnancy must be avoided during their use. In addition, IMiDs are prothrombotic, and patients must take aspirin or full warfarin anticoagulation when they are on IMiDs. IMiDs also have cardiac effects; thalidomide has been reported to cause bradycardia, and lenalidomide has been noted recently to raise the BNP level. IMiDs can also produce worsening azotemia in patients with amyloid renal disease.[25] These agents are used at lower doses in AL than in multiple myeloma, and patients must be monitored closely for the earlier-mentioned and other side effects.

Bortezomib has a different spectrum of toxicities, with neuropathy being a common dose-related side effect. The cardiac side effects of bortezomib are less well understood, although exacerbations of CHF and arrhythmia have been seen and cardiotoxicity has been replicated in animal models.[26] These agents should still be considered to be investigational in patients with AL.

HEREDITARY TTR AMYLOIDOSIS

Variant ATTR arises from point mutations in exons 1 to 4 of the TTR exons on chromosome 18, resulting in more than 100 identified single amino acid substitutions. Disease prevalence is estimated at 1 in 100,000 people in the United States, giving ATTR orphan disease status (<200,000 affected in the United States). One ATTR mutation, V122I, is found in 3.9% of the African American population; however, the rate of clinical expression is undefined, and African Americans are still more likely to present with symptomatic AL CMP than FAC.[27] In contrast, the ATTR carrier frequency in northern Portugal is 100 times more than the prevalence in the United States, and in certain northern Swedish communities, ATTR affects 3% to 5% of the population.

The clinical spectrum of ATTR is variable and dependent on the nature of the mutation. Most TTR mutations induce peripheral and/or autonomic neuropathy (FAP), followed by amyloid CMP (FAC) and, less frequently, renal disease. V30 M typically induces neuropathy and rarely affects the heart, whereas T60A and V122I almost exclusively produce CMP and infrequently affect peripheral nerves. FAC is predominant for approximately 40 ATTR variants. The course of TTR FAC differs from AL-related heart dysfunction. In contrast to the rapidly deteriorating course of AL CMP, FAC develops slowly and patients are often asymptomatic until the amyloid involvement of the myocardium is advanced in late stages of disease. Although oligomeric LCs themselves seem to be deleterious on myocardial contractility, variant TTR does not seem to affect heart function (L. W. Connors, PhD, personal communication, 2010). However, ATTR CMP more often presents with conduction delays or complete heart block than AL CMP.

TTR is almost exclusively produced by the liver, with minor quantities made by the choroid plexus and retinal epithelium. In an effort to eliminate variant TTR production and prevent continued amyloid fibril formation, liver transplant was first performed in Sweden in 1990. To date, more than 1700 liver transplants have been undertaken in patients with ATTR (see the Familial Amyloidotic Polyneuropathy World Transplant Registry at http://www.fapwtr.org/). Although well tolerated, liver transplants have not proven the panacea they were predicted to be. Once fibril formation has begun, it seems that in some cases wild-type TTR made by the transplanted liver can be incorporated into the amyloid deposits and the disease can progress.[28,29] These findings led to recommendations to limit liver transplant in ATTR to patients with early neurologic disease and minimal signs of cardiac amyloid deposition. For those with ATTR CMP, 2 therapeutic options remain: heart and liver transplant or experimental medical therapies.

Over the past decade, experiments examining the thermodynamic landscape of ATTR fibril formation determined that disaggregation of native TTR tetramer represented the critical and rate-limiting steps. Small molecules occupying the thyroid-binding sites raised the activation barrier for TTR tetramer dissociation. Using x-ray crystallography to characterize the thyroid-binding site and high throughput modeling, Dr Jeffery Kelly (The Scripps Research Institute) identified a nonsteroidal antiinflammatory drug (NSAID), diflunisal, as a candidate small-molecule inhibitor of ATTR fibril formation. At the same time, FoldRx Pharmaceutical (Cambridge, MA, USA) developed a proprietary small-molecule inhibitor, tafamidis, designed to maximize ATTR tetramer binding and eliminate potential NSAID toxicities. Both agents inhibit ATTR fibril formation in vitro. These independent investigational programs led to separate international multicenter randomized placebo-controlled studies; results are pending. Small-molecule inhibitors, RNA interference, or protein stabilizers appear to be the future of ATTR management, particularly in patients with amyloid CMP at disease presentation in whom liver transplant may not halt progression.

MANAGEMENT OF HF AND ARRHYTHMIAS IN PATIENTS WITH ACMP

Regardless of the specific treatment directed against the plasma cell dyscrasia, supportive care to decrease symptoms and support organ function plays an important role in the management of disease and requires coordinated care by specialists in multiple disciplines.

The mainstay of the treatment of HF in ACMP is sodium restriction and the use of diuretics; higher doses may be required if the serum albumin level is low as a result of concomitant nephrotic syndrome. Furthermore, achieving a balance between HF and intravascular volume depletion is particularly challenging, especially in patients with autonomic nervous system involvement or nephrotic syndrome. Diuretic resistance is common in patients with severe nephrotic syndrome, and metolazone or spironolactone may be required in conjunction with loop diuretics. In a patient with anasarca, intravenous diuresis is often needed because absorption of diuretics may be impaired. Diuretic-resistant large pleural effusions may indicate the presence of pleural amyloid.[30] Such effusions can be managed with repeated thoracenteses or placement of indwelling pleural catheters for continuous drainage; pleurodesis is often ineffective and is frequently complicated by pneumothorax because of friable pleural tissue.

In contrast to other types of HF, in ACMP, there is no evidence that drugs such as β-blockers or angiotensin-converting enzyme (ACE) inhibitors are beneficial; in fact, their use can be quite dangerous. Any of these drugs should be used cautiously in ACMP, starting with a low dose administered in a monitored setting because even small doses may result in profound hypotension. β-Blockers and calcium channel blockers may produce hypotension because of their negative inotropic effect.[31–33] Patients with ACMP may be hypersensitive to ACE inhibitors because in the setting of amyloid-induced autonomic dysfunction, there may be increased reliance on the renin-angiotensin system for maintenance of adequate blood pressure. There are no published data on the use of intravenous inotropic or vasodilator drugs in patients with severe HF resulting from amyloidosis. Renal-dose dopamine (1–3 μg/kg/min) can be helpful for the treatment of anasarca, provided that renal function is unimpaired. Patients may be particularly prone to dysrhythmias at higher doses of dopamine or with dobutamine therapy.

Digoxin is also not generally useful in amyloidosis, and patients may be at an increased risk of digoxin toxicity, despite therapeutic serum digoxin levels. Digoxin has been shown to bind avidly to amyloid fibrils,[34] leading to high local levels of the drug in the myocardium.

Thus, options for medical management of patients with severe ACMP are limited. In highly selected cases, orthotopic heart transplant may be considered. Early experience with cardiac transplant in AL suggested that mortality did not differ from that in other disorders,[35] but with longer follow-up, greater mortality than expected was observed, usually because of disease progression in the heart or other organs.[36] As a result of these observations, many solid organ transplantation centers consider AL a contraindication to heart transplant. However, with the advent of high-dose chemotherapy and stem cell transplant, it is possible to transplant the heart and perform chemotherapy 6 to 12 months later to eliminate the underlying plasma cell dyscrasia, preventing amyloid deposition in the transplanted heart and other organs. Several patients have been treated successfully with this combined approach and have an actuarial survival that is similar to that of patients undergoing heart transplant for other indications.[37,38]

Arrhythmias occur frequently in patients with ACMP,[22] yet the optimal management of arrhythmias in these patients with ACMP remains controversial. Atrial fibrillation can often be suppressed with amiodarone. Patients who fail amiodarone or do not tolerate it may be candidates for ablation procedures. Patients with atrial fibrillation should be anticoagulated if possible, although patients who have amyloidosis are often prone to bleeding because of capillary fragility or deficiency of circulating clotting factors. Furthermore, in severe ACMP, the atria as well as the ventricles are infiltrated, and atrial contractile dysfunction may be present even during sinus rhythm, predisposing to atrial thrombus formation.[39] It is therefore prudent to anticoagulate patients with amyloidosis if there is defective left atrial mechanical activity on echocardiography, even in the absence of fibrillation.[40]

Management of ventricular arrhythmias is challenging, and evidence-based guidelines are lacking. Patients with recurrent syncope or symptomatic ventricular arrhythmias may also be treated with amiodarone, which can suppress ectopy but has not been proved to reduce mortality from sudden death because of ventricular fibrillation or PEA. Implantable defibrillators have been used, again without clear proof of efficacy. The infiltrated myocardium may be difficult to cardiovert. Nonetheless, anecdotal evidence supports the use of implantable defibrillators in selected cases.

SUMMARY

ACMP occurs in the setting of genetic diseases, blood dyscrasias, chronic infections and inflammation, and advanced age. Cardiologists are on the front lines of diagnosis of ACMP when evaluating patients with unexplained dyspnea, CHF, or arrhythmias. Noninvasive detection of diastolic cardiac dysfunction and unexplained left ventricular hypertrophy should be followed by biopsy to demonstrate the presence of amyloid deposits and appropriate genetic, biochemical, and immunologic testing to accurately define the type of amyloid. Growing treatment options exist for these diseases, and timely diagnosis and institution of therapy is essential for preservation of cardiac function.

REFERENCES

1. Girnius S, Dember L, Doros G, et al. The changing face of AA amyloidosis: a single centre experience. Amyloid 2010;17(Suppl 1): 72.
2. Connors LH, Richardson AM, Theberge R, et al. Tabulation of transthyretin (TTR) variants as of 1/1/2000. Amyloid 2000;7:54.
3. Gustavsson A, Jahr H, Tobiassen R, et al. Amyloid fibril composition and transthyretin gene structure in senile systemic amyloidosis. Lab Invest 1995; 73:703.
4. Ruberg FL, Appelbaum E, Davidoff R, et al. Diagnostic and prognostic utility of cardiovascular magnetic resonance imaging in light-chain cardiac amyloidosis. Am J Cardiol 2009;103:544.
5. Hawkins PN, Aprile C, Capri G, et al. Scintigraphic imaging and turnover studies with iodine-131 labeled serum amyloid P component in systemic amyloidosis. Eur J Nucl Med 1998;25:701.
6. Libbey CA, Skinner M, Cohen AS. Use of abdominal fat tissue aspirate in the diagnosis of systemic amyloidosis. Arch Intern Med 1983;143:1549.
7. Dubrey SW, Cha K, Skinner M, et al. Familial and primary (AL) cardiac amyloidosis: echocardiographically similar diseases with distinctly different clinical outcomes [see comments]. Heart 1997;78:74.
8. Ng B, Connors LH, Davidoff R, et al. Senile systemic amyloidosis presenting with heart failure: a comparison with light chain-associated amyloidosis. Arch Intern Med 2005;165:1425.
9. Brenner DA, Jain M, Pimentel DR, et al. Human amyloidogenic light chains directly impair cardiomyocyte function through an increase in cellular oxidant stress. Circ Res 2004;94:1008.
10. Liao R, Jain M, Teller P, et al. Infusion of light chains from patients with cardiac amyloidosis causes diastolic dysfunction in isolated mouse hearts. Circulation 2001;104:1594.
11. Shi J, Guan J, Jiang B, et al. Amyloidogenic light chains induce cardiomyocyte contractile dysfunction and apoptosis via a non-canonical p38alpha MAPK pathway. Proc Natl Acad Sci U S A 2010; 107:4188.
12. Biolo A, Ramamurthy S, Connors LH, et al. Matrix metalloproteinases and their tissue inhibitors in cardiac amyloidosis: relationship to structural,

functional myocardial changes and to light chain amyloid deposition. Circ Heart Fail 2008;1:249.

13. Obici L, Perfetti V, Palladini G, et al. Clinical aspects of systemic amyloid diseases. Biochim Biophys Acta 2005;1753:11.

14. Gertz MA, Comenzo R, Falk RH, et al. Definition of organ involvement and treatment response in immunoglobulin light chain amyloidosis (AL): a consensus opinion from the 10th International Symposium on Amyloid and Amyloidosis, Tours, France, 18-22 April 2004. Am J Hematol 2005;79:319.

15. Palladini G, Campana C, Klersy C, et al. Serum N-terminal pro-brain natriuretic peptide is a sensitive marker of myocardial dysfunction in AL amyloidosis. Circulation 2003;107:2440.

16. Dispenzieri A, Gertz MA, Kyle RA, et al. Serum cardiac troponins and N-terminal pro-brain natriuretic peptide: a staging system for primary systemic amyloidosis. J Clin Oncol 2004;22:3751.

17. Dispenzieri A, Kyle RA, Gertz MA, et al. Survival in patients with primary systemic amyloidosis and raised serum cardiac troponins. Lancet 2003;361:1787.

18. Apridonidze T, Comenzo R, Hoffman J, et al. Troponin as a prognostic marker in cardiac amyloidosis. Amyloid 2010;17:167a.

19. Gertz M, Merlini G. Definition of organ involvement and response to treatment in AL amyloidosis: an updated consensus opinion. Amyloid 2010;17:48a.

20. Jaccard A, Moreau P, Leblond V, et al. High-dose melphalan versus melphalan plus dexamethasone for AL amyloidosis. N Engl J Med 2007;357:1083.

21. Skinner M, Sanchorawala V, Seldin DC, et al. High-dose melphalan and autologous stem-cell transplantation in patients with AL amyloidosis: an 8-year study. Ann Intern Med 2004;140:85.

22. Goldsmith YB, Liu J, Chou J, et al. Frequencies and types of arrhythmias in patients with systemic light-chain amyloidosis with cardiac involvement undergoing stem cell transplantation on telemetry monitoring. Am J Cardiol 2009;104:990.

23. Meier-Ewert HK, Sanchorawala V, Berk J, et al. Regression of cardiac wall thickness following chemotherapy and stem-cell transplantation for AL amyloidosis. Amyloid 2010;17(Suppl 1):150.

24. Palladini G, Perfetti V, Obici L, et al. Association of melphalan and high-dose dexamethasone is effective and well tolerated in patients with AL (primary) amyloidosis who are ineligible for stem cell transplantation. Blood 2004;103:2936.

25. Specter R, Sanchorawala V, Seldin DC, et al. Kidney dysfunction during lenalidomide treatment for AL amyloidosis. Nephrol Dial Transplant 2011;26:881.

26. Nowis D, Maczewski M, Mackiewicz U, et al. Cardiotoxicity of the anticancer therapeutic agent bortezomib. Am J Pathol 2010;176:2658.

27. Connors LH, Prokaeva T, Lim A, et al. Cardiac amyloidosis in African Americans: comparison of clinical and laboratory features of transthyretin V122I amyloidosis and immunoglobulin light chain amyloidosis. Am Heart J 2009;158:607.

28. Dubrey SW, Davidoff R, Skinner M, et al. Progression of ventricular wall thickening after liver transplantation for familial amyloidosis. Transplantation 1997;64:74.

29. Liepnieks JJ, Benson MD. Progression of cardiac amyloid deposition in hereditary transthyretin amyloidosis patients after liver transplantation. Amyloid 2007;14:277.

30. Berk JL, Keane J, Seldin DC, et al. Persistent pleural effusions in primary systemic amyloidosis: etiology and prognosis. Chest 2003;124:969.

31. Gertz MA, Falk RH, Skinner M, et al. Worsening of congestive heart failure in amyloid heart disease treated by calcium channel-blocking agents. Am J Cardiol 1985;55:1645.

32. Gertz MA, Skinner M, Connors LH, et al. Selective binding of nifedipine to amyloid fibrils. Am J Cardiol 1985;55:1646.

33. Pollak A, Falk RH. Left ventricular systolic dysfunction precipitated by verapamil in cardiac amyloidosis. Chest 1993;104:618.

34. Rubinow A, Skinner M, Cohen AS. Digoxin sensitivity in amyloid cardiomyopathy. Circulation 1981;63:1285.

35. Hosenpud JD, Uretsky BF, Griffith BP, et al. Successful intermediate-term outcome for patients with cardiac amyloidosis undergoing heart transplantation: results of a multicenter survey. J Heart Transplant 1990;9:346.

36. Hosenpud JD, DeMarco T, Frazier OH, et al. Progression of systemic disease and reduced long-term survival in patients with cardiac amyloidosis undergoing heart transplantation. Follow-up results of a multicenter survey. Circulation 1991;84:III338.

37. Dey BR, Chung SS, Spitzer TR, et al. Cardiac transplantation followed by dose-intensive melphalan and autologous stem-cell transplantation for light chain amyloidosis and heart failure. Transplantation 2010;90:905.

38. Lacy MQ, Dispenzieri A, Hayman SR, et al. Autologous stem cell transplant after heart transplant for light chain (AL) amyloid cardiomyopathy. J Heart Lung Transplant 2008;27:823.

39. Modesto KM, Dispenzieri A, Cauduro SA, et al. Left atrial myopathy in cardiac amyloidosis: implications of novel echocardiographic techniques. Eur Heart J 2005;26:173.

40. Feng D, Syed IS, Martinez M, et al. Intracardiac thrombosis and anticoagulation therapy in cardiac amyloidosis. Circulation 2009;119:2490.

Interventional Strategies to Manage Heart Failure in Patients with Cancer

Charles Porter, MD[a],*, David Slosky, MD[b]

KEYWORDS

- Heart failure • Cancer • Cardiovascular disease
- Interventional strategies

THE INCREASING IMPORTANCE OF CONSIDERING PATIENTS WITH CANCER FOR CARDIAC INTERVENTION

Cancer survivors and those being treated for cancer comprise a significant segment of the population and continue to grow largely because of the success of cancer therapy and the aging population. In 2006, more than 11 million Americans were alive after having ever been diagnosed with some form of invasive cancer. Approximately 1.7 million (14.5%) who had been diagnosed with cancer were longer-term survivors who had been diagnosed at least 20 years earlier.[1] As a result of improved treatment for cancer, these conditions are not typically rapidly lethal and effectively cancer has been converted into a chronic condition that needs to be managed. Additionally, patients commonly manifest cardiovascular (CV) disease during a more protracted treatment for cancer and thus require a careful evaluation for underlying or resultant CV disease.

THE CHANGING FACES OF CANCER SURVIVAL VARIES BY TUMOR

The recent striking declines in the 2 major causes of death in the United States, heart disease and cancer, require the clinician to keep abreast of how changes in mortality impact bedside decision making in patients with both conditions. There has been a 30% decline in 5-year mortality rates from all cancers between periods ending in 1984 to 1986 and 1999 to 2005[2] with a 29.5% decline in cardiovascular disease mortality rate in the decade between 1996 and 2006.[3] As treatments and outcomes have improved with both diseases, it is important and challenging for both the oncologist and cardiologist to stay current with recommended guidelines and approaches to patient care.

When considering how the prognosis of a malignancy should be balanced against the morbidity and benefits of a cardiac intervention, guidance may be gained from the statement in the current American Heart Association/American College of Cardiology guideline for heart failure regarding cardiac resynchronization therapy: "Placement of an implantable cardioverter-defibrillator is reasonable in patients with LVEF [left ventricular ejection fraction] of 30% to 35% of any origin with NYHA [New York Heart Association] functional class II or III symptoms who are taking chronic optimal medical therapy and who have reasonable expectation of survival with good functional status of more than 1 year."[4] Extrapolating the 1-year survival expectation with good functional status precedent to other cardiac interventions must consider the relative morbidity and complication risks of other cardiovascular interventions being contemplated. Identifying the least invasive option when considering cardiac therapies in patients with cancer may be the most important principle.

Although the future of the allocation of health care resources seems less predictable now than

a University of Kansas Medical Center in Kansas City, Kansas City, MO, USA
b Vanderbilt University, Nashville, TN, USA
* Corresponding author. 828 West, 56 Street, Kansas City, MO 64113-1111.
E-mail address: cbporter@mac.md

Heart Failure Clin 7 (2011) 395–402
doi:10.1016/j.hfc.2011.03.010
1551-7136/11/$ – see front matter © 2011 Elsevier Inc. All rights reserved.

previously, the increasing numbers of patients with cancer who have 5-year survival rates significantly greater than 50% mandates that cardiologists dealing with such patients should be actively considering the use of mechanical, electrical, or surgical interventions when the potential cardiovascular benefit may improve quality of life or survival by preventing or treating heart failure.

CASE STUDIES

The care of patients with a malignancy, from a cardiologist's perspective, is immensely challenging. In addition to attention to the ischemic, valvular, and hypertensive forms of heart disease, the cardiologist must also be knowledgeable about the many ways in which cancer and the treatment modalities affect the heart. A delicate balance exists to manage 2 diseases to achieve an ideal outcome for the individual patient. It is important for cardiovascular specialists to have a significant understanding of the prevention, identification, and treatment of cardiac disease, specifically heart failure, in patients with cancer to optimize clinical outcomes. This review focuses on some examples of these challenges with an emphasis on cardiac dysfunction in patients with cancer with valvular, pericardial, and ischemic heart disease.

Case 1: Clinical Decision Making Associated with Atrial Fibrillation, Severe Mitral Regurgitation, and Metastatic Melanoma

A 67-year-old man returned for follow-up in a cardiology clinic in October, 2009 reporting recent onset progressive exertional dyspnea. Over the prior 2 months his symptoms progressed to the point of NYHA class III symptoms with dyspnea while showering, requiring 10 minutes rest to recover. He was unable to continue his work as an outdoor event photographer or to play golf as he had been doing without limitations 2 months earlier. Examination confirmed a holosystolic murmur of mitral regurgitation. Echo-Doppler study showed left ventricular (LV) enlargement with LV end diastolic dimension (LVEDD) of 83 mm and LV end systolic dimension (LVESD) of 55 mm, whereas his LVEF was 65% with right ventricular systolic pressure estimated at 54 mm Hg. The posterior mitral valve leaflet prolapsed severely with the appearance of a flail leaflet subsection.

Past history included ocular melanoma detected during refraction in 2003 and was treated with proton therapy. In 2006, metastatic disease to the lung and liver was detected and over the next 2 years he was treated with a series of

chemotherapies, including dacarbazine, temozolamide, carboplatin, and paclitaxel (Taxol).

In September 2007, he presented with asymptomatic atrial fibrillation with ventricular response 45 and blood pressure 130/80. At that time, Echo-Doppler study revealed LV enlargement with an LVESD of 53 mm with an estimated LVEF of 45% and the estimated right ventricular systolic pressure was 35 mm Hg. He had moderate to severe mitral regurgitation at that time. Warfarin was withheld because of concerns about intracranial hemorrhagic risks with metastatic melanoma and cardioversion was not attempted. In September 2008, biochemotherapy with cisplatin, vinblastine, dacarbazine, interleukin (IL)-2, and interferon was begun with doses limited by respiratory and marrow intolerance. He then received cisplatin, vinblastine, and dacarbazine (no IL-2 or interferon) until April 2009 when progression of disease led to initiation of temozolomide and thalidomide. Warfarin was begun at this time because of the risks of venous thromboembolism with temozolomide and thalidomide combination.

With the rapid onset of class III symptoms and well-preserved LV systolic performance in October 2009, the patient was thought to be a candidate for mitral valve repair and was referred to cardiothoracic surgery. Coronary angiography revealed mild coronary atherosclerosis. In November 2009, he underwent robotic mitral valve repair and internal ligation of the left atrial appendage. He was dismissed on the sixth postoperative day. He subsequently completed cardiac rehabilitation and returned to his work and recreational activities. He noted complete resolution of exertional dyspnea. Postoperative echo-Doppler revealed mild to moderate mitral regurgitation, LVEDD of 58 mm, and LVEF of 35%. Fifteen months after his mitral valve repair the patient is receiving sorafenib for intracranial metastases with minimal complaints of dyspnea.

In March 2010, enlargement of hepatic and pulmonary metastases were seen and brain magnetic resonance imaging (MRI) revealed multiple metastatic lesions. Temozolomide, thalidomide, and warfarin were discontinued and sorafenib was initiated, and the patient received 39 Gy whole brain irradiation. In May 2010, an MRI showed no growth of tumors or new lesions.

This single case illustrates many complexities that a cardiologist and an oncologist may face while caring for patients with advanced cancer.

Atrial fibrillation and anticoagulation in patients with cancer

Oncologists routinely face difficult issues with anticoagulation in patients with cancer who are at increased risk for venous or arterial thrombosis. In the setting of atrial fibrillation and its attendant risk for heart failure, the cardiologist has to evaluate the risk and benefits of adding anticoagulation. The CHADS2 scoring system commonly used to determine the advisability of initiating warfarin does not include tumor or treatment-specific risk factors for hemorrhage that might identify those patients with cancer with increased risk of warfarin.[5] The risk of warfarin-related hemorrhage has been reported to be as much as 6 times higher than for patients without malignancy, although rigorous monitoring can provide reasonably safe and effective international normalized ratio results.[6] At least 27 antineoplastic agents or combination drug regimens have been reported as interacting with warfarin, including drugs, such as trastuzumab, sorafenib, imatinib and erlotinib, that are in newer classes of targeted therapies, and more are likely to be developed. It seems crucially important that any new agents will have to have potential interactions with anticoagulation defined.[7]

Before making a firm recommendation for the use of warfarin in patients with cancer based solely on a CHADS2 score, the managing cardiologist must consider the increased risks of hemorrhage in patients with cancer. Certainly this assessment includes the risk factors that will increase the chance of warfarin-related bleeding, such as multiple drug interactions, malnutrition, vomiting, and hepatic dysfunction.[8] Additional factors to consider include the risk of intracranial hemorrhage. In fact, the highest incidence of intracranial hemorrhage has been reported in patients whose primary tumors are melanoma, choriocarcinoma, thyroid carcinoma, and renal cell carcinoma. The risk of spontaneous brain hemorrhage is less common with brain metastases from primary lung or breast tumors.[9] Although there are no trials of warfarin versus other antithrombotic therapy in patients with cancer with atrial fibrillation, there are some comparison studies for shorter periods of up to 6 months. The use of the low molecular weight heparin (LMWH) dalteparin, was found to be no more hazardous than a coumarin and was superior in the prevention of deep venous thrombosis (DVT), pulmonary embolus (PE), or both after initial 5 to 7 days dalteparin (200 IU/kg body weight) in both groups. Recurrent DVT was less common on the dalteparin group than the coumarin group with no increase in bleeding (6% dalteparin vs 4% warfarin, p = not significant).[10] Based on these data guidelines for patients with cancer with DVT or PE now call for 3 to 6 months of treatment with LMWH and chronic anticoagulation indefinitely with either an oral vitamin K

antagonist or LMWH thereafter as long as the cancer is active.[11] However, no specific guidance is offered on patients with cancer with atrial fibrillation being considered for antithrombotic therapy. If extrapolation from DVT/PE data is reasonable, then patients being considered for warfarin because of atrial fibrillation who are at high risk, the use of LMWH may be reasonable. Although oral alternatives to warfarin have been extensively evaluated and dabigatran has now been approved by the Food and Drug Administration (FDA) for use in atrial fibrillation; published[12] clinical experience in patients with malignancies is still forthcoming.

Evidence-based management of valve disease in patients with cancer can create therapeutic dilemmas

The clinical course of the patient previously discussed illustrates the array of therapeutic options that can be offered to patients with advanced malignancy. The improved tolerability and success of these newer regimens may allow patients to have a high quality of life during therapy even with extensive disease and intensive therapy. Although the absolute number of patients may be small who can continue vigorous professional and recreational activities during therapy for metastatic disease, such as this patient who had hepatic, pulmonary, and brain metastases, these patients are increasingly present. With off-label indications or with patients who have failed to respond to other regimens, there is no evidence base upon which to determine the duration of benefit that can be expected. Cardiologists accustomed to making recommendations for the management of valvular heart disease based on published guidelines[13] face uncertainty about what should be recommended, and close collaboration with the oncologist is necessary for estimating the overall prognosis.

How should patients' malignancy be determined to override an evidence-based guideline recommendation for intervention for valvular heart disease?

With such limited evidence available, the experience of the cardiologist and the oncologist, the opinion of patients, and the evolution of both the cancer and the heart disease become the major factors for both the initial decision and subsequent reevaluations of any situation. In this case summarized herein, the uncertainty of the prognosis from the malignancy and an asymptomatic patient created a consensus of oncologists, cardiologists, and the patient that deferring mitral surgery was the preferred decision. The possibility that severe LV dysfunction would develop more rapidly than the spreading of melanoma was a recognized possibility.

When the patient developed symptoms of heart failure in 2009, unfavorable remodeling had occurred (increase LVESD) and the mitral valve anatomy appearing suitable for valve repair, making a less invasive option that did not require long-term anticoagulation feasible. Even with the metastatic melanoma, his heart failure symptoms were severely limiting although he had no direct symptoms from his metastatic melanoma. The patient and the providers agreed that surgical intervention to reduce or eliminate heart failure symptoms and to prevent further cardiovascular deterioration was warranted to improve quality of life.

How do newer, less invasive procedures for valve repair or replacement influence decisions to intervene?

The development of several less invasive and better-tolerated transthoracic and percutaneous interventions for valvular heart disease should be considered highly attractive options for patients with concurrent valve disease and underlying co-morbidity, such as cancer. Aortic valve replacement using modified transthoracic approaches has been under development for several years. Port access techniques involving right thoracic inframammary incision are principally used with evolving approaches to cardioplegia, cardiopulmonary bypass, and mode of infusing cardioplegia with either antegrade or retrograde cardioplegia being used.[14,15] The results of minimally invasive aortic valve replacement are also encouraging with one randomized trial of 120 patients receiving either conventional versus minimally invasive aortic valve replacements reporting that minimally invasive techniques were associated with earlier postoperative extubation, less postoperative analgesia, less transfusion requirement, and fewer supraventricular arrhythmias. Survival rates assessed an average of 294 days after surgery were equivalent.[16] For physicians caring for patients with cancer with increased risks of leukopenia and infection, the reduced infection rates reported in some series of minimally invasive valve repair seem promising. The outcomes of 109 consecutive patients undergoing port-access approaches compared with 88 matched patients previously undergoing conventional techniques reported in 2001 showed a striking reduction in infection rate in the minimally invasive group with a 0.9% incidence of sepsis versus a 5.7% incidence in the conventional group ($P = .05$). Transfusion requirements were less (52.3% vs 64.8%, $P = .05$), as was overall length of hospital stay

(7 days median vs 9 days, $P = .001$). Hospital mortality was similar in both groups (3.7% vs 3.4%, $P = .62$), whereas cardiopulmonary bypass time was longer with the minimally invasive approach (139 minutes vs 110 minutes, $P<.001$).[17]

The same group's 10-year experience with minimally invasive mitral valve repair has subsequently been reported with confirmation of the previously reported reduction in incidence of surgical site sepsis. Surgical site sepsis occurred in 0.5% in the minimally invasive group versus 2.1% in the conventionally treated sternotomy group ($P = .01$). Overall hospital mortality was 1.3% for isolated mitral valve pair with either minimally invasive or standard sternotomy groups. Perioperative atrial fibrillation occurred less frequently in the minimally invasive group compared with the sternotomy group (22.8% vs 37.2% $P = .001$), whereas the stroke and endocarditis rates were no different.[18] Overall, the low rate of infection in these studies indicate that the risk of infection as a relative contraindication to valve surgery has been declining and may be particularly favorable when minimally invasive transthoracic techniques are used in experienced centers. Another single-center experience of minimally invasive mitral valve surgery using propensity-matching methods reported outcomes in 590 pairs undergoing isolated mitral valve surgery; similar hospital mortality (0.17% minimally invasive vs 0.85% conventional $P = .2$) was reported, with nonsignificant differences between stroke infection, renal failure, and myocardial infarction. A reduction in patients transfused (30% vs 37% $P<.001$), an increase in the number of patients extubated in the operating room (18.0% vs 5.7% $P<.0001$), and lower pain scores all favored the minimally invasive surgical cohort. No apparent detriments were reported.[19] Fully robotic approaches to valve repair and replacement of both aortic and mitral valves have been reported but randomized trials or even case-controlled studies are insufficient to determine their benefits over minimally invasive techniques.[20]

Percutaneous mitral valve repair using a novel clip that attaches segments of regurgitant mitral valve leaflets in a manner that reduces regurgitation without thoracic incision or cardiopulmonary bypass is currently being evaluated in clinical trials comparing results to those with surgical repair or replacement. The device lacks FDA approval but early results are encouraging.[21] Reductions in mitral regurgitation and left ventricular volumes and improvements in quality of life and functional class versus baseline were reported in the Endovascular Valve Edge-to-Edge Repair Study (EVEREST) II trial of 279 subjects treated at

37 sites. A total of 9.6% of subjects receiving the MitraClip and 57.0% of control subjects experienced the primary endpoint (death) or 1 of 11 other complications included in the major adverse events safety endpoint. The overall clinical success rate evaluated with a noninferiority hypothesis was comparable at 1 year, although the trend for clinical success favored surgery (87.8% clinical success) versus the mitral valve clip (72.4% clinical success). The deep wound infection rate was zero in both groups.[22] Percutaneous treatment of severe aortic valve stenosis has been performed in more than 4000 patients worldwide using one of two models of valve. Although neither valve has received FDA approval, it appears that midterm outcomes show no evidence of restenosis or prosthetic valve dysfunction. Procedural mortality and acute complication rates appear highly encouraging. Further randomized trials are needed before the technique becomes available for noninvestigative applications.[23]

Case 2: Percutaneous Management of Pericardial Disease in a Patient with Cancer

A 56-year-old woman, diagnosed with stage III breast cancer in April 1999 (T2N2, 3-cm tumor, more than 10 lymph nodes positive) that was high grade and estrogen receptor/progesterone receptor (ER/PR) positive but HER2 negative, underwent bilateral mastectomies with a left axillary dissection and reconstructive surgery. This procedure was followed by adjuvant chemotherapy with accelerated high-dose doxorubicin hydrochloride (Adriamycin), cyclophosphamide (Cytoxan), and paclitaxel (Taxol). She then had radiation therapy to the chest wall and lymph node bearing areas. Subsequently, she was given paclitaxel (Taxol) for 5 years followed by letrozole for 2 years, which was completed in 2006. The patient was asymptomatic until June 2010, when she presented with rapidly progressive dyspnea on exertion. She was found to have a large pericardial effusion and underwent a pericardiocentesis with drainage of the effusion. The cytology of the fluid was positive for neoplastic cells, which were compatible with a diagnosis of adenocarcinoma. A staging computed tomography (CT) scan revealed large bilateral pleural effusions and a 1.8-cm apical lung nodule. A diagnostic biopsy of the lung lesion was consistent with adenocarcinoma, which was ER/PR and HER2 negative. A follow-up echocardiogram 2 weeks after presentation demonstrated no recurrence of the pericardial effusion. She is currently being treated with a platinum-based chemotherapeutic regimen.

Pericardial manifestations of cancer commonly present with metastases that arise from direct tumor extension or lymphatic spread of an intrathoracic tumor

The size of the implant generally determines the magnitude of the effect. A small area may lead to focal, acute pericarditis while multiple pericardial lesions can produce varying severity of pericardial effusion. Any hemodynamic effect that is cause by the effusion is most commonly responsible for the clinical symptoms in these patients. Tumors arising in the lung account for approximately 60% of these clinical presentations, which manifest as effusive pericarditis or tamponade. Malignant pericardial effusions are more common than pericarditis without effusion. The pericardial fluid is either serous, sanguinous, or hemorrhagic. The volume of fluid is variable ranging from 300 mL to more than 1 L. Cytology should be routinely performed and is abnormal in approximately 50% of patients. Therefore, the quality of the fluid and microscopic examination may not always be used to distinguish benign from malignant pericardial effusions. In addition, many patients have received radiation therapy to the chest, which may promote constrictive pericardial disease. The development of symptoms in patients with malignant pericardial effusions is commonly insidious and therefore leads to a delay in diagnosis. In a series of 189 patients, only 55% of individuals with malignant pericardial effusions had symptoms before death.[24] In a second study, 42% of 36 patients with cardiac tamponade who were part of a cohort of 215 patients with malignant pericardial effusions did not have the diagnosis of cardiac tamponade before echocardiography.[25] This finding is relevant because the reason for referral was commonly heart failure, myocardial infarction, or shock. Most patients with pericardial manifestations of cancer are symptomatic. Detection of these symptoms requires a careful history and physical examination. Critical signs and symptoms include dyspnea, chest discomfort, pulsus paradoxus, and elevated jugular venous pressure. These findings can be nonspecific and require that the etiology of the symptoms be differentiated from other conditions. Other physical findings that may suggest a clinically significant pericardial effusion include unexplained tachycardia, tachypnea, and reduction in the intensity of heart sounds. The presence of coexisting hypertension does not mitigate against cardiac tamponade. The amount of pericardial fluid does not determine the presence or absence of the pericardial friction rub.

The majority of patients with malignant pericardial effusions have an abnormal chest radiograph.

The most common abnormality is cardiomegaly. In addition, one may observe a hilar mass or mediastinal widening if patients have an intrathoracic malignancy. The diagnosis may not be apparent initially, or confused with heart failure because patients may have symptoms of left ventricular dysfunction, such as dyspnea and edema. However, in the presence of cardiomegaly and absent pulmonary venous congestion on chest radiograph, typical heart failure is less likely. The electrocardiogram is generally abnormal but nonspecific in the presence of a pericardial effusion with or without tamponade. The QRS amplitude in the limb or precordial leads is usually low and there may be nonspecific ST segment changes. Electrical alternans of the QRS complex is rare; however, it is thought to be diagnostic of cardiac tamponade. Pericardial effusion and tamponade are commonly diagnosed with echo-Doppler. The hemodynamics can then be confirmed with a right heart catheterization, which can support the diagnosis of tamponade and allow the clinician to determine if therapeutic intervention is appropriate.

The traditional procedures that have been used to treat malignant pericardial effusions include pericardiocentesis with in-dwelling catheter drainage, subxiphoid pericardial windows, installation of sclerosing or chemotherapeutic agents in the pericardial space,[26] and pericardiotomy. Echocardiographic guidance has reduced the risk of the procedure significantly. Pericardioscopy, balloon pericardiotomy, and pericardial biopsy may be used to obtain fluid, relieve tamponade, and obtain pericardial tissue for microscopic analysis.[27] Surgical intervention may be necessary if the fluid is loculated or a pericardial window is necessary.

Case 3: Acute Coronary Syndrome in a Patient with Cancer Undergoing Active Cancer Treatment

A 55-year-old man with a history of rectal carcinoma was admitted to the hospital with dyspnea, cough, and sputum production in November 2010. He had radiographic findings of a right lower-lobe pneumonia. While being treated with antibiotics, a metastatic lesion was subsequently discovered by CT and positron emission tomography involving the sacrum. He was scheduled to receive leucovorin/5-FU/oxaliplatin/irinotecan (FOLFIRI) therapy.

Past history
He was diagnosed with stage T4N2 adenocarcinoma of the rectum in October 2000 and was treated with anterior resection and received adjuvant radiation and chemotherapy, initially with oxaliplatin, followed by bevacizumab (Avastin) until March 2009. He had multiple surgical complications, including wound dehiscence and multiple fistulas. He also had hypertension after starting therapy with bevacizumab (Avastin) that was controlled with an angiotensin-converting enzyme inhibitor.

During his treatment for pneumonia, he developed anterior chest tightness radiating to his left arm associated with diaphoresis. He had a newly developed abnormal electrocardiogram with 2-mm ST depression in the anterior leads and was treated with aspirin, heparin, beta-blockers, and nitrates and his pain resolved. Cardiac biomarkers were abnormal with a troponin I of 1.6 pg/mL. A CT scan demonstrated no evidence of a pulmonary embolism or dissection. After stabilization, a cardiac catheterization was performed that revealed multivessel disease with significant stenosis in the proximal portion of all 3 epicardial coronary arteries with overall normal LV function. An extensive discussion took place between the patient, family, cardiologist, cardiovascular surgeon, and oncologist. Overall it was agreed that this patient was a candidate for revascularization and it was determined that a nonsurgical approach might be reasonable. He then had 3 bare metal stents uneventfully placed in each of the proximal coronary arteries. He was discharged 2 days later on aspirin, clopidogrel, simvastatin, and a beta-blocker.

The management of ischemic heart disease involves several basic strategies
These strategies include management of risk factors; nonpharmacologic attention to lifestyle; medications to treat angina; and revascularization procedures, including percutaneous and surgical techniques. Special consideration should be made based on patients' long-term prognosis and bleeding risk. Bare metal stents may be preferable in many situations because of the unpredictability of the patients' response to cancer therapy and subsequent risks of bleeding and infection. Some patients may require chronic anticoagulation therapy for their malignancy or cardiac disease and have increased risk for long-term dual antiplatelet therapy. Consequently, evidence-based recommendations for the management of patients with cancer with asymptomatic and symptomatic CV disease are lacking and close collaboration with oncology is a must. Ultimately, arriving at a reasonable clinical decision that allows optimal cancer therapy and maximal control of CV disease is the goal.

There are many factors in patients with CV disease and cancer that predispose to thrombotic complications
These factors include a general state of hypercoagulability; potentially adverse effects of chemotherapy;

platelet activation (mediated by several mechanisms ranging from increased expression of platelet adhesion molecules to direct platelet activation by contact with molecules on the surface of the tumor cell membrane); and increased platelet adhesion to fibrinogen, especially in metastatic disease.[28,29] Furthermore, surgical wounds of previously irradiated tissues are prone to vascular alterations associated with increased incidence of microvascular occlusion and delayed wound healing. The adverse effects of radiation on tissues can be acute, usually occurring within 4 to 6 weeks after exposure, and late effects, which may occur months to years after irradiation and are linked to endothelial dysfunction.[30] The activated endothelium is prone to atherosclerosis[31] and has prothrombotic properties, by promoting leukocyte or platelet endothelial cell adherence, leukocyte infiltration into tissue, and thrombus formation.[32] Nitric oxide-mediated, endothelial-dependent relaxation is impaired in human cervical arteries 4 to 6 weeks after irradiation; thus, vascular tissues are more prone to vasoconstriction and occlusion.[33] Furthermore, sustained inflammation caused by NF-kB activation in human radiated arteries may explain CV disease years after radiation.[34]

SUMMARY

The unique clinical circumstances that are typically encountered by cardiology providers when caring for patients undergoing treatment for cancer require an in-depth understanding of the recommended treatments for the diagnosis and management of heart failure and ischemic heart disease. It is also recognized that there is not a broadly described clinical research basis from which to provide guidance when specific clinical decision making is required. Thus, it is imperative that cardiology and oncology closely collaborate when difficult patient decisions arise. Ultimately, engaging each discipline together with active patient involvement in clinical care will undoubtedly provide optimal care for our patients.

REFERENCES

1. Cancer trends progress report-2009/2010 Update. Bethesda (MD): National Cancer Institute, NIH, DHHS; 2010.

2. Cancer facts and figures 2010. Atlanta (GA): American Cancer Society; 2010.

3. Heart disease and stroke statistics 2010 Update at a glance. American Heart Association; 2010.

4. Hunt SA, Abraham WT, Chin MH, et al. ACC/AHA 2005 Guideline Update for the Diagnosis and Management of Chronic Heart Failure in the Adult: a report of the American College of Cardiology/American Heart Association Task Force on Practice Guidelines (Writing Committee to Update the 2001 Guidelines for the Evaluation and Management of Heart Failure): developed in collaboration with the American College of Chest Physicians and the International Society for Heart and Lung Transplantation: endorsed by the Heart Rhythm Society. Circulation 2005;112:e154–235.

5. Rietbrock S, Heeley E, Plumb J, et al. Chronic atrial fibrillation: incidence, prevalence, and prediction of stroke using the congestive heart failure, Hypertension, Age >75, Diabetes mellitus, and prior Stroke or transient ischemic attack (CHADS2) risk stratification scheme. Am Heart J 2008;156:57–64.

6. Hutten BA, Prins MH, Gent M, et al. Incidence of recurrent thromboembolic and bleeding complications among patients with venous thromboembolism in relation to both malignancy and achieved international normalized ratio: a retrospective analysis. J Clin Oncol 2000;18:3078–83.

7. Pangilinan JM, Pangilinan PH Jr, Worden FP. Use of warfarin in the patient with cancer. J Support Oncol 2007;5:131–6.

8. Zacharski LR, Prandoni P, Monreal M. Warfarin versus low-molecular-weight heparin therapy in cancer patients. Oncologist 2005;10:72–9.

9. Mandybur TI. Intracranial hemorrhage caused by metastatic tumors. Neurology 1977;27:650–5.

10. Lee AY, Levine MN, Baker RI, et al. Low-molecular-weight heparin versus a coumarin for the prevention of recurrent venous thromboembolism in patients with cancer. N Engl J Med 2003;349:146–53.

11. Kearon C, Kahn SR, Agnelli G, et al. Antithrombotic therapy for venous thromboembolic disease: American College of Chest Physicians Evidence-Based Clinical Practice Guidelines (8th Edition). Chest 2008;133:454S–545S.

12. Petersen P, Grind M, Adler J. Ximelagatran versus warfarin for stroke prevention in patients with nonvalvular atrial fibrillation. SPORTIF II: a dose-guiding, tolerability, and safety study. J Am Coll Cardiol 2003;41:1445–51.

13. Bonow RO, Carabello BA, Chatterjee K, et al. ACC/AHA 2006 guidelines for the management of patients with valvular heart disease: a report of the American College of Cardiology/American Heart Association Task Force on Practice Guidelines (writing Committee to Revise the 1998 guidelines for the management of patients with valvular heart disease) developed in collaboration with the Society of Cardiovascular Anesthesiologists endorsed by the Society for Cardiovascular Angiography and Interventions and the Society of Thoracic Surgeons. J Am Coll Cardiol 2006;48:e1–148.

14. Cosgrove DM 3rd, Sabik JF, Navia JL. Minimally invasive valve operations. Ann Thorac Surg 1998; 65:1535–8 [discussion: 1538–9].

15. Byrne JG, Karavas AN, Cohn LH, et al. Minimal access aortic root, valve, and complex ascending aortic surgery. Curr Cardiol Rep 2000;2:549–57.

16. Machler HE, Bergmann P, Anelli-Monti M, et al. Minimally invasive versus conventional aortic valve operations: a prospective study in 120 patients. Ann Thorac Surg 1999;67:1001–5.

17. Grossi EA, Galloway AC, Ribakove GH, et al. Impact of minimally invasive valvular heart surgery: a case-control study. Ann Thorac Surg 2001;71:807–10.

18. Galloway AC, Schwartz CF, Ribakove GH, et al. A decade of minimally invasive mitral repair: long-term outcomes. Ann Thorac Surg 2009;88:1180–4.

19. Iribarne A, Russo MJ, Easterwood R, et al. Minimally invasive versus sternotomy approach for mitral valve surgery: a propensity analysis. Ann Thorac Surg 2010;90:1471–7 [discussion: 7–8].

20. Smith JM, Stein H, Engel AM, et al. Totally endoscopic mitral valve repair using a robotic-controlled atrial retractor. Ann Thorac Surg 2007;84:633–7.

21. Feldman T, Kar S, Rinaldi M, et al. Percutaneous mitral repair with the MitraClip system: safety and midterm durability in the initial EVEREST (Endovascular Valve Edge-to-Edge REpair Study) cohort. J Am Coll Cardiol 2009;54:686–94.

22. Mauri L, Garg P, Massaro JM, et al. The EVEREST II Trial: design and rationale for a randomized study of the evalve mitraclip system compared with mitral valve surgery for mitral regurgitation. Am Heart J 2010;160:23–9.

23. Zajarias A, Cribier AG. Outcomes and safety of percutaneous aortic valve replacement. J Am Coll Cardiol 2009;53:1829–36.

24. Thurber DL, Edwards JE, Achor RW. Secondary malignant tumors of the pericardium. Circulation 1962;26:228–41.

25. Markiewicz W, Borovik R, Ecker S. Cardiac tamponade in medical patients: treatment and prognosis in the echocardiographic era. Am Heart J 1986; 111:1138–42.

26. Martinoni A, Cipolla CM, Cardinale D, et al. Long-term results of intrapericardial chemotherapeutic treatment of malignant pericardial effusions with thiotepa. Chest 2004;126:1412–6.

27. Maisch B, Ristic A, Pankuweit S. Evaluation and management of pericardial effusion in patients with neoplastic disease. Prog Cardiovasc Dis 2010;53: 157–63.

28. Nash GF, Turner LF, Scully MF, et al. Platelets and cancer. Lancet Oncol 2002;3:425–30.

29. Sarkiss MG, Yusuf SW, Warneke CL, et al. Impact of aspirin therapy in cancer patients with thrombocytopenia and acute coronary syndromes. Cancer 2007; 109:621–7.

30. Quarmby S, Kumar P, Kumar S. Radiation-induced normal tissue injury: role of adhesion molecules in leukocyte-endothelial cell interactions. Int J Cancer 1999;82:385–95.

31. Panes J, Anderson DC, Miyasaka M, et al. Role of leukocyte-endothelial cell adhesion in radiation-induced microvascular dysfunction in rats. Gastroenterology 1995;108:1761–9.

32. Salame MY, Verheye S, Mulkey SP, et al. The effect of endovascular irradiation on platelet recruitment at sites of balloon angioplasty in pig coronary arteries. Circulation 2000;101:1087–90.

33. Sugihara T, Hattori Y, Yamamoto Y, et al. Preferential impairment of nitric oxide-mediated endothelium-dependent relaxation in human cervical arteries after irradiation. Circulation 1999;100: 635–41.

34. Halle M, Gabrielsen A, Paulsson-Berne G, et al. Sustained inflammation due to nuclear factor-kappa B activation in irradiated human arteries. J Am Coll Cardiol 2010;55:1227–36.

Long-Term Cardiac and Pulmonary Complications of Cancer Therapy

Joachim Yahalom, MD[a],*, Carol S. Portlock, MD[b]

KEYWORDS

- Anthracyclines • Cardiac toxicity • Pulmonary toxicity
- Radiotherapy • Taxanes • Trastuzumab

Many systemically administered chemotherapeutic and biologic agents may cause late cardiovascular complications.[1,2] Late cardiac effects are most commonly related to cancer treatment by anthracyclines, mitoxantrone, paclitaxel, docetaxel, and trastuzumab. The cardiotoxicity that results from mediastinal radiotherapy is discussed in detail. Pulmonary complications of chemotherapy and radiotherapy are discussed separately.

ANTHRACYCLINE-RELATED CARDIAC TOXICITY

Anthracyclines are a group of important potent drugs used in the treatment of many pediatric and adult malignancies. Anthracycline cardiomyopathy is characterized by a dose-dependent progressive decrease in systolic left ventricular function often leading to congestive heart failure. Abnormalities in left ventricular size and function measured by noninvasive testing can be detected before the development of overt congestive heart failure. Patients who have abnormal heart function following treatment with anthracyclines may or may not have clinical symptoms.

The delayed cardiomyopathy associated with anthracycline therapy presents clinically as classic congestive heart failure, including fatigue, shortness of breath, dyspnea on exertion, sinus tachycardia, S3 gallop rhythm, pedal edema/pleural effusions, and elevated jugular venous distention. These may be subtle at onset and progress gradually.

Anthracycline cardiomyopathy risk depends on the cumulative total dose.[3] At 450 mg/m^2 for doxorubicin there is a 5% risk, and for other anthracyclines this cumulative dose is: 900 mg/m^2 for daunorubicin, 935 mg/m^2 for epirubicin, and 223 mg/m^2 for idarubicin. Mediastinal irradiation that includes the heart, older (particularly >70 years) or younger (<15 years) age, coronary artery disease, other valvular or myocardial conditions, and hypertension are cofactors in cardiomyopathy risk. When administered concurrently, trastuzumab may potentiate anthracycline cardiotoxicity. Other agents with known cardiotoxic effects may be additive.

Cardiac dysfunction is established by comparing baseline with serial left ventricular function studies. Left ventricular ejection fraction (LVEF) may be measured by echocardiography or nuclear imaging and 50% or more is considered within the normal range. A low LVEF contraindicates the use of anthracyclines.

Typical findings on echocardiograms are left ventricular diastolic/systolic dysfunction and later septal wall motion dysfunction. The left ventricle is initially not enlarged or only moderately enlarged.

This article originally appeared in *Hematology/Oncology Clinics of North America*, volume 22, number 2.

[a] Department of Radiation Oncology, Memorial Sloan-Kettering Cancer Center, 1275 York Avenue, New York, NY 10021, USA

[b] Department of Medicine, Memorial Sloan-Kettering Cancer Center, 1275 York Avenue, New York, NY 10021, USA

* Corresponding author.

E-mail address: yahalomj@mskcc.org

Heart Failure Clin 7 (2011) 403–411

doi:10.1016/j.hfc.2011.04.002

Global hypokinesis and muscle wall thinning is seen with late cardiomyopathy. Sinus tachycardia, low voltage, poor R-wave progression, and nonspecific T wave changes are noted on EKG, but these are late findings and can be nonspecific.

In pediatrics, subclinical cardiomyopathy is more common than in adults at comparable doses, resulting in progressive loss of ventricular mass, reduced cardiac output, and restrictive cardiomyopathy. There does not seem to be a threshold cumulative dose below which left ventricular dysfunction is not seen.[4–7]

Prevention of late cardiomyopathy requires the recognition of early dysfunction during chemotherapy. A decrease in ejection fraction, changes in diastolic function, and changes in troponins/brain natriuretic peptide have all been studied and are predictive in small series. The simplest is serial LVEF in susceptible patients, and discontinuing anthracycline with a significant decrease from baseline.[8–10] For doxorubicin, a repeat study should be performed at 200 mg/m^2, and all patients should have a follow-up study at 300 to 400 mg/m^2 and every 50 to 100 mg/m^2 thereafter.

Anthracycline strategies to reduce cardiovascular risk include: analogs, low-dose or infusional drug schedules, and the use of liposomal formulations.[11,12] Dexrazoxane decreases the risk for clinical cardiomyopathy with doxorubicin doses of 300 mg/m^2 or more.[13] Its role in upfront treatment regimens remains under investigation.

Anthracycline cardiomyopathy is managed like other causes of dilated cardiomyopathy with ACE inhibitors, β-blockers, and diuretics. These measures are palliative rather than curative and, unfortunately, the dysfunction may be progressive despite these agents. Cardiac transplantation provides the only curative option.

Selective cardiomyocyte apoptosis seems to play a major role in the development of anthracycline cardiomyopathy.[14] Cardiomyocyte metabolism of the anthracycline generates free radicals resulting in membrane lipid peroxidation with the consequent activation of the extrinsic and intrinsic apoptotic pathways, and cardiomyocyte intrinsic antioxidant defense is more limited than that of other organs.

Mitoxantrone is an anthracenedione, structurally related to the anthracyclines, and also causes a dose-related cardiomyopathy. Mitoxantrone cardiomyopathy is rarely seen before 100 mg/m^2 cumulative dose. LVEF should be monitored regularly thereafter and a total dose of 140 mg/m^2 should not be exceeded. Sequential use of doxorubicin followed by mitoxantrone raises cardiomyopathy risk.[15] The mechanism of cardiac damage with mitoxantrone is not fully understood.

TAXANES-RELATED CARDIAC TOXICITY

The taxanes, paclitaxel and docetaxel, are important antimicrotubule agents derived from the yew tree and their cardiotoxicity seems to be related to the taxane ring structural similarities to yew taxine.

Most of paclitaxel's cardiovascular effects are acute/subacute (asymptomatic bradycardia, hypersensitivity reactions, and life-threatening atrial or ventricular rhythm disturbances or conduction abnormalities in approximately 0.5% of patients).[16]

Congestive heart failure does not seem to be caused by paclitaxel, whereas it does seem to potentiate doxorubicin-associated cardiac dysfunction. The sequencing of paclitaxel and doxorubicin are critical in the development of cardiotoxicity [17–20] and is believed to be attributable to an interaction that results in reduced doxorubicin elimination and higher plasma levels.[21] Doxorubicin clearance is therefore paclitaxel schedule–dependent, occurring most prominently when paclitaxel immediately precedes doxorubicin or follows it by less than 1 hour. The taxane docetaxel does not seem to enhance doxorubicin cardiac dysfunction.[22] Although both taxanes increase toxic cardiomyocyte doxorubicinol production in vitro, only paclitaxel seems to be clinically cardiotoxic.

TRASTUZUMAB-RELATED CARDIAC TOXICITY

Trastuzumab is a humanized monoclonal antibody targeting p185^{HER2} (ErbB2 or HER2 receptor), a transmembrane receptor tyrosine kinase of the epidermal growth factor family. This receptor protein is overexpressed or amplified in 20% to 30% of breast cancer and trastuzumab is an important agent in the management of Her2-positive breast cancer.

Cardiac ErbB2 is essential for normal adult cardiac function; in a mouse model it has been shown that cardiac ErbB2-deficient mice develop a dilated cardiomyopathy beginning in the second postnatal month through adulthood. In addition, ErbB2-deficient cardiomyocytes are more susceptible to anthracycline toxicity.[23,24]

Trastuzumab is specific for the human ErbB2 receptor and cannot be studied directly in mice. A two-hit model, in which hemodynamic overload or anthracycline exposure with trastuzumab promotes the development of cardiomyopathy, has been proposed.[25] In a recent prospective human study, trastuzumab preceding anthracycline-based adjuvant therapy revealed no cardiac toxicity, supporting this hypothesis.[26]

Trastuzumab cardiotoxicity is well studied and a 4% to 10% incidence of cardiac dysfunction overall is reported.[27,28] Concurrent trastuzumab with paclitaxel or anthracycline-based regimens increases the incidence up to 25%. The degree of cardiac dysfunction is greatest with concurrent trastuzumab/anthracycline as compared with trastuzumab/paclitaxel. Cardiomyopathy without recovery is seen in approximately half of affected trastuzumab/anthracycline-treated patients, whereas most trastuzumab/paclitaxel-treated patients recover. Older age, cumulative doxorubicin greater than or equal to 300 mg/m[2], and concurrent anthracycline are risk factors.

Like anthracycline cardiomyopathy, tachycardia and decrease in LVEF may be early indicators with later progression to a full-blown cardiomyopathy. Unlike anthracyclines, trastuzumab cardiac toxicity is not antibody cumulative dose dependent, and is more treatable and reversible.[27] Once reversed, trastuzumab can often be safely reintroduced with close monitoring.

Trastuzumab scheduling seems key to preventing cardiac toxicity. When used before anthracycline, the cardiac stress signals that precipitate toxicity may be eliminated.[25] Most importantly, avoidance of concurrent anthracycline exposure and identifying high-risk patients are essential.

RADIATION-RELATED CARDIOVASCULAR COMPLICATIONS

Radiotherapy of lymphomas involving the mediastinum, or radiation for lung and breast cancers, may expose some (or rarely all) of the heart to potential radiation damage. Of the most concern is the potential acceleration of coronary artery disease that could lead to myocardial infarction or even sudden death. Other long-term complications of cardiac irradiation include chronic pericarditis, valvular damage, arrhythmias, and conduction disturbances. Some data suggest that anthracycline-induced congestive heart failure may be enhanced in patients who received mediastinal irradiation in addition to anthracyclines.

Much of the information available on late complications of mediastinal radiation comes from children treated for Hodgkin lymphoma (HL). These patients received curative radiation treatment at a young age and thus provide many years of follow-up that is required for a chronic disease to develop.[29] Most of the studies reported in recent years on long-term cardiac complication include primarily patients who were treated in the 1960s through the mid-1980s; this is the era when most patients who had HL, including children, received radiation as a single modality. In those pioneer days of radiotherapy, radiation in high doses was given to very large volumes (often including all or most of the heart) using radiation technology that is now outdated.[29]

Similar to the gradual progressive nature of anthracycline-related cardiac toxicity that may remain latent to up to 20 years and is diagnosed only by special testing as a subclinical disease, radiation-related damage may be slow to develop and patients who have various degrees of damage remain asymptomatic for years. Often more than one cardiac structure is affected and it is not unusual to find patients who have coronary artery disease and valvular disease (clinical or subclinical).

Coronary Heart Disease in Patients Who Have Hodgkin Lymphoma

Experiments in laboratory animals,[30–32] analysis of pathologic specimens,[33] clinical observations, and, in the 1990s, long-term risk analysis in large series of patients treated for HL all indicate that mediastinal irradiation may facilitate the development of coronary heart disease (CHD) (**Table 1**).[35–41]

Stenosis at the origin of the coronary arteries seems to be a common finding for radiation-associated CHD.[39,42,43] After mediastinal irradiation, there is a greater likelihood for right coronary or left main or left anterior descending coronary artery lesions as opposed to circumflex lesions, which might be because the former vessels, particularly at their origin, receive more radiation.[34]

The studies that analyzed the risk for mortality from myocardial infarction in patients who were treated for HL are summarized in **Table 1**. Although only approximately 1% to 2% of patients who had HL in these series died of myocardial infarction, the observed risk in all seven series was higher than expected.

The current involved-field radiotherapy concept, better fractionation schemes, modern equipment, and improved planning result in lower exposure of radiation to the coronary arteries and may have a lower risk for promoting CHD.[44] In a study by Boivin and colleagues,[34] the relative risk for acute myocardial infarction was reduced from 6.33 for patients treated during the years 1940 to 1966 to 1.97 (with no significant difference from unity) for patients irradiated from 1967 to 1985.

Hancock and colleagues[35] analyzed the risk for cardiac disease in patients who had HL who were treated at Stanford from 1961 to 1991. In patients who were irradiated before age 21 years the relative risk for death from acute myocardial infarction was 41.5 and the actuarial risk for fatal or nonfatal myocardial infarction at 22 years was 8.1%. Of note, all deaths in this study occurred in patients

Table 1
Relative risk for mortality from myocardial infarction after mediastinal irradiation for Hodgkin lymphoma

Study	Center	Patients (n)	Lethal Myocardial Infarctions	Relative Risk	95% CI
Boivin et al[34]	Multiple	4665	68	2.6	1.1–5.9
Hancock et al[35]	Stanford	2232	55	3.2	1.5–5.8
Henry-Amar et al[36]	European Organization for Treatment and Research on Cancer	1449	17	8.8	5.1–14.1
Mauch et al[37]	Joint Center for Radiation Therapy (Boston)	636	15[a]	2.2[a]	1.2–3.6
Glanzmann et al[38]	Zurich	352	8	4.2	1.8–8.3
Reinders et al[39]	Rotterdam	258	12[b]	5.3	2.7–9.3
Swerdlow et al[40]	Britain	7033	168	2.5	2.1–2.9

[a] Includes one patient who died of cardiomyopathy.
[b] Myocardial infarction or sudden death.

who received relatively high doses of radiation (42–45 Gy) to the mediastinum. When the Stanford analysis was extended to include 2232 patients of all age groups who had HL, the relative risk for death from acute myocardial infarction was 3.2.[35] This study showed that patients younger than 20 years who received high-dose irradiation had the highest relative risk, that the risk decreases with increasing age, and that patients older than 50 years of age had no increased risk. These results contrast with data published by other investigators,[34] however, suggesting an increased risk for acute myocardial infarction for the older age groups. The small number of patients in the Stanford study who received radiation doses of less than 30 Gy did not allow an adequate analysis of the dose effect. The average interval between HL treatment and death from acute myocardial infarction was 10.3 years, but risk was already significant during the first 5 years after treatment and remained elevated throughout the follow-up period (more than 20 years).[35]

Two European studies analyzed the risk for ischemic heart disease in patients who had HL who received standard fractions and dose (30–42 Gy) of mediastinal irradiation.[38,39] Both studies demonstrated an increase of ischemic heart disease after mediastinal irradiation. Of importance, a multivariate analysis of risk factors in the Rotterdam study showed that increasing age, gender (male), and a pretreatment cardiac medical history were significant for developing ischemic heart disease in irradiated patients.[39] In a study from Zurich, a detailed analysis of the effect of other CHD risk factors on the radiation-induced risk was performed. The study showed that,

although the risk for CHD after irradiation increased by 4.2 for all patients, in irradiated female patients and in all irradiated patients who did not have other cardiovascular risk factors (smoking, hypertension, obesity, hypercholesterolemia, diabetes) the risk remained as expected in the normal population.[38] In a recent study of 1474 HL survivors treated mostly with radiation with or without chemotherapy, hypercholesterolemia was the most significant independent risk factor for developing CHD.[41] These data suggest that aggressive modification of CHD risk factors, such as hypercholesterolemia, is warranted in patients who received mediastinal radiation therapy or anthracycline-containing chemotherapy.

Although radiation was considered by some to be the only culprit in the induction of CHD in patients who had lymphoma and chemotherapy-alone regimens were supposed to avoid CHD, it was of surprise and concern to learn recently that anthracycline-containing regimens, such as ABVD (doxorubicin, bleomycin, vinblastine, dacarbazine) and R-CHOP (rituximab, cyclophosphamide, doxorubicin, vincristine, prednisone), even if given without radiotherapy, are associated with increased CHD risk.[40,45] Aviles studied 476 patients who had HL treated with anthracycline-containing chemotherapy and no radiation.[45] At a median follow-up of 11.5 years, 9% of patients who received ABVD had a clinical cardiac event and 7% had a cardiac-related death. The standard mortality ratio for cardiac death for patients who received doxorubicin was 46.4 (95% CI: 28.9–70.1) and the absolute excess risk (AER) was 39.[45]

The largest and most recent analysis of myocardial infarction (MI) mortality risk after treatment of

HL is from a collaborative British cohort study of 7033 patients.[40] This study included 3590 patients who received radiotherapy without anthracyclines, 3052 patients who received chemotherapy with supradiaphragmatic radiation, and 1744 patients who received anthracycline regimens and no radiotherapy. For the whole group of HL survivors, the death from MI was significantly more than expected; SMR was 2.5 with an AER of 125.8. The risk was higher for males. The relative risk for death from MI decreased sharply with older age at first treatment, but as expected the AER increased with age. The 20-year cumulative risk for MI mortality for patients treated at age younger than 35 years was 1.8%. The risk for death during the first year after treatment was fourfold compared with the general population and it was higher for patients treated before 1980.[40]

Of particular concern are the new data regarding chemotherapy alone.[40,45] In the British study,[40] the risk for death from MI was statistically significantly increased for patients who had received anthracyclines (SMR of 2.9) and especially those treated with ABVD (SMR of 9.5). These data remained significantly elevated for patients who received those chemotherapy regimens and no radiation therapy (SMR of 7.8). The authors suggested that the risk was particularly high for ABVD (compared with other doxorubicin-containing regimens) because ABVD alone was virtually always given for a full six cycles. The increased risk for patients treated with anthracyclines was primarily during the first year after treatment and the highest risk was in young patients (≤35 years). MI mortality risk was also significantly increased for treatment with vincristine with or without radiation.[40]

Heart Disease Following Radiation of Breast Cancer

Long-term mortality data from three trials that randomized patients who had breast cancer to receive postmastectomy radiotherapy as opposed to no additional treatment demonstrated a higher incidence of cardiac death in the irradiated group.[46–48] The excess in mortality did not appear until after 10 years posttreatment.[47,48] In one study, the increase in mortality risk was significant only in women who were irradiated for tumors in the left breast. It was also increased in patients treated with orthovoltage irradiation, as opposed to those treated with more modern supervoltage equipment.[48]

A recent study from the Netherlands of 4414 10-year breast cancer survivors who were treated from 1970 through 1986 recorded cardiovascular morbidity and mortality events.[49,50] It showed that radiation to the breast alone is not associated with increased risk for cardiovascular disease. Similar to other studies,[51,52] it also documented that the increased risk for MI that was noted in patients treated before 1980 has disappeared with more recent radiation therapy techniques.

Techniques that reduce the risk for irradiating the coronary arteries have been developed; they include the prone breast technique[53] and use of three-dimensional CT planning and intensity-modulated radiation therapy.[54] Patients who have breast cancer irradiated with modern techniques are unlikely to receive a significant dose of radiation to the coronary arteries.

In patients who have breast cancer, conventional-dose doxorubicin-containing chemotherapy used as an adjuvant in combination with local-regional irradiation was not associated with a significant increase in the risk for cardiac events. Higher doses of adjuvant doxorubicin were associated with a three to fourfold increased risk for cardiac events, however. This finding seems to be especially true in patients treated with higher dose volumes of cardiac irradiation.[55] In one recent large-scale study, patients who had breast cancer who were treated with CMF (cyclophosphamide, methotrexate, 5-fluorouracil) and radiotherapy had a significantly higher risk for congestive heart failure compared with patients treated with radiotherapy alone.[49]

Detection of Coronary Heart Disease in Asymptomatic Patients and Prevention Options

Monitoring and reduction of other contributing CHD risk factors in patients who received mediastinal irradiation should be part of the follow-up of patients who underwent mediastinal irradiation. The value of routine noninvasive or invasive cardiac studies in asymptomatic patients has not been fully determined, however.[36,56–59] In a recent screening study of 294 patients who received mediastinal radiation (median dose of 44 Gy) from 1960 to 1995, 21% of screened patients had abnormal ventricular images at rest.[59] During stress testing that included echocardiography and radionuclide perfusion 14% showed abnormalities in one or both tests. Based on these tests, 40 patients underwent coronary angiography and 55% of them (7% of the screened population) had 50% or greater stenosis. The risk for a cardiac event in those patients was significantly related to abnormal stress testing, older age, radiotherapy given in early period, and higher radiation therapy dose given to the mediastinum.

Early detection of CHD should be encouraged, particularly in patients irradiated with high radiation therapy dose (practiced mostly in the past) and those who have other CHD risk factors,[56,57] because angioplastic or surgical intervention may be indicated in special anatomic or clinical situations.[60] Successful treatment of radiation-induced coronary disease with bypass surgery and with stenting or angioplasty has been reported.[43,60,61] In some cases, surgery may be technically difficult because of mediastinal and pericardial fibrosis.[33]

RADIATION-INDUCED DELAYED PERICARDITIS

Late radiation-induced pericarditis that may occur between 4 months to several years after treatment is a relatively uncommon complication today.[62,63] Most cases of radiation-induced pericarditis and pericardial effusion resolve spontaneously, usually within 16 months. Rarely, patients who have delayed pericarditis progress within 5 to 10 years to develop symptomatic constriction requiring pericardiectomy. Occult constrictive pericarditis requires no surgical intervention and usually has a good prognosis.

RADIATION-INDUCED MYOCARDIAL DYSFUNCTION

When myocardial dysfunction is detected after standard-dose mediastinal irradiation, it is typically mild or subclinical.[38,64,65] Noninvasive studies using echocardiography and radionuclide angiography detected subtle left ventricular dysfunction in patients who had HL evaluated a few years after mediastinal irradiation.[56] A study of asymptomatic patients who were treated with mediastinal irradiation for HL at a young age showed reduced average left ventricular dimension and mass suggestive of restricted cardiomyopathy in 42% of patients.[66] Most patients who have abnormal ventricular function findings, however, do not have clinical heart failure.[66] The magnitude of the potential contribution of cardiac irradiation to the risk for doxorubicin-induced cardiomyopathy is not well established. Some data suggest potentiation of anthracycline-induced cardiotoxicity when combined with radiotherapy. Yet, the histopathologies of radiation heart disease and anthracycline heart disease are different, and the combined effects are probably additive rather than synergistic.[65] It was reported that doxorubicin-induced decrease in LVEF was aggravated with concurrent mediastinal irradiation.[67,68] In programs of combined modality

therapy for HL that included relatively low doses of doxorubicin (up to 300 mg/m^2) and mediastinal irradiation of 20 to 40 Gy, no significant clinical myocardial dysfunction was detected.[69]

Symptomatic myocardial dysfunction after a radiation dose that does not exceed 60 Gy is rare.[51,52] The few cases described with intractable heart failure had myocardial fibrosis as part of pancarditis, a generalized process with damage to all three layers of the heart. The hemodynamic pattern is usually of restrictive cardiomyopathy and is difficult to distinguish from constrictive pericarditis.[64]

RADIATION-INDUCED VALVULAR DISEASE

Clinically significant valvular heart disease resulting from mediastinal irradiation is relatively uncommon.[64] Analysis of 635 patients treated for HL before the age of 21 years revealed 29 patients in whom new murmurs of indeterminate significance developed. Of those, 14 received mediastinal doses of 44 Gy or more, and 2 patients who received high-dose irradiation died of valvular heart disease.[35] When echocardiographic studies were performed in asymptomatic patients who had HL more than 7 years after mediastinal irradiation, valvular abnormalities were detected in 25% to 33% of the patients, although there was rarely any clinical significance. An echocardiographic study of 294 asymptomatic patients who received mediastinal irradiation disclosed moderate or severe regurgitation of the aortic valve in 5.0% of patients, of the mitral valve in 3.4%, and of the tricuspid valve in 1.4%. Four percent of the patients had aortic stenosis.[70] Valvular disease, particularly involving the aortic valve, increased with time after irradiation. Of 73 asymptomatic patients evaluated more than 20 years after mediastinal irradiation, 60% had mild or more aortic regurgitation and 16% had aortic stenosis. Radiation dose, volumes, and technique of radiation delivery have markedly changed over the last 3 decades, and the lower prevalence of valvular disease in patients treated at less than 20 years may reflect those changes.[71] In a retrospective study of 415 patients who were irradiated from 1962 to 1998, 6.2% of patients developed clinically significant valvular dysfunction at a median of 22 years.[68] Of interest is a report from Norway that showed a significantly higher risk for cardiopulmonary complications for female subjects after radiation for HL.[44,72] The mean interval from irradiation to detection of valvular disease in asymptomatic and symptomatic patients was 11.5 and 16.5 years, respectively.[73] Patients who received mediastinal radiotherapy and an anthracycline-containing chemotherapy had significantly more valvular disorders than patients receiving radiation therapy with no anthracyclines.[41]

LATE CHEMOTHERAPY- OR RADIATION-INDUCED PULMONARY TOXICITY

Although many chemotherapeutic agents and radiation of the lungs may cause acute pulmonary toxicity, chronic pulmonary complications in cancer survivors are relatively rare. Bleomycin, the chemotherapy drug notorious for acute pneumonitis, is the most-studied agent. It is often used for germ cell tumors and for Hodgkin and non-Hodgkin lymphomas. Risk factors for bleomycin toxicity are bleomycin cumulative dose, age, smoking, renal dysfunction, mediastinal radiotherapy, and administration of oxygen.[74,75] Most patients who have acute bleomycin-induced pneumonitis recover with discontinuation of the drug or corticosteroid treatment. Only a minority progress to pulmonary fibrosis.[74]

Radiation pneumonitis has been reported mostly in patients irradiated for lung cancer, Hodgkin or non-Hodgkin lymphoma involving the mediastinum, breast cancer, or other tumors involving the thorax. In patients who received radiotherapy for lung cancer, the risk for radiation pneumonitis is in the range of 5% to 15%. The risk is increased with concomitant chemotherapy, previous history of lung irradiation, and withdrawal of corticosteroids.[76] In a retrospective multivariate analysis of a large group of patients who had both chemotherapy and radiation, higher daily radiation fractions and the total radiation dose were associated with a significantly higher risk for pneumonitis. The overall risk was 7.8%.[77]

The risk for pneumonitis after radiation for Hodgkin lymphoma involving the mediastinum or after radiation for breast cancer is markedly lower than in patients who have lung cancer. With modern techniques, lower doses, and conformation of the radiation field to the postchemotherapy residual mass, the risk for posttreatment subacute pneumonitis is less than 3% in lymphomas and less than 1% in breast cancer. The vast majority of patients who experience posttreatment radiation pneumonitis have a self-limited course with complete resolution of the process and the clinical symptoms. Patients who develop acute bleomycin pneumonitis or subacute radiation pneumonitis are followed with pulmonary function tests and most show significant improvement over time.[78]

REFERENCES

1. Jones RL, Swanton C, Ewer M. Anthracycline cardiotoxicity. Expert Opin Drug Saf 2006;5(6):791–809.

2. Jones RL, Ewer MS. Cardiac and cardiovascular toxicity of nonanthracycline anticancer drugs. [review]. Expert Rev Anticancer Ther 2006;6(9):1249–69.

3. Keefe DL. Anthracycline-induced cardiomyopathy. Semin Oncol 2001;28(12):2–7.

4. Giantris A, Abdurrahman L, Hinkle A, et al. Anthracycline-induced cardiotoxicity in children and young adults. Crit Rev Oncol Hematol 1998;27(1):53–68.

5. Massin MM, Dresse MF, Schmitz V, et al. Acute arrhythmogenicity of first-dose chemotherapeutic agents in children. Med Pediatr Oncol 2002;39:93–8.

6. Kremer LCM, van der Pal HJH, Offringa M, et al. Frequency and risks factors of subclinical cardiotoxicity after anthracycline therapy in children: a systematic review. Ann Oncol 2002;13:819–29.

7. Lipshultz SE, Lipsitz SR, Sallan SE, et al. Chronic progressive cardiac dysfunction years after doxorubicin therapy for childhood acute lymphoblastic leukemia. J Clin Oncol 2005;23(12):2629–36.

8. Nousiainen T, Jantunen E, Vanninen E, et al. Early decline in left ventricular ejection fraction predicts doxorubicin cardiotoxicity in lymphoma patients. Br J Cancer 2002;86:1697–700.

9. Mitani I, Jain D, Joska TM, et al. Doxorubicin cardiotoxicity: prevention of congestive heart failure with serial cardiac function monitoring with equilibrium radionuclide angiocardiography in the current era. J Nucl Cardiol 2003;10:132–9.

10. Suter TM, Meier B. Detection of anthracycline-induced cardiotoxicity: is there light at the end of the tunnel? Ann Oncol 2002;13(5):647–9.

11. van Dalen EC, Michiels EM, Caron HN, et al. Different anthracycline derivates for reducing cardiotoxicity in cancer patients. Cochrane Database Syst Rev 2006;4:CD005006.

12. van Dalen CD, van der Pal HJH, Caron HN, et al. Different dosage schedules for reducing cardiotoxicity in cancer patients receiving anthracycline chemotherapy [review]. Cochrane Database Syst Rev 2006;4:CD005008.

13. Swain SM, Whaley FS, Gerber MC, et al. Cardioprotection with dexrazoxane for doxorubicin-containing therapy in advanced breast cancer. J Clin Oncol 1997;15:1318–32.

14. Minotti G, Menna P, Salvatorelli E, et al. Anthracyclines: molecular advances and pharmacologic developments in antitumor activity and cardiotoxicity. [review]. Pharmacol Rev 2004;56(2):185–229.

15. Clark GM, Tokaz LK, Von Hoff DD, et al. Cardiotoxicity in patients treated with mitoxantrone on Southwest Oncology Group phase II protocols. Cancer Treatment Symposia 1984;3:25–30.

16. Arbuck SG, Strauss H, Rowinsky E, et al. A reassessment of cardiac toxicity associated with Taxol. J Natl Cancer Inst Monogr 1993;15:117–30.

17. Giordano SH, Booser DJ, Murray JL, et al. A detailed evaluation of cardiac toxicity: a phase II study of doxorubicin and one- or three-hour-infusion paclitaxel in patients with metastatic breast cancer. Clin Cancer Res 2002;8:3360–8.

18. Biganzoli L, Cufer T, Bruning P, et al. Doxorubicin-paclitaxel: a safe regimen in terms of cardiac toxicity in metastatic breast carcinoma patients. Results from a European organization for research and treatment of cancer multicenter trial. Cancer 2003;97: 40–5.

19. Gianni L, Dombernowsky P, Sledge G, et al. Cardiac function following combination therapy with paclitaxel and doxorubicin: an analysis of 657 women with advanced breast cancer. Ann Oncol 2001;12: 1067–73.

20. Tan-Chiu E, Yothers G, Romond E, et al. Assessment of cardiac dysfunction in a randomized trial comparing doxorubicin and cyclophosphamide followed by paclitaxel, with or without trastuzumab as adjuvant therapy in node-positive, human epidermal growth factor receptor 2-overexpressing breast cancer: NSABP B-31. J Clin Oncol 2005;23(31):7811–9.

21. Holmes FA, Madden T, Newman RA, et al. Sequence-dependent alteration of doxorubicin pharmacokinetic by paclitaxel in a phase I study of paclitaxel and doxorubicin in patients with metastatic breast cancer. J Clin Oncol 1996;14(10):2713–21.

22. Chan S, Friedrichs K, Noel D, et al. Prospective randomized trial of docetaxel versus doxorubicin in patients with metastatic breast cancer. J Clin Oncol 1999;17(8):2341–54.

23. Crone SA, Zhao YY, Fan L, et al. ErbB2 is essential in the prevention of dilated cardiomyopathy. Nat Med 2002;8(5):459–65.

24. Ozcelik C, Erdmann B, Pilz B, et al. Conditional mutation of the ErbB2 (HER2) receptor in cardiomyocytes leads to dilated cardiomyopathy. Proc Natl Acad Sci U S A 2002;99(13):8880–5.

25. Chien KR. Herceptin and the heart—a molecular modifier of cardiac failure. N Engl J Med 2006; 354(8):789–90.

26. Joensuu H, Kellokumpu-Lehtinen PL, Bono P, et al. Adjuvant docetaxel or vinorelbine with or without trastuzumab for breast cancer. N Engl J Med 2006;354(8):809–20.

27. Smith K, Dang C, Seidman AD. Cardiac dysfunction associated with trastuzumab. Expert Opin Drug Saf 2006;5(5):619–29.

28. Seidman A, Hudis C, Pierri MK, et al. Cardiac dysfunction in the trastuzumab clinical trials experience. J Clin Oncol 2002;20(5):1215–21.

29. Carver JR, Shapiro CL, Ng A, et al. American Society of Clinical Oncology Clinical Evidence Review on the Ongoing Care of Adult Cancer Survivors: cardiac and pulmonary late effects. J Clin Oncol 2007;25:3991–4008.

30. Amronim GD, Solomon RD. Production of arteriosclerosis in the rabbit: a quantitative assessment. Arch Pathol 1965;75:219.

31. Gold H. Production of arteriosclerosis in the rat: effect of X-ray and high-fat diet. Arch Pathol 1961; 71:268.

32. Artom C, Lofton HB, Clarkson TB. Ionizing radiation atherosclerosis and lipid metabolism in pigeons. Radiat Res 1965;26:165.

33. McEniery PT, Dorosti K, Schiavone WA, et al. Clinical and angiographic features of coronary artery disease after chest irradiation. Am J Cardiol 1987;60:1020.

34. Boivin JF, Hutchison GB, Lubin JH, et al. Coronary artery disease mortality in patients treated for Hodgkin's disease. Cancer 1992;69:1241.

35. Hancock SL, Tucker MA, Hoppe RT. Factors affecting late mortality from heart disease after treatment of Hodgkin's disease. JAMA 1993;270:1949.

36. Henry-Amar M, Hayat M, Meerwaldt JH. Causes of death after therapy for early stage Hodgkin's disease entered on EORTC protocols. Int J Radiat Oncol Biol Phys 1990;19:1155.

37. Mauch P, Kalish L, Marcus KC, et al. Long-term survival in Hodgkin's disease. Cancer J Sci Am 1995;1:33.

38. Glanzmann C, Kaufmann P, Jenni R, et al. Cardiac risk after mediastinal irradiation for Hodgkin's disease. Radiother Oncol 1998;46:51.

39. Reinders JG, Heijmen BJ, Olofsen-van Acht MJ, et al. Ischemic heart disease after mantlefield irradiation for Hodgkin's disease in long-term follow-up. Radiother Oncol 1999;51:35.

40. Swerdlow AJ, Higgins CD, Smith P, et al. Myocardial infarction mortality risk after treatment for Hodgkin disease: a collaborative British cohort study. J Natl Cancer Inst 2007;99:206–14.

41. Aleman BM, van del Belt-Dusebout AW, De Bruin M, et al. Late cardiotoxicity after treatment for Hodgkin lymphoma. Blood 2007;109:1878–86.

42. Handler CE, Livesey S, Lawton PA. Coronary ostial stenosis after radiotherapy: angioplasty or coronary artery surgery? Br Heart J 1989;61:208.

43. Orzan F, Brusca A, Conte MR, et al. Severe coronary artery disease after radiation therapy of the chest and mediastinum: clinical presentation and treatment. Br Heart J 1993;69:496.

44. Lund MB, Kongerud J, Boe J, et al. Cardiopulmonary sequelae after treatment for Hodgkin's disease: increased risk in females? Ann Oncol 1996;7:257.

45. Aviles A, Neri N, Nambo MJ, et al. Late cardiac toxicity secondary to treatment in Hodgkin's disease. A study comparing doxorubicin, epirubicin and mitoxantrone in combined therapy. Leuk Lymphoma 2005;46:1023–8.

46. Host H, Brennhoud IO, Loeb M. Post-operative radiotherapy in breast cancer: long-term results from the Oslo study. Int J Radiat Oncol Biol Phys 1986;12:727.

47. Jones JM, Ribeiro GG. Mortality patterns over 34 years of breast cancer patients in a clinical trial of post-operative radiotherapy. Clin Radiol 1989;40:204.

48. Haybittle JL, Brinkley D, Houghton J, et al. Postoperative radiotherapy and late mortality: evidence from the Cancer Research Campaign trial for early breast cancer. BMJ 1989;298:1611.

49. Hooning MJ, Berthe A, Aleman MP, et al. Long-term risk of cardiovascular disease in 10-year survivors of breast cancer. J Natl Cancer Inst 2007;99:365–75.

50. Giordano SH, Hortobagyi GN. Local recurrence of cardiovascular disease: pay now or later. J Natl Cancer Inst 2007;99:340–1.

51. Darby SC, McGale P, Taylor CW, et al. Long-term mortality from heart disease and lung cancer after radiotherapy breast cancer: prospective cohort study of about 300,000 women in US SEE registries. Lancet Oncol 2005;6:539–40.

52. Giordano SH, Juo YF, Freeman JL, et al. Risk of cardiac death after adjuvant radiotherapy for breast cancer. J Natl Cancer Inst 2005;97:406–7.

53. Stegman LD, Beal KP, Hunt MA, et al. Long-term clinical outcomes of whole-breast irradiation delivered in the prone position. Int J Radiat Oncol Biol Phys 2007;68:73–81.

54. Landau D, Adams EJ, Webb S, et al. Cardiac avoidance in breast radiotherapy: a comparison of simple shielding techniques with intensity-modulated radiotherapy. Radiother Oncol 2001;60:247.

55. Shapiro CL, Hardenbergh PH, Gelman R, et al. Cardiac effects of adjuvant doxorubicin and radiation therapy in breast cancer patients. J Clin Oncol 1998;16:3493.

56. Savage DE, Constine LS, Schwartz RG, et al. Radiation effects on left ventricular function and myocardial perfusion in long-term survivors of Hodgkin's disease. Int J Radiat Oncol Biol Phys 1990;19:721.

57. Pierga JY, Maunoury C, Valette H, et al. Follow-up thallium-201 scintigraphy after mantle field radiotherapy for Hodgkin's disease. Int J Radiat Oncol Biol Phys 1993;25:871.

58. Pihkala J, Happonen JM, Virtanen K, et al. Cardiopulmonary evaluation of exercise tolerance after chest irradiation and anticancer chemotherapy in children and adolescents. Pediatrics 1995;95:755.

59. Piovaccari G, Ferretti RM, Prati F, et al. Cardiac disease after chest irradiation for Hodgkin's disease: incidence in 108 patients with long follow-up. Int J Cardiol 1995;49:39.

60. Reber D, Birnbaum DE, Tollenaere P. Heart disease following mediastinal irradiation: surgical management. Eur J Cardiothorac Surg 1995;9:202–5.

61. Van Son JA, Noyez L, van Asten WN. Use of internal mammary artery in myocardial revascularization after mediastinal irradiation. J Thorac Cardiovasc Surg 1992;104:1539.

62. Adams MJ, Lipshutz SE, Schwartz C, et al. Radiation-associated cardiovascular disease: manifestations and management. Semin Radiat Oncol 2003;13:346.

63. Ruckdeschel JC, Chang P, Martin RG, et al. Radiation-related pericardial effusions in patients with Hodgkin's disease. Medicine 1975;54:245.

64. Arsenian MA. Cardiovascular sequelae of therapeutic thoracic radiation. Prog Cardiovasc Dis 1991;33:299.

65. Lagrange JL, Darcourt J, Benoliel J, et al. Acute cardiac effects of mediastinal irradiation: assessment by radionuclide angiography. Int J Radiat Oncol Biol Phys 1992;22:897.

66. Adams MJ, Lipsitz SR, Colan SD, et al. Cardiovascular status in long-term survivors of Hodgkin's disease treated with chest radiotherapy. J Clin Oncol 2004;22:3139–48.

67. Clements IP, Davis BJ, Wiseman GA. Systolic and diastolic cardiac dysfunction early after the initiation of doxorubicin therapy: significance of gender and concurrent mediastinal radiation. Nucl Med Commun 2002;23:521.

68. Hequet Q, Le QH, Moullet I, et al. Subclinical late cardiomyopathy after doxorubicin therapy for lymphoma in adults. J Clin Oncol 2004;22:1864–71.

69. Glanzmann C, Huguenin P, Lutolf UM, et al. Cardiac lesions after mediastinal irradiation for Hodgkin's disease. Radiother Oncol 1994;30:43.

70. Heidenreich PA, Hancock SL, Lee BK, et al. Asymptomatic cardiac disease following mediastinal irradiation. J Am Coll Cardiol 2003;42:743.

71. Byrd BF III, Mendes LA. Cardiac complications of mediastinal radiotherapy. The other side of the coin. J Am Coll Cardiol 2003;42:750.

72. Gustavsson A, Eskilsson J, Landberg T, et al. Late cardiac effects after mantle radiotherapy in patients with Hodgkin's disease. Ann Oncol 1990;1:355.

73. Carlson RG, Mayfield WR, Normann S, et al. Radiation-associated valvular disease. Chest 1991;99:538.

74. Sleijfer S. Bleomycin-induced pneumonitis. Chest 2001;120:617–24.

75. O'Sullivan JM, Huddar RA, Norman AR, et al. Predicting the risk of bleomycin lung toxicity in patients with germ-cell tumors. Ann Oncol 2003;14:91–6.

76. McDonald S, Rubin P, Phillips TL, et al. Injury to the lung from cancer therapy: clinical syndromes, measurable endpoints, and potential scoring systems. Int J Radiat Oncol Biol Phys 1995;31:1187–203.

77. Roach M III, Gandara DR, Yuo HS, et al. Radiation pneumonitis following combined modality therapy for lung cancer: analysis of prognostic factors. J Clin Oncol 1995;13:2606–12.

78. Hirsch A, Vander Els N, Straus DJ, et al. Effect of ABVD chemotherapy with and without mantle or mediastinal irradiation on pulmonary function and symptoms in early-stage Hodgkin's disease. J Clin Oncol 1996;14:1297–305.

Preoperative Evaluation of the Oncology Patient

Sunil K. Sahai, MD[a,b], Ali Zalpour, PharmD, BCPS[a],
Marc A. Rozner, MD, PhD[c],*

KEYWORDS

- Cancer • Preoperative evaluation • Surgery
- Chemotherapy

Although surgery remains the mainstay of cancer care, the advent of multidisciplinary approaches and the use of multiple therapeutic modalities has increased treatment complexity.[1] In patients with solid tumor malignancies, 75% undergo a surgical procedure for a cure. Some 90% will have surgery for other reasons,[2,3] which include diagnostic or palliative procedures, brachytherapy (the implanting of radiation seeds or devices), or surgery unrelated to cancer (eg, vascular surgery or hysterectomy for postmenopausal bleeding). The increasing age of patients with cancer, the increasing number of comorbid conditions, and the complexity of care before surgery often affect their perioperative course. A previous article in this publication addressed these issues from the internist's view point,[4] and reviews have also been written for anesthesiologists.[5,6] This article provides an update for all providers involved in the delivery of perioperative medical care for patients with cancer. Even today, there remains no set of guidelines for these patients. This review focuses primarily on perioperative aspects of chemotherapy, because it is unique to cancer medicine. Because many of the chemotherapeutic agents discussed herein have been used for many decades, some of the references to these agents are old.

GOALS OF PREOPERATIVE ASSESSMENT

Ideally, the preoperative assessment serves as a roadmap to guide the patient safely through surgery and the perioperative period. For the medically complex patient whose cancer is complicated by comorbid conditions, this guidance often requires close cooperation between internal medicine consultants, anesthesiologists, critical care physicians, and the surgeons. Sometimes, other medical needs of these patients are ignored because of their cancer treatment. For example, in a study of 161 patients with cancer and a pacemaker presenting for cancer surgery, 32% had not undergone interrogation of their devices for more than 1 year.[7]

In many settings, preoperative patients are routed to an internal medicine consultant before surgery. In general, nonsurgical medical comorbidities should be identified at this visit, and targeted preoperative testing and other consultations should be ordered with attention to appropriate optimization and perioperative risk assessment. Many patients are then evaluated at a preoperative anesthesiology clinic that provides anesthetic risk assessment for a variety of surgical and nonsurgical procedures requiring anesthesia.[6]

This article originally appeared in *Medical Clinics of North America*, volume 94, number 2.

[a] Department of General Internal Medicine, The University of Texas M.D. Anderson Cancer Center, 1515 Holcombe Boulevard, Unit 1465, Houston, TX 77030, USA

[b] Internal Medicine Perioperative Assessment Center, Department of General Internal Medicine, The University of Texas M.D. Anderson Cancer Center, 1515 Holcombe Boulevard, Unit 1465, Houston, TX 77030, USA

[c] The University of Texas M.D. Anderson Cancer Center, Department of Anesthesiology and Perioperative Medicine, 1400 Holcombe Boulevard, Unit 0409, Houston, TX 77030, USA

* Corresponding author. The University of Texas M.D. Anderson Cancer Center, 1400 Holcombe Boulevard, Unit 0409, Houston, TX 77030.

E-mail address: mrozner@mdanderson.org

Heart Failure Clin 7 (2011) 413–426
doi:10.1016/j.hfc.2011.04.003

Probably the most difficult issue surrounding cancer surgery is its timing, because cancer surgery often is neither truly elective nor truly emergent. Delaying cancer surgery to embark on an extended diagnostic evaluation of a new finding, or to achieve ideal medical optimization of a comorbid condition can render surgical intervention impossible because of tumor growth or extension.[8] As a result, customary perioperative guidelines might not be applicable to patients with cancer who are undergoing surgery.

CANCER, CANCER TREATMENT, AND PERIOPERATIVE IMPLICATIONS

In its most fundamental form, cancer represents a disruption of the body's homeostasis, and chemotherapy and/or radiation therapy can further disrupt this homeostasis from the subcellular level to the functional level. Many patients who were functionally vigorous before their cancer diagnosis become unable to achieve an adequate exercise tolerance as a result of the effects of treatment. Therefore, preoperative evaluation must take into account all previous treatments and their effects on the patient. An updated list of the most commonly used chemotherapy agents, their mechanisms of action, and perioperative implications of their side effects is given in **Table 1**. Common combinations of chemotherapeutic and adjunctive agents are listed in **Table 2** because many patients with cancer will be able to identify their protocols but not the specific agents. Many chemotherapy combinations involve administration of steroids (see **Table 2**), which can produce immunosuppression and glucose intolerance. Throughout this document, common brand/index names are shown in the text.

CARDIOVASCULAR EFFECTS AND EVALUATION

A variety of chemotherapeutic agents directly affect the heart and the cardiovascular system, and these effects often outlast the acute treatment stage. Although most practitioners are aware of the link between doxorubicin (Adriamycin) and the development of heart failure, many are unaware that the anthracycline class includes daunorubicin, epirubicin, idarubicin, mitoxantrone, and valrubicin. All of these drugs are similar to doxorubicin except for their potency.[9] The risk of developing cardiomyopathy increases greatly if the total dose is more than 550 mg/m^2 for daunorubicin and doxorubicin, and 900 mg/m^2 for epirubicin.[10–12] The likelihood of developing cardiomyopathy further depends on the presence of preexisting cardiac disease, concomitant administration of other chemotherapeutic agents

(particularly cyclophosphamide [Cytoxan], paclitaxel [Taxol], and trastuzumab [Herceptin]), chest irradiation, and extremes of age. In addition, any preexisting cardiomyopathy can exacerbate the cardiotoxicity of other agents in these patients.[13,14]

Other chemotherapeutic agents have been associated with cardiomyopathy, including taxanes such as paclitaxel and docetaxel (Taxotere). In addition, newer agents such as the tyrosine kinase inhibitors (see **Table 1**) have been associated with cardiomyopathy.[15]

Cardiac effects are not limited to cardiomyopathy; some agents can produce myocardial ischemia from coronary artery spasm or bradyarrhythmias.[16] The pyrimidine analogue 5-fluorouracil (5-FU) is used to treat several cancers, and it has the potential to induce myocardial ischemia, with or without progression to myocardial infarction. Co-administration of 5-FU with cisplatin seems to increase the incidence of ischemic events.[11] Capecitabine (Xeloda) is an oral, prodrug formulation of 5-FU. Because activation of the drug takes place mainly in cancer cells, the toxicity profile of capecitabine is believed to be lower than that of 5-FU.[17] Nevertheless, capecitabine use has produced myocardial ischemia and infarction, presumably by mechanisms similar to that of 5-FU.[10]

Electrocardiographic changes as well as chest pain have been found in patients during the administration of 5-FU. Any patient experiencing chest pain during 5-FU administration should be referred to a cardiologist to identify any underlying coronary artery disease,[18] although some might have normal coronary anatomy.[19]

Some other agents deserve mention: thalidomide can cause severe bradycardia necessitating pacemaker implantation.[20] In addition, co-administration of doxorubicin and vincristine has been reported to change pacing threshold.[21]

Radiation therapy to the thorax or mediastinum might damage the heart and its associated vascular structures. The potential adverse effects of mediastinal or mantle irradiation include coronary artery disease, pericarditis, cardiomyopathy, valvular disease, and conduction abnormalities.[22] A significantly higher risk of death as a result of ischemic heart disease has been reported for patients treated with radiation therapy to the chest for Hodgkin disease and breast cancer,[23] although not all investigators agree that breast irradiation leads to increased heart disease.[24] Coronary artery endothelial cell damage from radiation has been proposed as one mechanism for heart disease after chest irradiation. Factors affecting development of coronary artery disease include the percentage of the left ventricle irradiated, concurrent hormonal treatment, and a history of hypercholesterolemia.[25] As noted earlier, the risk of cardiomyopathy increases when radiation therapy is combined with doxorubicin (or any of the anthracyclines), because there seems to be a synergistic toxic effect on the myocardium.[23]

For the perioperative cardiac evaluation of the patient with cancer undergoing noncardiac surgery, many practitioners rely on the latest *Guidelines for Perioperative Evaluation* from the American College of Cardiology/American Heart Association (ACC/AHA).[26] However, the multiple toxicities associated with previous cancer treatment, along with decreases in a patient's functional status, increase the importance of a complete history of the patient's symptoms. The patient who presents with fatigue and dyspnea on exertion may have symptoms consistent with a particularly vigorous course of chemotherapy or cardiomyopathy secondary to prior chemotherapy or radiation therapy. As a result, application of the ACC/AHA guidelines may lead to unnecessary testing based on the use of functional status. In these patients, their functional status before the onset of treatment becomes an important factor in their planned preoperative course. The patient with cancer with cardiomyopathy probably benefits from beta blocker therapy.[27] In the absence of significant contraindications, these patients should be treated according to the ACC/AHA guidelines for heart failure.[16,28] These patients can be followed with serial echocardiography or repeated evaluations of serum B-type natriuretic peptide.[16]

As previously mentioned, complications from cancer and cancer care can include cardiomyopathy, ischemic heart disease, congestive heart failure, hypertension, hypotension, pericarditis, and bradyarrhythmias. In high-risk patients, noninvasive testing might be useful to predict postoperative cardiac complications.[29] Any decision to delay surgery in high-risk patients should be made in consultation with the patient's other physicians, because preoperative angiography and coronary artery stent placement can lead to significant surgical delay,[30] which might render a previously resectable cancer unresectable.

PULMONARY AND AIRWAY EFFECTS AND EVALUATION

As in the cardiovascular system, previous chemotherapy and radiation treatment can adversely affect the lungs. Bleomycin (BLM), an antitumor antibiotic used in treatment of germ cell tumors and certain hematological malignancies, causes interstitial pneumonitis followed by pulmonary fibrosis. BLM-induced pneumonitis occurs in 3% to 5% of patients receiving cumulative doses of less than 300 mg. At doses greater than 500 mg,

20% of patients experience pneumonitis. Lung fibrosis can develop even 10 years after cessation of therapy.[31] Advanced age, preexisting lung disease, or previous radiation therapy to the chest seems to predispose patients to pulmonary fibrosis.[32] In addition to BLM, other chemotherapeutic agents can cause interstitial pneumonia or pulmonary fibrosis in up to 25% of patients, including busulfan; chlorambucil; cyclophosphamide; melphalan; methotrexate; the nitrosoureas (carmustine [BCNU], lomustine [CCNU], or semustine-methyl [CCNU]), and vinca alkaloids with mitomycin. Many of these agents have also been associated with other pulmonary toxic effects including bronchiolitis obliterans with organizing pneumonia, pulmonary infiltrates with eosinophilia, noncardiac pulmonary edema, and pleural effusion. Vinca alkaloids with mitomycin have been reported to induce or exacerbate asthma.[33]

During the preoperative evaluation of patients with agents known to cause pulmonary toxicities, signs and symptoms of pulmonary compromise (dyspnea, nonproductive cough, pleurisy, crackles on examination) must be thoroughly vetted, because postoperative pulmonary complications are common. Although routine pulmonary testing is not usually warranted, chest radiograph, spirometry, arterial blood gases, and assessment of diffusing capacity should be considered if the patient will benefit from medical optimization before surgery.[34] Patients found to have restrictive lung disease, an increased alveolar-arterial oxygen gradient, and/or a decreased diffusing capacity may require special pulmonary care in the perioperative period.[35]

Pulmonary function testing may be indicated in those patients with known pulmonary fibrosis who have a poor functional status and have received radiation to the chest and/or BLM therapy if the treatment plan will be modified based on untoward results. A preoperative therapeutic thoracentesis for a pleural effusion may increase a patient's pulmonary reserve during surgery. In addition, patients with chronic obstructive pulmonary disease may benefit from pulmonary rehabilitation before surgery.[36] For appropriate patients with pulmonary compromise who will undergo neoadjuvant therapy before their surgical intervention, referral to a pulmonary rehabilitation program can make good use of this interval.

Radiation therapy to the head and neck area can compromise the airway. Many patients who undergo head and neck radiation develop trismus, limited mouth opening, limited neck extension, and limited mobility of pharyngeal structures, all of which can complicate the anesthesiologist's access to the airway for intubation. Even though

Table 1
Common chemotherapeutic agents

Class	Agents	Mechanism	Perioperative Implications
Alkylating Agents			
Nitrosoureas	Carmustine (BiCNU) Lomustine (CeeNU)	Inhibits DNA and RNA synthesis	Pulmonary fibrosis
Methylating agents	Procarbazine (Matulane)	Methylation of nucleic acid that leads to DNA and RNA synthesis inhibition	Hemorrhage Seizure Hemolysis Ototoxicity Edema Tachycardia
	Dacarbazine (DTIC-Dome)		Hepatic necrosis and occlusion Hepatic vein thrombosis
	Temozolamide (Temodar)		Seizure and gait abnormality Peripheral edema
Platinums	Cisplatin (Platinol; Platinol-AQ) Carboplatin (Paraplatin) Oxaliplatin (Eloxatin)	Inhibition of DNA replication	Acute renal tubular necrosis Magnesium wasting Peripheral sensory neuropathy Paresthesias Ototoxicity
Nitrogen mustards	Cyclophoshamide (Cytoxan; Neosar) Ifosfamide (Ifex)	Cross-linking DNA strands	Pericarditis Pericardial effusions Pulmonary fibrosis Hemorrhagic cystitis Water retention
	Melphalan (Alkeran) Chlorambucil (Leukeran)		Anemia SIADH SIDAH Seizures

Antimetabolites

Anthracyclines/ anthraquinolones	Doxorubicin (Adriamycin PFS; Adriamycin RDF), Daunorubicin (Cerubidine), Epirubicin (Ellence), Idarubicin (Idamycin), Mitoxantrone (Novantrone), Valrubicin (Valstar)	Interruption of DNA synthesis; Inhibition of topisomerase type II	Cardiomyopathy, ECG changes
Antitumor antibiotics: natural product	Bleomycin (Blenoxane), Mitomycin C (Mutamycin)	Inhibition of DNA and RNA synthesis	Pulmonary fibrosis, Pneumonitis, Pulmonary hypertension
Pyrimidine analogue	Capecitabine (Xeloda), Cytarabine (Ara-C), Fluorouracil (5-FU) Adrucil; Efudex), Gemcitabine (Gemzar)	Pyrimidine antimetabolite that interferes with DNA synthesis	Myocardial ischemia/infarction, Coronary vasospasm, Edema, Proteinuria
Purine analog	Thioguanine (6-TG; 6-thioguanine; TG; tioguanine), Pentostatin (Nipent; 2'-deoxycoformycin; DCF)	Purine antimetabolite that interferes with DNA synthesis	Hepatotoxicity, Pulmonary toxicity, Deep vein thrombophlebitis, Chest pain, Edema, AV block, Arrhythmia, Hypo and hypertension, Thrombosis, Tachycardia, Acute renal failure, Tumor lysis syndrome
	Cladribine (Leustatin, 2-CdA)		CVA/TIA, Angina, Thrombosis, Arrhythmia, CHF
	Fludarabine (Fludara)		Acute renal failure, Tumor lysis syndrome
	Mercaptopurine (Purinethol; 6-mercaptopurine; 6-MP)		Intrahepatic cholestasis and focal centralobular necrosis

(continued on next page)

Table 1
(continued)

Class	Agents	Mechanism	Perioperative Implications
Folate antagonist	Methotrexate (Mexate; Rheumatrex)	Methotrexate is a folate antimetabolite that inhibits DNA synthesis	Elevated liver enzymes Pulmonary edema Pleural effusions Encephalopathy Meningismus Myelosuppression
Substituted urea	Hydroxyurea (Hydrea)		Seizure Edema
Microtubule Assembly Inhibitors			
Taxanes	Paclitaxel (Taxol) docetaxel (Taxotere)	Microtubule assembly Inhibitor	Peripheral neuropathy Bradycardia Autonomic dysfunction Hypertension Angina Cerebrovascular accident Coronary ischemia ECG abnormalities, Raynaud phenomenon SIADH
Alkaloids	Vinblastine (Vincaleukoblastine; VLB)		GI bleed Paresthesias Recurrent laryngeal nerve palsy Autonomic dysfunction Orthostasis Hypo and hypertension
	Vincristine (Vincasar)		SIADH

Biologic Agents

	Drug	Mechanism	Side Effects
Monoclonal antibodies	Alemtuzumab (Campath)	Binding to immune cells to accelerate antibody dependent lysis of tumor cells	Dysrhythmia/tachycardia/SVT Hypotension and hypertension Pulmonary bleeding Hypertension Thromboembolic events Cardiopulmonary arrest Tumor lysis syndrome Electrolyte abnormality Cardiomyopathy Thrombus formation Pulmonary toxicity Tachycardia Hypertension Chest pain Hyper and hypotension Thrombosis Peripheral edema Arrhythmia Tachycardia Hyper and hypotension
	Bevacizumab (Avastin)		
	Cetuximab (Erbitux) Rituximab (Rituxan)		
	Trastuzumab (Herceptin)		
	Daclizumab (Zenapax)		
	Ibritumomab (Zevalin) Palivizumab (Synagis) Muromonab-CD3 (Orthoclone OKT3)		

Biologic Response Modulators

	Drug	Mechanism	Side Effects
Interleukins	Aldesleukin (IL-2; Proleukin) Denileukin diftitox (Ontak)	Promotes proliferation and differentiation of T and B cells	Capillary leak syndrome Peripheral edema Hypotension ECG changes
Interferon	Interferon alfa-2b (Intron A) Interferon alfacon-1 (Infergen)	Alteration in cellular differentiation	Arrhythmia Chest pain Pulmonary pneumonitis Ischemic disorders Hyperthyroidism Hypothyroidism Pulmonary infiltrates Ischemic disorders Hyperthyroidism Hypothyroidism
	Peginterferon alfa-2a (Pegasys) Peginterferon alfa-2b (PEG-Intron)		

(continued on next page)

Table 1
(continued)

Class	Agents	Mechanism	Perioperative Implications
Vascular Endothelial Growth Factor (VEGF) Inhibitor			
Tyrosine kinase inhibitors	Imatinib (Gleevec)	Inhibition of angiogenesis through VEGF receptor blockade	Edema Left ventricular dysfunction
	Sorafenib (Nexavar)		Cardiac ischemia and infarction Hypertension Thromboembolism
	Sunitinib (Sutent)		Cardiac ischemia and infarction Thromboembolism Adrenal insufficiency Pulmonary hemorrhage Hypertension Hypothyroidism Cardiomyopathy QT prolongation
	Dasatinib (Sprycel)	BCR-ABL tyrosine kinase inhibitor	Torsade de pointes Fluid retention Cardiomyopathy QT prolongation Pulmonary hemorrhage Platelet dysfunction
	Nilotinib (Tasigna)		QT prolongation Hypertension Peripheral edema
Epidermal Growth Factor Receptor (EGFR) Inhibitor			
	Erlotinib (Tarceva)	Epidermal growth factor receptor (HER1/EGFR)-tyrosine kinase	Deep venous thrombosis Arrhythmia Pulmonary toxicity Cerebrovascular accidents Myocardial ischemia, Syncope Edema
	Lapatinib (Tykerb)		Cardiomyopathy Pulmonary toxicity QT prolongation Pulmonary fibrosis
	Panitumumab (Vectibix)		Peripheral edema

Angiogenesis Inhibitors

Immunomodulators	Thalidomide (Thalomid) Lenalidomide (Revlimid)	Blocks tissue necrosis factor (TNF), suppression of angiogenesis, prevention of free-radical–mediated DNA damage, and increased cell-mediated cytotoxic effects	Thromboembolism Edema Bradycardia

Enzymes

	Asparginase (Elspar; Kidrolase)	Inhibits protein synthesis by hydrolyzing asparagine to aspartic acid and ammonia	Thrombosis Glucose intolerance Coagulopathy

Miscellaneous

Topoisomerase I inhibitor	Irinotecan (Camptosar, CPT-11) Topotecan (Hycamtin) Rubitecan (Orathecin)	Inhibits topoisomerase I and causes DNA breakdown	Neutropenia Diarrhea Cholinergic syndrome
Epipodophyllotoxin topoisomerase II inhibitor	Etoposide (Vepesid, VP-16)	Inhibits topoisomerase II and causes DNA breakdown	Neutropenia Stevens-Johnson syndrome Toxic epidermal necrolysis Myocardial infarction Congestive heart failure

Generic and brand names are used in this table. Some chemotherapy agents have Index names that are used as well.
Data from Refs. [51–54]

Table 2
Common chemotherapeutic combinations

Combination Abbreviation	Chemotherapy Components	Steroids
A-CMF	Doxorubicin, cyclophosphamide, methotrexate, 5-fluorouracil	
ABVD	Bleomycin, doxorubicin, vinblastine, dacarbazine	
BEP	Bleomycin, etoposide, cisplatin	
BEACOPP	Bleomycin, etoposide, vincristine, cyclophosphamide, vincristine, procarbazine	Prednisone
CAPP	Cyclophosphamide, doxorubicin, cisplatin	Prednisone
CAPOX	Capecitabine, oxaliplatin;	
CHOP ± rituximab[a]	Cyclosphosphamide, doxorubicin, vincristine	Prednisone
CHOEP ± rituximab[a]	Cyclosphosphamide, doxorubicin, etoposide, vincristine	Prednisone
CHOP-Bleo	Cyclosphosphamide, doxorubicin, vincristine, bleomycin	Prednisone
DHAP	Cisplatin, cytarabine	Dexamethasone
ESHAP	Cisplatin, cytarabine, etoposide	Methylprednisolone
FAC	5-Fluorouracil, cyclophosphamide, doxorubicin	
FEC	5-Fluorouracil, cyclophosphamide, epirubicin	
FOLFIRI	5-Fluorouracil, irinotecan, leucovorin	
FOLFOX	5-Fluorouracil, leucovorin, oxaliplatin	
hyper-CVAD	Course A: cyclophosphamide, doxorubicin, methotrexate, vincristine (± MESNA) Course B: cytarabine, leucovorin, methotrexate	Dexamethasone (course A only)
M-VAC	Methotrexate, vinblastine, doxorubicin, cisplatin	
R-CHOP	Rituximab + CHOP	
TAC	Cyclophosphamide, docetaxel, doxorubicin	
TCG	Paclitaxel, cisplatin, gemcitabine	
VAD	Doxorubicin, vincristine	Dexamethasone
VIM	Etoposide, ifosfamide, methotrexate	
VIP	Etoposide, ifosfamide, cisplatin, MESNA	

Only generic names are used in this table. Commonly, the brand name Adriamycin is used for the drug doxorubicin. Another generic name is hydroxydaunorubicin, and this name is the source of the "H" in many abbreviations that include this drug.
[a] CHOP or CHOEP plus rituximab are often abbreviated R-CHOP or R-CHOEP.
Data from LEXI-Comp ONLINE. Available at: http://www.crlonline.com. Accessed February 15, 2010.

many patients continue to demonstrate a normal external airway on physical examination, they might be difficult to ventilate or intubate after induction of general anesthesia or during a medical emergency. Thus, alternatives to direct laryngoscopy must be readily available for use in these patients.

GASTROINTESTINAL AND HEPATOBILIARY CONCERNS

Although all patients with cancer are at risk for malnutrition, patients with gastrointestinal (GI) tract malignancies are especially vulnerable. Radiation therapy to the abdomen can cause radiation-induced enteritis, leading to malabsorption and diarrhea. Low serum albumin levels are a marker for malnutrition, and an albumin level less than 3.0 g/dL has been shown to increase the risk of postoperative pneumonia according to a recent meta-analysis.[37] However, there seems to be no effective short-term treatment of this problem at this time.

Cancer that involves the liver, either as a primary site or through metastatic disease, as well as chemotherapy, may complicate the perioperative course through coagulopathy, biliary dysfunction, and malnutrition. Agents known to cause liver dysfunction are methotrexate, L-asparaginase, cytosine arabinoside, plicamycin, streptozocin, and 6-mercaptopurine.

GENITOURINARY AND RENAL

Several chemotherapeutic agents can cause renal insufficiency. In addition, tumor location can affect renal function, either through direct tumor invasion (eg, a primary urologic malignancy) or through mechanical issues leading to obstructive hydronephrosis. Cisplatin, used in a variety of head and neck, GI, genitourinary, and gynecologic malignancies can produce a dose-related nephrotoxicity, which represents its major dose-limiting toxicity. Toxicity occurs in 28% to 36% of patients after a single 50 mg/m^2 dose, manifested by increases in blood urea nitrogen, serum creatinine, and serum uric acid levels. A significant number of patients receiving cisplatin (and other platinum-based agents) develop magnesium wasting and hypomagnesemia,[38,39] and magnesium supplementation might ameliorate the sensory peripheral neuropathy that can develop with cisplatin[40] or oxaliplatin.[41]

Cyclophosamide, used to treat breast cancer and hematogenous malignancies, can cause hemorrhagic cystitis, producing obstructive uropathy from blood clot accumulation in the bladder. Treatment can require emergent cystoscopy or placement of percutaneous nephrostomy tubes. Hematuria from bladder cancer can influence perioperative anticoagulation strategies, especially in the patient with a cardiac stent; concern about bleeding from the antiplatelet therapy must be balanced with the protection conferred against stent stenosis. Tumor lysis syndrome can cause renal insufficiency.[42]

HEMATOLOGY

Cancer produces a hypercoagulable state caused by higher levels of cytokines, clotting factors, and cancer procoagulant.[43,44] Some chemotherapy agents, especially thalidomide, can exacerbate this issue.[10] As a result, venous thromboembolism (VTE) prophylaxis in the perioperative period should be used in all patients with cancer unless a specific contraindication is present.[45]

Patients who are undergoing chemotherapy and multiple laboratory draws often have wide variability in blood counts. Anemia has been treated with erythropoietin agents, but their use has been associated with shorter survival,[46] and controversy exists about the role of erythropoietin receptors on tumor cells.[47] Pancytopenia, thrombocytosis, and polycythemia are common, either as a result of treatment, or the disease itself. Phlebotomy and/or transfusions may be needed depending on the specific situation. Some patients may be taking hydroxyurea and/or anagrelide (Agrylin) to assist in the management of the thrombocytosis. In general, hydroxyurea inhibits platelet formation and may be safely continued throughout the perioperative period. Anagrelide inhibits platelet formation and aggregation and may need to be stopped in the perioperative period to avoid bleeding complications.[48]

NEUROLOGY

Tumors or metastatic disease of the brain or spinal cord may complicate postoperative VTE prophylaxis. In addition, many of these patients take steroids to limit or reduce cerebral swelling and pressure, and their blood sugar levels can be increased, leading to steroid-induced diabetes. Myasthenia gravis occurs as a paraneoplastic syndrome in about 30% of those with thymomas.[49] Eaton-Lambert syndrome, another paraneoplastic event, is associated with small cell lung cancer, and appropriate perioperative precautions need to be considered in both conditions.[50] The presence of a neurologic malignancy can complicate anticoagulation therapy (ie, coumadin for atrial fibrillation, clopidogrel for coronary athersclerosis) and VTE prophylaxis in these patients.

ENDOCRINOLOGY

Cushing syndrome resulting from ectopic production of adrenocorticotropic hormone has been associated with small cell lung cancer, pancreatic cancer, carcinoid, and thymic tumors. The syndrome of inappropriate secretion of antidiuretic hormone (SIADH) can accompany several types of lung cancer, including small cell, large cell, and adenocarcinoma. SIADH can be found in patients with pancreatic and duodenal cancers. Many of these patients will have mild, asymptomatic hyponatremia, which is generally not a contraindication to surgery.

Several conditions can lead to hypercalcemia, including ectopic production of parathyroid hormone, prostaglandins, and metastatic bone disease. Patients with elevated calcium levels should be investigated for occult hyperparathyroidism. Tumors associated with hypercalcemia include breast cancer, non–small cell lung cancer, and multiple myeloma.

Hypoglycemia can accompany mesenchymal tumors, adrenocortical tumors, pancreatic non–islet cell tumors, and hepatocellular cancer. Treatment is symptomatic, and some of these patients will need glucose supplementation on the day of their surgery in view of their nil-per-os status.

Hyperglycemia often accompanies chemotherapy, especially when steroids are co-administered. Many of these patients also have multiple risk factors for diabetes, and a glycosylated hemoglobin determination can be used to help determine the extent of the disease. Standard recommendations for diabetes management in the perioperative period also apply to patients with cancer, although special attention is required for the patient who requires a multiple day preoperative diet/caloric restriction regimen.

Adrenal insufficiency is common in patients who have received steroids in the course of their cancer care, and, as noted earlier, hypothyroidism can develop in those patients who have received radiation for head and neck cancers.

SPECIAL CONSIDERATIONS

Patients with complex head and neck cancers need careful evaluation by an anesthesiologist for any potential airway issues. Those patients undergoing head and neck surgery with obstructive sleep apnea and who have already obtained a positive pressure mask might benefit from evaluation by a pulmonologist, because their mask might not fit correctly after surgery, or its position might jeopardize any skin or tissue grafts placed for reconstructive procedures.

With regard to traditional laboratory testing, most practitioners realize that perioperative medicine has moved away from the comprehensive metabolic screening panel before surgery. However, selective laboratory testing (eg, electrolyte, renal function, and magnesium determination for the patient exposed to recent steroid therapy or nephrotoxic chemotherapy) may uncover secondary metabolic or hematologic issues that need to be addressed in the perioperative period. Chest radiograph and electrocardiographic evaluation might be indicated for those with a history of thoracic cancer, previous thoracic surgery, or radiotherapy to the chest wall. Thyroid function screening before surgery in a patient with a history of irradiation to the neck and the chest seems warranted, as these patients can develop occult thyroid insufficiency. In this cost conscious era, many of these studies may have been obtained during the work-up of a patient with cancer and need not be repeated for the planned surgical procedure if the test values have been obtained recently and there seems no change in a patient's status.

SUMMARY

Although the perioperative care of the patient with cancer is, in many ways, unchanged from the usual patient without a history of cancer, the broad systemic effects of cancer and cancer therapy pose challenges that need to be addressed. The role of physicians familiar with cancer, cancer treatment, and cancer-related comorbidities can play an integral part in the management of the patient who has cancer in the perioperative period.

REFERENCES

1. Geraci JM, Escalante CP, Freeman JL, et al. Comorbid disease and cancer: the need for more relevant conceptual models in health services research. J Clin Oncol 2005;23(30):7399–404.
2. Daly JM, Decosse JJ. Principles of surgical oncology. In: Calabrese P, Schein PS, Rosenberg SA, editors. Medical oncology. Toronto: Macmillan; 1995. p. 261.
3. Fox KR. Surgery in the patient with cancer. In: Goldmann DR, Brown FH, Guarnieri DM, editors. Perioperative medicine: medical care of the surgical patient. 2nd edition. New York: McGraw-Hill; 1994. p. 283–93.
4. Manzullo EF, Weed HG. Perioperative issues in patients with cancer. Med Clin North Am 2003; 87(1):243–56.
5. Davis MM, Rozner MA. Effects of cancer treatment on perioperative anesthetic care. In: Lake CL, Johnson JO, McLoughlin TM, editors. Advances in anesthesia. New York: Mosby; 2004. p. 121–42.
6. Andrabi TR, Rozner MA. Preoperative anesthesia evaluation. In: Shaw AD, Riedel BJ, Burton AW, et al, editors. Acute care of the cancer patient. Boca Raton (FL): Taylor and Francis; 2005. p. 243–58.
7. Rozner MA, Nguyen AD, Roberson JC. Inadequate pacemaker follow-up detected at the preanesthetic visit. Anesthesiology 2002;96:A1071.
8. Ewer MS. Specialists must communicate in complex cases. Int Med World Rep 2001;16(5):17.
9. Gharib MI, Burnett AK. Chemotherapy-induced cardiotoxicity: current practice and prospects of prophylaxis. Eur J Heart Fail 2002;4(3):235–42.
10. Micromedix(R) Healthcare Series. Thompson Healthcare: Greenwood Village (CO); 2008. Available at: http://www.micromedex.com/about_us/legal/cite/. Accessed February 15, 2010.
11. Ewer MS, Benjamin RS. Cardiac complications. In: Bast RC, Kufe DW, Pollock RE, et al, editors. Cancer medicine. 5th edition. London: B.C. Decker, Incorporated; 2000. p. 2324–39.
12. Zambetti M, Moliterni A, Materazzo C, et al. Long-term cardiac sequelae in operable breast cancer patients given adjuvant chemotherapy with or without doxorubicin and breast irradiation. J Clin Oncol 2001;19(1):37–43.
13. Philips JA, Marty FM, Stone RM, et al. Torsades de pointes associated with voriconazole use. Transpl Infect Dis 2007;9(1):33–6.

14. Bdair FM, Graham SP, Smith PF, et al. Gemcitabine and acute myocardial infarction–a case report [review]. Angiology 2006;57(3):367–71.

15. Chu TF, Rupnick MA, Kerkela R, et al. Cardiotoxicity associated with tyrosine kinase inhibitor sunitinib. Lancet 2007;370(9604):2011–9.

16. Youssef G, Links M. The prevention and management of cardiovascular complications of chemotherapy in patients with cancer [review]. Am J Cardiovasc Drugs 2005;5(4):233–43.

17. Kaklamani VG, Gradishar WJ. Role of capecitabine (Xeloda) in breast cancer. Expert Rev Anticancer Ther 2003;3(2):137–44.

18. Anand AJ. Fluorouracil cardiotoxicity. Ann Pharmacother 1994;28(3):374–8.

19. Akpek G, Hartshorn KL. Failure of oral nitrate and calcium channel blocker therapy to prevent 5-fluorouracil-related myocardial ischemia: a case report. Cancer Chemother Pharmacol 1999;43(2):157–61.

20. Kaur A, Yu SS, Lee AJ, et al. Thalidomide-induced sinus bradycardia. Ann Pharmacother 2003;37(7–8):1040–3.

21. Wilke A, Hesse H, Gorg C, et al. Elevation of the pacing threshold: a side effect in a patient with pacemaker undergoing therapy with doxorubicin and vincristine. Oncology 1999;56(2):110–1.

22. Adams MJ, Hardenbergh PH, Constine LS, et al. Radiation-associated cardiovascular disease. Crit Rev Oncol Hematol 2003;45(1):55–75.

23. Basavaraju SR, Easterly CE. Pathophysiological effects of radiation on atherosclerosis development and progression, and the incidence of cardiovascular complications. Med Phys 2002;29(10):2391–403.

24. Vallis KA, Pintilie M, Chong N, et al. Assessment of coronary heart disease morbidity and mortality after radiation therapy for early breast cancer. J Clin Oncol 2002;20(4):1036–42.

25. Lind PA, Pagnanelli R, Marks LB, et al. Myocardial perfusion changes in patients irradiated for left-sided breast cancer and correlation with coronary artery distribution. Int J Radiat Oncol Biol Phys 2003;55(4):914–20.

26. Fleisher LA, Beckman JA, Brown KA, et al. ACC/AHA 2007 guidelines on perioperative cardiovascular evaluation and care for noncardiac surgery: a report of the American College of Cardiology/American Heart Association Task Force on practice guidelines (Writing Committee to revise the 2002 guidelines on perioperative cardiovascular evaluation for noncardiac surgery). Published 9-27-2007. Available at: http://circ.ahajournals.org/cgi/content/short/116/17/e418. Accessed November 18, 2008.

27. Mukai Y, Yoshida T, Nakaike R, et al. Five cases of anthracycline-induced cardiomyopathy effectively treated with carvedilol. Intern Med 2004;43(11):1087–8.

28. Hunt SA. ACC/AHA 2005 guideline update for the diagnosis and management of chronic heart failure in the adult: a report of the American College of Cardiology/American Heart Association Task Force on practice guidelines (Writing Committee to update the 2001 guidelines for the evaluation and management of heart failure). J Am Coll Cardiol 2005;46(1):1116–43.

29. Chang K, Sarkiss M, Won KS, et al. Preoperative risk stratification using gated myocardial perfusion studies in patients with cancer. J Nucl Med 2007;48(3):344–8.

30. Grines CL, Bonow RO, Casey DE Jr, et al. Prevention of premature discontinuation of dual antiplatelet therapy in patients with coronary artery stents: a science advisory from the American Heart Association, American College of Cardiology, Society for Cardiovascular Angiography and Interventions, American College of Surgeons, and American Dental Association, with representation from the American College of Physicians. Circulation 2007;115(6):813–8.

31. Tashiro M, Izumikawa K, Yoshioka D, et al. Lung fibrosis 10 years after cessation of bleomycin therapy. Tohoku J Exp Med 2008;216(1):77–80.

32. Einhorn L, Krause M, Hornback N, et al. Enhanced pulmonary toxicity with bleomycin and radiotherapy in oat cell lung cancer. Cancer 1976;37(5):2414–6.

33. Copper JA Jr. Drug-induced lung disease. Adv Intern Med 1997;42:231–68.

34. Smetana GW. Preoperative pulmonary evaluation: identifying and reducing risks for pulmonary complications. Cleve Clin J Med 2006;73(Suppl 1):S36–41.

35. Klein DS, Wilds PR. Pulmonary toxicity of antineoplastic agents: anaesthetic and postoperative implications. Can Anaesth Soc J 1983;30(4):399–405.

36. Sekine Y, Chiyo M, Iwata T, et al. Perioperative rehabilitation and physiotherapy for lung cancer patients with chronic obstructive pulmonary disease. Jpn J Thorac Cardiovasc Surg 2005;53(5):237–43.

37. Smetana GW, Lawrence VA, Cornell JE. Preoperative pulmonary risk stratification for noncardiothoracic surgery: systematic review for the American College of Physicians. Ann Intern Med 2006;144(8):581–95.

38. Stohr W, Paulides M, Bielack S, et al. Nephrotoxicity of cisplatin and carboplatin in sarcoma patients: a report from the late effects surveillance system. Pediatr Blood Cancer 2007;48(2):140–7.

39. Kintzel PE. Anticancer drug-induced kidney disorders. Drug Saf 2001;24(1):19–38.

40. Lajer H, Daugaard G. Cisplatin and hypomagnesemia. Cancer Treat Rev 1999;25(1):47–58.

41. Grothey A. Oxaliplatin-safety profile: neurotoxicity [review]. Semin Oncol 2003;30(4:Suppl 15):5–13.

42. Coiffier B, Altman A, Pui CH, et al. Guidelines for the management of pediatric and adult tumor lysis

syndrome: an evidence-based review. J Clin Oncol 2008;26(16):2767–78.

43. Adcock DM, Fink LM, Marlar RA, et al. The hemostatic system and malignancy. Clin Lymphoma Myeloma 2008;8(4):230–6.

44. Gouin-Thibault I, Achkar A, Samama MM. The thrombophilic state in cancer patients. Acta Haematol 2001;106(1–2):33–42.

45. Lyman GH, Khorana AA, Falanga A, et al. American Society of Clinical Oncology guideline: recommendations for venous thromboembolism prophylaxis and treatment in patients with cancer. J Clin Oncol 2007;25(34):5490–505.

46. Tovari J, Pirker R, Timar J, et al. Erythropoietin in cancer: an update [review]. Curr Mol Med 2008; 8(6):481–91.

47. Fandrey J. Erythropoietin receptors on tumor cells: what do they mean? [review]. Oncologist 2008; 13(Suppl 3):16–20.

48. Harrison CN. Essential thrombocythaemia: challenges and evidence-based management. Br J Haematol 2005;130(2):153–65.

49. Maggi L, Andreetta F, Antozzi C, et al. Thymoma-associated myasthenia gravis: outcome, clinical and pathological correlations in 197 patients on a 20-year experience. J Neuroimmunol 2008; 201–202:237–44.

50. O'Neill GN. Acquired disorders of the neuromuscular junction. Int Anesthesiol Clin 2006;44(2): 107–21.

51. MICROMEDEX Healthcare Series. Available at: http://www.thomsonhc.com/home/dispatch. Accessed February 15, 2010.

52. LEXI-Comp ONLINE. Available at: http://www.crlonline. com. Accessed February 15, 2010.

53. Skeel RT. Biologic and pharmacologic basis of cancer chemotherapy. In: Lippincott's handbook of cancer chemotherapy. 6th edition. Philadelphia (PA): Lippincott Williams and Wilkins; 2003.

54. Balmer CM, Valley AW, Lannucci A. Cancer treatment and chemotherapy. In: DiPiro JT, Talbert RL, Yee GC, et al, editors. Pharmacotherapy: a pathophysiologic approach. 6th edition. New York: McGraw-Hill Book Co; 2005. p. 2279–328.

Chemotherapy-Induced Cardiotoxicity in Women

Kelli S. Dempsey, MSN, APRN-BC, AOCNP

KEYWORDS

- Breast cancer • Bevacizumab • Cardiotoxicity
- Chemotherapy • Doxorubicin • Trastuzumab

Chemotherapy-induced cardiotoxicity (CIC) can cause treatment dilemmas, decreased survival, increased morbidity, and complicated psychosocial issues. The purpose of this article is threefold: to define CIC; to discuss a model for evaluation and treatment; and to present a case study.

Heart disease is the leading cause of death in the United States, with cancer a very close second. The American Cancer Society estimates that 678,060 women were diagnosed with cancer and 270,100 women died of cancer in the United States during 2007. The three most common sites of cancer in women are breast (26%), lung (15%), and colon (11%).[1] Every 3 minutes a women in the United States is diagnosed with breast cancer.[2] In 2007, more than 176,000 women were diagnosed with breast cancer, and more than 40,000 in the United States died of this disease.[1] The incidence of breast cancer in women has increased from 1 in 20 in 1960 to one in eight in 2007.[2] Although CIC is not unique to women, some of the most common cardiotoxic agents are chemotherapy drugs used to treat breast cancer. In the United States, 99% of patients who have breast cancer are female.[3] Therefore the scope of this article is limited to CIC in women who have breast cancer.

The median age for women at diagnosis of breast cancer is 61 years, and the median age of death caused by breast cancer is 69 years. The overall 5-year survival rate for women who have breast cancer is 88%. In 2004, there were more than 2 million women alive in the United States who had a history of breast cancer.[4] Improvements in the detection and treatment of breast cancer have resulted in a 24% decrease in mortality from breast cancer since 1990.[5] Breast cancer is becoming a manageable chronic disease, comparable in its chronicity to diabetes or hypertension.[6] Many survivors of breast cancer actually are at greater risk of death from cardiovascular disease than from cancer.[6]

CHEMOTHERAPY-INDUCED CARDIOTOXICITY

Cardiotoxicity is defined as a poisonous or deleterious effect upon the heart.[7] CIC is cardiotoxicity that develops as a result of chemotherapy administration. CIC can manifest on a continuum ranging from asymptomatic, transient arrhythmias to fatal cardiomyopathy resulting from permanent left ventricular dysfunction. CIC may occur acutely during treatment or years later and varies for different chemotherapy drugs.[8] **Table 1** summarizes the cardiotoxic manifestations of various chemotherapy drugs, and **Box 1** offers related definitions.

The signs and symptoms of cardiotoxicity vary widely. Signs of cardiac dysfunction may include changes in blood pressure or heart rate, irregular heart rhythms, murmurs, carotid bruits, distended jugular veins, decreased pulses, edema, and changes in skin color.[9] The most common symptoms of cardiac problems associated with cardiotoxicity are pain, dyspnea, weight gain, edema, weakness, fatigue, palpitations, dizziness, syncope and swelling of an extremity with deep venous thromboembolism.[10]

The quality of pain varies with the cardiac disorder present. Ischemic pain often presents as pressing, squeezing, or a weight-like pressure

This article originally appeared in *Critical Care Nursing Clinics of North America*, volume 20, number 3.
Deaconess Clinic, 4055 Gateway Boulevard, Newburgh, IN 47630, USA
E-mail address: kellidempsey@insightbb.com

Heart Failure Clin 7 (2011) 427–435
doi:10.1016/j.hfc.2011.04.004

Table 1
Chemotherapy agents associated with cardiotoxicity

Condition	Chemotherapeutic Agent
Angina	Cytarabine; fludarabine
Arrhythmias	All-trans retinoic acid (ATRA); arsenic trioxide; aldesleukin; busulfan (tamponade); capecitabine; cisplatin; cyclophosphamide (high dose); cytarabine; daunorubicin (acute); dimethyl sulfoxide; doxorubicin (acute); epirubicin (acute); fluorouracil; idarubicin (acute); ifosfamide; interferons; decitabine; methotrexate; mitoxantrone; paclitaxel; rituximab; thalidomide
Cardiogenic shock	Fluorouracil
Cardiomyopathy	Cyclophosphamide; daunorubicin; epirubicin (chronic); trastuzumab
Chronic heart failure	Aldesleukin; ATRA; alemtuzumab (chronic); bevacizumab; capecitabine; cisplatin; cytarabine; daunorubicin (chronic); decitabine; doxorubicin (chronic); epirubicin (chronic); fluorouracil; idarubicin (chronic); ifosfamide; imatinib; interferon (high-dose); mitomycin; mitoxantrone; paclitaxel; pentostatin; trastuzumab
Deep venous thromboembolism	Bevacizumab; thalidomide
Edema	Imatinib; thalidomide
Effusion	ATRA; imatinib
Endomyocardial fibrosis	Busulfan
Heart block	Cyclophosphamide; cisplatin; interferon
Hypertension	Bevacizumab; bleomycin; cisplatin; mitomycin; procarbazine; vinblastine
Hypotension	Aldesleukin; alemtuzumab; ATRA; carmustine; cetuximab dacarbazine; denileukin diftitox; etoposide; fludarabine; interferon; paclitaxel; rituximab; tamoxifen; thalidomide; vincristine
Ischemia/infarction	ATRA; bevacizumab; bleomycin; capecitabine; cisplatin; dactinomycin; epirubicin (chronic); etoposide
Left ventricular dysfunction	Interferon; trastuzumab
Myocarditis/pericarditis	ATRA; bleomycin; cyclophosphamide; cytarabine; doxorubicin; etoposide; mitoxantrone
Possible cardiac toxicity	Altretamine; amifostine; aminoglutethimide; anagrelide; anastrazole; bevacizumab; bexarotene; campath; cytarabine (liposomal); estramustine; etoposide; exemestane; flutamide; gosrelin; leuprolide; megesterol acetate; oprelvekin; oxaliplatin; tamoxifen; teniposide; thalidomide; tretinoin
Vasospasm	Interferon; trastuzumab

From: Mays, Theresa. 2007 Oncology Preparatory Review Course Handbook. Used with permission from the American College of Clinical Pharmacy and the American Society of Health-System Pharmacists; with permission.

on the chest and possibly radiating to the neck, arm, or jaw. Pericardial inflammatory pain feels like burning or stabbing and worsens with coughing or lying down. Pulmonary embolism pain typically is pleuritic and usually is associated with dyspnea.[10] Dyspnea is uncomfortable or labored breathing which worsens with exertion and when lying down. Palpitations are the perception of heart action and may be associated with increased weakness, fatigue, and dizziness.[10] Patients receiving potentially cardiotoxic chemotherapy

agents and their family members/caregivers should be educated about the signs and symptoms of cardiotoxicities and about the need to notify health care personnel when signs or symptoms of these conditions occur.

MODEL OF EVALUATION AND TREATMENT
Evaluation

The general model for the evaluation and treatment of CIC is similar to that used to evaluate

Box 1
Definitions of cardiotoxicity-related terms

Angina: acute pain in the chest

Arrhythmias: variation from the normal heart rhythm

Cardiogenic shock: acute peripheral circulatory failure secondary to primary cardiac problem

Cardiomyopathy: primary myocardial disease

Edema: accumulation of excess fluid

Effusion, pericardial: accumulation of fluid in the pericardium

Fibrosis: formation of fibrous tissue

Heart block: impairment of conduction in heart excitation

Hypertension: high blood pressure, typically > 140/80

Hypotension: low blood pressure, typically < 100 systolic

Infarction: interruption of blood supply causing necrosis

Ischemia: deficiency of blood supply to the heart

Infarction: interruption of blood supply causing necrosis

Myocarditis: inflammation of the muscular wall of the heart

Pericarditis: inflammation of the pericardium

Thromboembolism: obstruction of blood vessel with thrombic material

Vasospasm: spasm of blood vessel decreasing caliber

From O'Toole M. Miller-Keane encyclopedia and dictionary of medicine, nursing, and allied health. 5th edition. Philadelphia: W.B.Saunders Company; 1992; with permission.

percentage of patients at diagnosis and the 5-year survival rates vary for the different stages of breast cancer (**Table 2**).[4,12]

Staging of breast cancer uses history, examination, surgery, imaging, and laboratory tests. Surgical interventions after initial biopsy may include lumpectomy, mastectomy, axillary dissection, sentinel lymph node biopsy, and biopsy at site of metastasis.[2,11] Imaging techniques for staging include radiography, CT scan, bone scan, MRI, and PET scans.[11] Laboratory testing with blood cell counts, chemistry panels, and tumor markers provides information on the patient's overall health and organ function and helps identify areas of possible metastasis, such as bone or liver.[11]

Once the need for treatment with chemotherapy, radiation, biologic, and/or hormonal therapy has been determined, evaluation for the patient's risk of developing CIC is indicated. Women who have breast cancer may have greater risk of developing cardiovascular disease because of risks associated with treatment as well as their prediagnosis risk stratification.[14] Women considering chemotherapy and/or hormone treatment after surgery and/or radiation therapy should be evaluated for pre-existing cardiovascular risk factors. These evaluations include the assessment of both modifiable and nonmodifiable risks. Modifiable risks (hyperlipidemia, smoking, sedentary lifestyle, high-caloric and/or high-fat diet, obesity, stress, hypertension, diabetes) and nonmodifiable risks (race, genetics, aging) should be assessed.[15]

Researchers from Duke University Medical Center recommend performing a formal cardiovascular risk assessment, using either the Framingham or Reynolds risk scores on all patients who have breast cancer before initiation of chemotherapy or hormonal therapy.[14] The Framingham

and design treatment regimens for patients who have breast cancer. An oncologist typically is consulted to see a patient who has a known diagnosis of breast cancer, often after biopsy and/or surgical intervention. To help guide prognosis and treatment choices, the oncology evaluation includes determination of the stage, grade, hormone receptor, and *HER2* status of the tumor.[11]

The treatment and prognosis of breast cancer depend on staging (extent of cancer) and tumor grade (pathologic features).[12,13] Staging tests determine whether the cancer is invasive or noninvasive, the size of the tumor, lymph node involvement, and whether there is distant spread (metastasis). Stages range from 0 to 4. The

Table 2
The percentage of patients at diagnosis and the associated 5-year survival rates for the stages of breast cancer

Stage	Diagnosis (%)	5-year Survival (%)
0 and 1 (localized)	61	98
2 (local spread)	31 (combined with stage 3)	81–92
3 (locally advanced)	31	54–67
4 (distant spread)	6	20–26

Heart Study prediction score takes into account age, high- and low-density cholesterol levels, blood pressure, smoking, and diabetes.[16] The Reynolds risk score considers age, smoking, systolic blood pressure, total and high-density cholesterol levels, C-reactive protein level, and parental history of myocardial infarction.[17]

Treatment

The chemotherapy and biologic therapy agents most commonly used for breast cancer are listed in **Table 3** along with their associated cardiotoxicities. The most common cardiotoxic agents are the anthracyclines (eg, doxorubicin and epirubicin) and the biologic agent, trastuzumab.[8,22] The incidence of clinical heart failure caused by anthracyclines is between 1% and 5% with asymptomatic decrease in left ventricular function ranging from 5% to 20%. Clinical heart failure increases when cardiotoxic drugs are used in combination.[23]

Doxorubicin is the major chemotherapy agent used for treating breast cancer.[24] Cardiotoxicity associated with doxorubicin ranges from early-onset sinus tachycardia to late-onset fatal cardiomyopathy.[8] Acute toxicities include arrhythmias, pericarditis, myocardial infarction, sudden

Table 3
Cardiotoxicity of chemotherapeutic agents used to treat breast cancer - synthesis of the literature [18,19,20,21]

Generic Name	Brand Name	Cardiotoxicity
Albumin-bound paclitaxel	Abraxane	None significant
Aromatase inhibitors	Arimidex, Aromasin, Faslodex, Femara	Angina, hypertension, infarction, thromboembolism
Bevacizumab	Avastin	Hypertension Ischemia Congestive heart failure
Capecitabine	Xeloda	Angina Congestive heart failure Ischemia
Carboplatin	Paraplatin	Ischemia
Cyclophosphamide	Cytoxan	Cardiomyopathy Myocarditis
Docetaxel	Taxotere	Edema
Doxorubicin	Adriamycin	See text
Epirubicin	Ellence	Arrhythmias Cardiomyopathy Congestive heart failure Ischemia
Fluorouracil	5-FU	Arrhythmias Congestive heart failure Ischemia
Gemcitabine	Gemzar	None significant
Lapatinib	Tykerb	Prolonged QT Decreased left ventricular ejection fraction
Methotrexate	Trexall	Arrhythmias Ischemia
Tamoxifen	Nolvadex	Thromboembolism
Trastuzumab	Herceptin	See text
Paclitaxel	Taxol	Arrhythmias Congestive heart failure Hypotension Ischemia
Pegylated liposomal doxorubicin	Doxil	CHF (must be included in measuring accumulated dose of athracycline)
Vinorelbine	Navelbine	Ischemia

cardiac death, congestive heart failure (CHF), and cardiomyopathy.[25] Chronic toxicity with anthracyclines includes cardiomyopathy and CHF.[25]

According to the Food and Drug Administration (FDA), a "black box" warning in the package insert alerts prescribers to the following serious potential problems [26]:

- An adverse reaction so serious in proportion to the potential benefit from the drug that it must be considered in assessing the risks and benefits of using the drug
- A serious adverse reaction that can be reduced or prevented
- FDA approval of drug that included restrictions to ensure safety.

The doxorubicin package insert contains a black box warning regarding "myocardial toxicity manifested in its most severe form by potentially fatal CHF," which may occur during treatment or months to years after treatment.[8]

Doxorubicin cardiotoxicity is related to the cumulative dosage a patient receives. The risk of cardiotoxicity ranges from 1% to 20% for doses of 300 mg/m^2 to 500 mg/m^2.[8] Doxorubicin cardiotoxicity also varies with the route of administration. Intravenous push (IVP) administration involves drug delivery over a matter of minutes. Continuous infusion, however, entails intravenous delivery of medication over a 48- or 96-hour time period. Findings from a landmark study published in 1989 involving 141 patients showed a 75% decrease in clinical CHF when patients received doxorubicin by continuous infusion as compared with IVP. Although this study demonstrated that administration of doxorubicin by continuous infusion decreased cardiotoxicity, this slower method of drug delivery did not affect treatment response rate, time to response, duration of response, or survival.[27]

Factors increasing the risk for anthracycline cardiotoxicity include prior mediastinal radiation, concurrent treatment with other cardiotoxic drugs, doxorubicin exposure at an early age, advanced patient age, and pre-existing heart disease.[8] A popular breast cancer regimen gives doxorubicin and cyclophosphamide for four cycles followed by paclitaxel with or without trastuzumab for four cycles.[24] Sequential administration of these drugs reduces cardiotoxicity.[22,24]

Cardiac monitoring is crucial for all women starting treatment with an anthracycline. The baseline ejection fraction should be determined with either a multigated radionuclide angiography (MUGA) or echocardiography (ECHO) study.[8] Clinical monitoring by history and examination is mandatory to find symptoms and signs of heart problems.

ECHO or MUGA is desirable at intervals during and after treatment.[8] Using the same technique for monitoring heart function provides consistency and improves recognition of deterioration in cardiac function.[8]

The doxorubicin package insert defines deterioration of cardiac function by left ventricular ejection fraction (LVEF) measurement as a 10% decline below the lower limit of normal (50%–70%), an LVEF of 45% or less, or a 20% decline from the baseline LVEF.[8] When CIC occurs, the benefit of further treatment must be weighed against the risk of developing irreversible cardiac damage.[8]

Her-2/Neu (*HER2*) is a gene that helps control cellular growth, division, repair, and helps control abnormal or defective cells.[28] The overamplification of *HER2* on a cell surface is thought to lead to increased cellular proliferation that can cause malignancy.[29] *HER2* is a poor prognostic indicator amplified in up to 30% of breast cancers and is associated with an increased risk of recurrence and death, increased incidence of positive lymph nodes, a 50% increased chance of brain metastases, and decreased response to hormonal therapy.[30,31] Conversely, *HER2*-positive breast cancers have a better response to anthracycline chemotherapy and thus have a better clinical prognosis.[32]

Trastuzumab is a monoclonal antibody biologic therapy that is effective in *Her2*-positive tumors. A monoclonal antibody is a type of protein synthesized in the laboratory that locates and binds to specific receptors in the body and on the surface of cancer cells.[28] Two studies enrolling more than 3000 patients showed a dramatic reduction of up to 52% in overall risk of recurrence in early invasive breast cancer with the addition of trastuzumab to the chemotherapy regimen.[33] The increased risk of CHF from adding trastuzumab to chemotherapy was approximately 4%, a risk most patients are willing to assume for the added benefit.[33] Most women developing CHF (68%) had resolution of symptoms by 6 months after completion of trastuzumab treatment.[33]

Trastuzumab includes a black box warning on the package insert regarding cardiomyopathy. The package insert notes that trastuzumab administration can result in left ventricular dysfunction and CHF, especially when administered with anthracyclines. Recommendations for decreasing the risk of CIC and improving detection of CIC include LVEF evaluation by ECHO or MUGA before beginning chemotherapy and frequently during treatment.[22] The large studies mentioned previously checked LVEF at baseline and at 3, 6, 9, 15, and 18 months.[33] Trastuzumab should be withheld or discontinued if there is a 16% or larger decrease from the baseline LVEF, an LVEF below normal with a 10% or greater decrease from baseline, persistent decreased LVEF for 8 weeks, and/or dosing interruptions on more than three occasions.[22]

Adjuvantonline.com is an excellent Web-based resource that stratifies the risks and benefits of various treatments for breast, lung, and colon cancer. This resource includes a slide presentation from the 2005 meeting of the American Society of Clinical Oncology that shows a table describing pretreatment LVEF values, patient age, and subsequent risk of developing cardiomyopathy with trastuzumab treatment. For women under age 50 years, the risk for developing CHF for baseline a LVEF of 50% to 54% was reported to be 6.3%, compared with 19.1% for women older than 50 years. A baseline LVEF higher than 65% decreased the risk of developing CHF to 0.6% for women younger than 50 years and 1.3% for women older than 50 years.

Bevacizumab is a monoclonal antibody used to treat breast, colon, and lung cancer. The package insert contains a black box warning for gastrointestinal perforation, wound-healing complications, and pulmonary hemorrhage.[34] The package insert states that 1.7% of patients in the manufacturer's clinical studies developed CHF.[34] When used in patients who had prior or concurrent anthracycline use and/or left chest wall radiation, the incidence increased to 4%.[34] Bevacizumab use is associated with arterial thromboembolic events (VTE) and hypertension.[34]

Thromboembolic events included stroke, transient ischemic attack (mini-stroke), myocardial infarction, and angina. Hypertension (> 150/100 mm Hg) and severe hypertension (> 200/110 mm Hg) were noted in as many as 18% of patients in clinical trials using bevacizumab. Patients treated with bevacizumab in oncology practices commonly develop hypertension that is manageable using antihypertensives.[34] The bevacizumab package insert recommends discontinuing or holding treatment until hypertension can be controlled.[34]

Thromboembolism affects approximately 15% of all patients who have cancer (personal communication, A. Kommareddy, 2007). Combined with smoking, implanted venous access devices, and chemotherapy agents that increase the risk of clotting, thromboembolism becomes a significant issue. Hormonal therapy with tamoxifen and aromatase inhibitors has improved breast cancer survival.[35,36] Tamoxifen has a black box warning for VTE including stroke, deep venous thromboembolism, infarction, and fatal pulmonary embolism.[35] The risk for developing VTE is present, but lower, with aromatase inhibitors.[36] As with chemotherapy, the risk of treatment with hormonal agents needs to be weighed against the benefits of treatment. Patients may have several pre-existing risks for developing clots, such as smoking, hypertension, irritable bowel syndrome, obesity, and/or personal or family history of clotting.[37] With multiple clotting risks, treatments other than hormones may be prudent.

Tests showing cardiac dysfunction may include EKG changes, decreased LVEF or anatomic disturbances on ECHO or MUGA, cardiomegaly (enlarged heart) on chest radiography, thromboembolism on Doppler imaging, hypokinesis of myocardium on stress imaging, and stenosed arteries with catheterization.[36] Laboratory findings may include abnormalities in arterial blood gases, complete blood cell counts, chemistry panels, troponins, brain natriuretic peptide, C-reactive protein, D-dimer, and homocysteine.[36–38]

Strategies for treatment and improvements in technology have diminished the long-term effects of CIC. Improved radiation therapy techniques that shield the heart, frequent cardiac screening, appropriate and prompt drug cessation or dose reductions, and intervention with cardioprotective medications help decrease CIC.[39] Dexrazoxane (Zinecard), a cardioprotectant chelating agent when infused with doxorubicin given by IVP, has been shown to decrease the development of CHF by 19%.[40] Dexrazoxane is not recommended for use at the beginning of anthracycline therapy because of the possibility that it might reduce the anticancer effects of the anthracycline.[6]

Stratification of risk factors is important in predicting the development of CIC when treatment using cardiotoxic chemotherapeutic and biologic agents is necessary. In patients who had elevated serum troponin I levels, 80% developed a 15% reduction in left ventricular dysfunction.[23] Cardinale and colleagues [41] randomly assigned 114 patients who had elevated troponin levels after treatment with high-dose chemotherapy (including anthracyclines) to receive either prophylactic enalapril, an angiotensin-converting enzyme (ace) inhibitor, or placebo for 1 year. The enalapril group had no left ventricular dysfunction but 43% of the placebo group developed a decrease in LV function of 10% or more.[41] Animal studies of the prophylactic use of erythropoietin and thrombopoietin to prevent or decrease the incidence of CIC development are ongoing.[42,43]

Once CIC occurs, treatment is directed at addressing specific symptom manifestations. The mainstays of treatment for left ventricular dysfunction, CHF, and cardiomyopathy are angiotensin-converting enzyme inhibitors, beta-blockers, and diuretics.[6] If venous thrombo-embolism occurs, treatment options include thrombolytic infusion, anticoagulation, use of compression stockings, and elevation of the affected extremity (A. Kommareddy, personal communication, 2007).

Case Study

A 47-year-old married white woman was diagnosed with stage IIIA right breast cancer in September 2005. Her tumor was estrogen-receptor (ER) and progesterone-receptor (PR) negative and *HER2*-receptor positive. Mild hypertension before diagnosis had been controlled with the angiotensin-converting enzyme inhibitor enalapril (Vasotec). Her baseline ejection fraction measured by ECHO was 55%. She had a right mastectomy followed by immediate reconstruction. Treatment with doxorubicin was started by continuous infusion to a total dose of 240 mg/m² and cyclophosphamide for four cycles. This regimen was followed by right chest radiation and then four cycles of paclitaxel with trastuzumab. The treatment was followed with maintenance trastuzumab beginning in May 2006.

The patient presented to the emergency department with new-onset dyspnea and viral pneumonia in March 2007. The ECHO showed an ejection fraction of 15% to 20%. Possible causes for the cardiomyopathy included doxorubicin treatment, trastuzumab treatment, viral pneumonia, and controlled hypertension. Given the low dose of doxorubicin and its administration by continuous infusion, doxorubicin was unlikely to be the cause of the CIC. Trastuzumab CIC was a possibility, but intercurrent infection or other conditions might have caused this cardiomyopathy. Cardiology treated and stabilized the patient with diuretics and beta-blockers. She was released on a regimen of carvedilol (Coreg) and aspirin. Over 8 months her ejection fraction improved to baseline.

When the patient complained of right upper quadrant pain in October 2007, she was diagnosed as having liver and right pelvic metastases. Further treatment for cancer was required. With her history of compromised cardiac function, she was treated with gemcitabine and albumin-bound paclitaxel, drugs with relatively low risk for CIC.[19,20] With her cancer now controlled, and at the patient's request, consideration is being given to rechallenging her with trastuzumab for maintenance treatment with careful cardiac monitoring and collaboration with her treating cardiologist. Although her disease is considered incurable, control of disease progression may enhance this patient's quality of life. Her survival depends on treatment sustaining long-term control of her ER-negative, PR-negative, and *HER2*-positive disease.

As with many chronic illnesses requiring complex treatment and rehabilitation, patients often are unable to work. The patient in the case study missed several weeks of work because of her illness, surgery, recovery, treatment, and complications, creating difficult socioeconomic issues affecting both the patient and her family. She ultimately lost her employment because of absenteeism exceeding that allowed by the Family Medical Leave Act. She continues to be insured through her husband's employment but does not have secondary coverage. She probably will be unlikely able to obtain insurance on her own in the future. Her disease has affected all facets of her and her family's life, physically, emotionally and financially.

REFERENCES

1. American Cancer Society. Cancer statistics 2007. Available at: http://www.cancer.org/docroot/PRO/content/PRO_1_1_Cancer_Statistics_2007_Presentation.asp. Accessed December 20, 2007.

2. About breast cancer: statistics, causes, symptoms, surgery options. Available at: http://www.breastcancer.org. Accessed December, 2007.

3. Facts for life breast cancer in men. Susan G. Komen for the Cure Web site. Available at: http://cms.komen.org/Komen/AboutBreastCancer/Resources. Updated 2007. Accessed December, 2007.

4. Surveillance Epidemiology and End Results Program. Available at: http://seer.cancer.gov. Accessed December, 2007.

5. Multiple hit hypothesis: how breast cancer treatment affects heart disease in women. Her2 Support Group Forum Web site. Available at: http://www.her2support.org. Accessed December, 2007.

6. Yeh ETH, Tong AT, Lenihan DJ, et al. Cardiovascular complications of cancer therapy: diagnosis, pathogenesis, and management. Circulation 2004; 109(25):3122–31.

7. O'Toole M. Miller-Keane encyclopedia and dictionary of medicine, nursing, and allied health. 5th edition. Philadelphia: W.B.Saunders Company; 1992.

8. Adriamycin [package insert]. Bedford (OH): Ben Venue Laboratories, Inc. and Bedford Laboratories; 2006.

9. Kozier B, Erb G, Olivieri R. Fundamentals of nursing concepts process and practice. 4th edition. Redwood City (CA): Benjamin/Cummings Publishing Co, Inc.; 1991. p. 408–11.

10. Beers MH, Berkow R. The Merck manual. 17th edition. Whitehouse (NJ): Merck Research Laboratories; 1999.

11. Singhal H. Breast cancer evaluation. Emedicine Web site. Available at: http://www.emedicine.com/med/topic3287.htm. Accessed January, 2008.

12. American Cancer Society. How is breast cancer staged? Available at: http://www.cancer.org. Updated September 13, 2007. Accessed December, 2007.

13. National Comprehensive Cancer Network. Practice guidelines in oncology—v.1.2008. Breast cancer. ST-1-3. National Comprehensive Cancer Network (NCCN) Web site. Available at: http://www.nccn.org/professionals/physician_gls/PDF/breast.pdf. Accessed December, 2007.

14. Jones LW, Haykowsky M, Pituskin EN, et al. Cardiovascular reserve and risk profile of postmenopausal women after chemoendocrine therapy for hormone receptor-positive operable breast cancer. Oncologist 2007;12(10):1156–64. Available at: http://theoncologist.alphamedpress.org/cgi/content/abstract/12/10/1156. Accessed January, 2008.

15. Oparil S. The importance of identifying and reducing cardiovascular risk factors in women. Available at: http://www.medscape.com/viewarticle/448971_5. Accessed January, 2008.

16. National Institutes of Health. Estimating coronary heart disease (CHD) risk using Framingham Heart Study prediction score sheets. Available at: http://www.nhlbi.nih.gov/about/framingham/riskabs.htm. Accessed January, 2008.

17. Calculating heart and stroke risk for women. Reynolds Risk Score Web site. Available at: http://www.reynoldsriskscore.org/. Accessed January 2008.

18. Mays T. Oncology Preparatory Review Course Handbook. The American College of Clinical Pharmacy and the American Society of Health-System Pharmacists; 2007.

19. Gemzar [package insert]. Indianapolis (IN): Eli Lilly and Company; 2006.

20. Abraxane [package insert]. Los Angeles (CA): Abraxis Oncology, Division of Abraxis BioScience, Inc.; 2007.

21. Doxil [package insert]. Bedford (OH): Ben Venue Laboratories, Inc.; 2006.

22. Herceptin [package insert]. South San Francisco (CA): Genentech, Inc.; 2006.

23. Granger CB. Prediction and prevention of chemotherapy-induced cardiomyopathy: can it be done? Circulation 2006;114(23):2432–3.

24. National Comprehensive Cancer Network. Practice guidelines in oncology—v.1.2008. Invasive breast cancer. BINV-I, BINV-J 1-5, BINV–M 1-6. Available at: http://www.nccn.org/professionals/physician_gls/PDF/breast.pdf. Updated January 2008. Accessed January 1, 2008.

25. Simbre VC II, Adams J, Deshpande SS, et al. Cardiomyopathy caused by antineoplastic therapies. Curr Treat Options Cardiovasc Med 2001;3:493–505. Available at: http://www.treatment-options.com. Accessed January, 2008.

26. US Food and Drug Administration. Guidance for industry. Available at: http://www.fda.gov/cber/gdlns/boxwarlb.htm. Updated January 20, 2006. Accessed December 28, 2007.

27. Hortobaygi GN, Frye D, Buzdar AU, et al. Decreased cardiac toxicity of doxorubicin administered by continuous intravenous infusion in combination chemotherapy for metastatic breast carcinoma. Cancer 1989;63(1):37–45.

28. National Cancer Institute. Dictionary of cancer terms. Available at: http://www.cancer/gov/Templates/db_alpha.aspx?expand=M. Accessed January 1, 2008.

29. The genes of cancer: oncogenes. HER-2/neu. Emory University Web site. Available at: http://www.cancerquest.org/index.cfm?page=325. Accessed January, 2008.

30. Hortobaygi GN. Trastuzumab in the treatment of breast cancer. N Engl J Med 2005;353(16):1734–6.

31. Smith M. SABCS: one-third of HER2-positive breast tumors metastasize to brain. MedPage Today Web site. Available at: http://www.medpagetoday.com/MeetingCoverage/SABCSMeeting/tb/7721. Accessed January, 2008.

32. Burstein HJ. The distinctive nature of HER2-positive breast cancers. N Engl J Med 2005;353(16):1652–4.

33. Romond E. Joint analysis of NSABP-B-31 and NCCTG–N9831. American Society of Clinical Oncology (ASCO) Web site. Available at: http://media.asco.org/player/default.aspx?LectureID=5817&conferenceFolder=VM2005&SessionFolder=ss11&slideonlu=yes&TrackIBN929&LectureTitle. Accessed December 10, 2007.

34. Avastin [package insert]. South San Francisco (CA): Genentech, Inc.; 2006.

35. Nolvadex [package insert]. Wilminton (DE): Astra Zeneca Pharmaceuticals; 2002.

36. Arimidex [package insert]. Wilmington (DE): Astra Zeneca Pharmaceuticals; 2006.

37. Heit JA. Prevention of deep venous thrombosis. In: Dalsing MC, editor. The vein handbook: a layman's versions of venous disorders. American Venous Forum Web site. Available at: http://www.venous-info.com/handbook/hbk10a.html. Accessed December 30, 2007.

38. Camp-Sorrell D. Cardiorespiratory effects in cancer survivors: cardiac and pulmonary toxicities may occur as late or long-term sequelae of cancer treatment. Am J Nursing 2006;106(Suppl 3):55–9.

39. Zinecard [package insert]. Kalamazoo (MI): Pharmacia and Upjohn; 1998.

40. Cardinale D, Sandri M, Colombo A, et al. Prognostic value of troponin I in cardiac risk stratification of cancer patients undergoing high-dose chemotherapy. Circulation 2004;109(22):2749–54.

41. Cardinale D, Colombo A, Sandri M, et al. Prevention of high-dose chemotherapy-induced cardiotoxicity in high-risk patients by angiotensin-converting enzyme inhibition. Circulation 2006;114(23):2474–81.

42. Li I, Takemura G, Li Y, et al. Preventative effect of erythropoietin on cardiac dysfunction in doxorubicin-induced cardiomyopathy. Circulation 2006;113(4):535–43.

43. Li K, Sung R, Huang W, et al. Thrombopoietin protects against in vitro and in vivo cardiotoxicity induced by doxorubicin. Circulation 2006;113(18):2211–20.

Index

heartfailure.theclinics.com

Moving?

Make sure your subscription moves with you!

To notify us of your new address, find your **Clinics Account Number** (located on your mailing label above your name), and contact customer service at:

Email: journalscustomerservice-usa@elsevier.com

800-654-2452 (subscribers in the U.S. & Canada)
314-447-8871 (subscribers outside of the U.S. & Canada)

Fax number: 314-447-8029

Elsevier Health Sciences Division
Subscription Customer Service
3251 Riverport Lane
Maryland Heights, MO 63043

*To ensure uninterrupted delivery of your subscription, please notify us at least 4 weeks in advance of move.

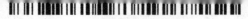

Printed in the United States
By Bookmasters